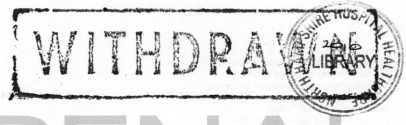

RENAL

Pathophysiology

■ The Essentials
THIRD EDITION

HELMUT G. RENNKE, M.D.

Professor of Pathology
Harvard Medical School and
Harvard–MIT Division of Health Sciences and Technology
Department of Pathology
Brigham & Women's Hospital
Boston, Massachusetts

BRADLEY M. DENKER, M.D.

Associate Professor of Medicine
Harvard Medical School
Renal Division, Department of Medicine
Brigham & Women's Hospital
Chief of Nephrology
Harvard–Vanguard Medical Associates
Boston, Massachusetts

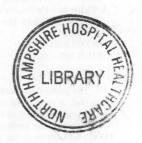

Wolters Kluwer
Health
Philadelphia · Baltim
Buenos Aires · Hong

Wilkins

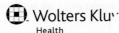

Acquisitions Editor: *Crystal Taylor*
Product Manager: *Stacey L. Sebring*
Marketing Manager: *Jennifer Kuklinski*
Designer: *Terry Mallon*
Compositor: *Aptara®, Inc.*
Printer: *C&C Offset Printing, Ltd*

Printed in China

First Edition, 1994
Second Edition, 2007

Library of Congress Cataloging-in-Publication Data

Rennke, Helmut G.
  Renal pathophysiology : the essentials / Helmut G. Rennke, Bradley M. Denker.—3rd ed.
    p. ; cm.
  Includes bibliographical references and index.
  ISBN 978-0-7817-9995-9
  1. Kidneys—Pathophysiology.   I. Denker, Bradley M.   II. Title.
  [DNLM: 1. Kidney Diseases—physiopathology.   2. Kidney—physiopathology. WJ 300
R416r 2010]
    RC903.9.R672 2010
    616.6'107—dc22

                                                                    2009013471

The publishers have made every effort to trace the copyright holders for borrowed material. If they have inadvertently overlooked any, they will be pleased to make the necessary arrangements at the first opportunity.
  To purchase additional copies of this book, call our customer service department at **(800) 638-3030** or fax orders to **(301) 223-2320**. International customers should call **(301) 223-2300.**
  Visit Lippincott Williams & Wilkins on the Internet: http://www.LWW.com.
Lippincott Williams & Wilkins customer service representatives are available from 8:30 am to 6:00 pm, EST.

To our families,
Stephanie and Christianne
Mary, Brendan, Jennifer, and Mackenzie

In this third edition of *Renal Pathophysiology: The Essentials*, we have maintained the general principles that guided us in the design and approach of the last two versions of the book. Over these last 15 years, we have received many comments and suggestions not only from our second-year medical students, but also from house staff, nephrology fellows, and colleagues; we are most grateful for their feedback and encouraging words. As a consequence of these suggestions, we have expanded the sections on molecular aspects of the mechanisms that result in kidney dysfunction and the morphologic expression of the major diseases that affect the kidney. The schematic illustrations are in two colors and the list of suggested readings has been updated. We have also added some color images that depict the histopathology changes of the major disease processes that affect the kidney. The core and the principal aim of the book remain unchanged: to provide the student with a solid understanding of the mechanisms that result in kidney dysfunction and disease and to serve as the basic reading material and text for a course in kidney pathophysiology.

HGR and BMD

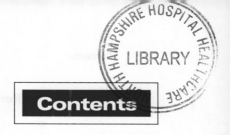

Contents

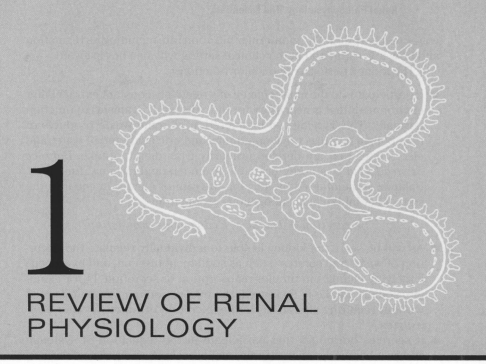

1

REVIEW OF RENAL PHYSIOLOGY

OBJECTIVES

By the end of this chapter, you should have an understanding of each of the following issues:

- The general mechanisms by which solute reabsorption and secretion occur in the different nephron segments.
- The factors regulating the glomerular filtration rate.
- The mechanisms by which the glomerular filtration rate is measured in patients.

Introduction

Although readers of this book should have already completed a course on normal renal physiology, a brief review of the basic principles involved is helpful in understanding the mechanisms by which disease might occur. Tubular functions will be discussed with a major emphasis on sodium and water reabsorption. The glomerular filtration rate including its regulation and how it is estimated in the clinical setting will also be reviewed.

The kidney performs two major functions:

■ It participates in the maintenance of a relatively constant extracellular environment that is necessary for the cells (and organism) to function normally. This is achieved by excretion of some waste products of metabolism (such as urea, creatinine, and uric acid) and of water and electrolytes that are derived primarily from dietary intake. *Balance* or *steady state* is a key principle in understanding renal functions. Balance is maintained by keeping the rate of excretion equal to the sum of net intake plus endogenous production:

$$Excretion = Intake + Endogenous\ production$$

■ As will be seen, the kidney is able to individually regulate the excretion of water and solutes (such as sodium, potassium, and hydrogen) largely by changes in tubular reabsorption or secretion. If, for example, sodium intake is increased, the excess sodium can be excreted without requiring alterations in the excretion of water or other electrolytes.

■ It secretes hormones that participate in the regulation of systemic and renal hemodynamics (renin, angiotensin II, and prostaglandins), red cell production (erythropoietin), and mineral metabolism [calcitriol, (1,25-OH dihydroxyvitamin D), the major active metabolite of vitamin D].

The kidney also performs a number of miscellaneous functions such as the catabolism of peptide hormones and the synthesis of glucose (gluconeogenesis) under fasting conditions.

Relation between Filtration and Excretion

The normal glomerular filtration rate (GFR) ranges from 130 to 145 L/day (90 to 100 mL/min) in women and from 165 to 180 L/day (115 to 125 mL/min) in men. This represents a volume that is more than 10 times that of extracellular fluid and approximately 60 times that of plasma; as a result, survival requires that virtually all of the filtered solutes and water be returned to the systemic circulation by tubular reabsorption.

Preventing excessive urinary sodium loss is essential to maintenance of the extracellular and plasma volumes (see Chapter 2). Figure 1.1 shows the organization of the nephron, and Table 1.1 lists the relative contribution of the different nephron segments to the reabsorption of filtered sodium and the neurohumoral factors involved in regulating transport at

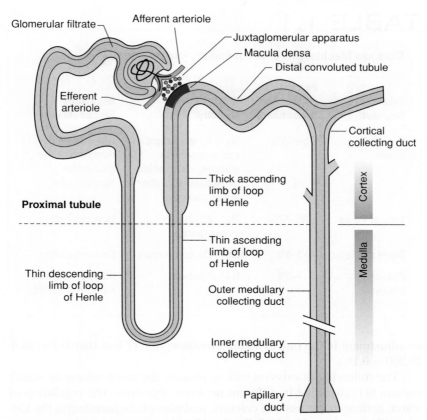

FIGURE 1.1. Anatomy of the nephron. Filtrate forms at the glomerulus and enters the proximal tubule. It then flows down the descending limb of the loop of Henle into the medulla, makes a hairpin turn, and then ascends back into the cortex. The next segment of the tubule is the distal convoluted tubule that becomes the cortical collecting duct and then the outer and inner medullary collecting duct before entering the papilla through the papillary duct. The sites and mechanisms of sodium reabsorption are summarized in Table 1.1.

that site. The bulk of the filtered sodium is reabsorbed in the proximal tubule and loop of Henle; however, day-to-day regulation primarily occurs in the collecting ducts, where the final composition of the urine is determined.

This regulatory system for solute excretion is highly efficient. For example, the filtered sodium load in a patient with a GFR of 180 L/day and a plasma water sodium concentration of 140 mEq/L is 25,200 mEq. Normal dietary sodium intake ranges from 80 to 250 mEq/day. Thus, more than 99% of the filtered sodium must be reabsorbed to remain in balance. Furthermore, increasing sodium intake by 25 mEq/day requires

TABLE 1.1

Sites and Mechanisms of Renal Sodium Reabsorption			
Tubule Segment	**Percent Filtered Na Reabsorbed**	**Mechanisms of Na Entry**	**Regulatory Factors (Major)**
Proximal tubule	50–55%	Na^+–H^+ exchange; cotransport with glucose, amino acids, phosphate, and other organic solutes	Angiotensin II; norepinephrine; glomerular filtration rate
Loop of Henle	35–40%	Na^+–K^+–$2Cl^-$ cotransport	Flow dependent
Distal tubule	5–8%	Na^+–Cl^- cotransport	Flow dependent
Collecting tubules	2–3%	Na^+ channels	Aldosterone; atrial natriuretic peptide

an adjustment in the rate of sodium reabsorption of less than 0.1% ($25 \div 25,200 = 0.1\%$).

The following discussion will emphasize the mechanisms by which sodium is reabsorbed in different nephron segments. The regulation of water, hydrogen, potassium, calcium, and phosphate handling in the kidney will be reviewed in the following chapters.

General Mechanism of Transtubular Sodium Reabsorption

The reabsorption of filtered sodium from the tubular lumen into the peritubular capillary occurs in two steps: Sodium must move from the lumen into the cell across the apical (or luminal) membrane; it must then move out of the cell into the interstitium and peritubular capillary across the basolateral (or peritubular) membrane.

As with any charged particle, sodium is unable to freely diffuse across the lipid bilayer of the cell membranes. Thus, transmembrane transporters or channels are required for sodium reabsorption to proceed. For example, the active transport of sodium out of the cell is mediated by the Na^+–K^+-ATPase pump in the basolateral membrane, which pumps three sodium ions out of the cell and two potassium ions into the cell.

A general model for transcellular sodium transport is shown in Figure 1.2. Sodium enters the cell via a transmembrane carrier (that may

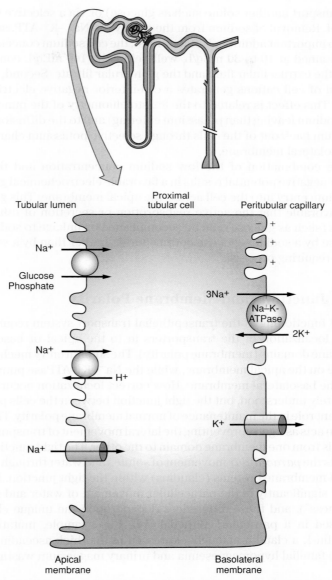

FIGURE 1.2. General model for transtubular sodium reabsorption and schematic model of ion transport in the proximal tubule. Filtered sodium enters the cell across the apical membrane via either (1) a transmembrane carrier that can also reabsorb (as with sodium–glucose or sodium–phosphate cotransport) or secrete (as with sodium–hydrogen exchange) another substance or (2) a selective sodium channel. This sodium is then returned to the systemic circulation by the Na^+–K^+-ATPase pump in the basolateral membrane. This pump also maintains the cell sodium concentration at a low level and creates a cell-interior negative potential, both of which result in a favorable electrochemical gradient that promotes passive sodium entry into the cell in all nephron segments.

also transport another solute such as glucose) or via a selective sodium channel. Removal of sodium from the cell by the Na^+–K^+-ATPase pump has two important additional effects. First, the cell sodium concentration is maintained at 10 to 30 mEq/L, well below the 140 mEq/L concentration in the extracellular fluid and the glomerular filtrate. Second, the net removal of cell cations generates a cell-interior negative electrical potential. This effect is related to the 3:2 stoichiometry of the pump (with more sodium leaving than potassium entering) and to the diffusion of the potassium back out of the cells through selective potassium channels in the basolateral membrane.

The combination of the low sodium concentration and the cell-interior negative potential results in a favorable electrochemical gradient for sodium entry into the cell across the apical membrane. This gradient is so favorable that the active reabsorption or secretion of other substances (such as glucose) can be accomplished by linkage to sodium (in this case by a sodium–glucose cotransporter) rather than by a separate energy-requiring process.

Tight Junctions and Membrane Polarity

Normal functioning of the transepithelial transport system requires the proper localization of the transporters in to the apical or basolateral membrane domains (membrane polarity). The sodium entry mechanisms must be on the apical membrane, while the Na^+–K^+-ATPase pump must be on the basolateral membrane. How correct localization occurs is not completely understood, but the tight junction between the cells plays an important role in the maintenance of normal membrane polarity. The tight junction acts as a gate, preventing the lateral movement of transporters or channels from one membrane domain to the other. The tight junction also prevents the *paracellular* movement of solutes and water through unique integral membrane proteins (claudins) within the tight junction. Epithelia vary significantly in the paracellular movement of water and solutes ("leakiness"), and these differences depend upon the unique claudins expressed in a particular epithelial cell. For example, mutations in paracellin-1, a claudin uniquely expressed in the thick ascending limb, leads to familial hypomagnesemia and urinary magnesium wasting.

Segmental Sodium Reabsorption

The major nephron segments (Fig. 1.1) reabsorb sodium by a mechanism similar to the general model in Figure 1.2. However, the apical membrane carrier or channel responsible for sodium entry into the cell is different in each segment (Figs. 1.2 to 1.5). An understanding of these different entry mechanisms in part explains some of the functions performed by each segment; it also assumes clinical importance with the use of diuretics, which inhibit tubular sodium reabsorption and lower the extracellular fluid volume in edematous states or in hypertension (see Chapter 4). The physiologic factors that regulate segmental sodium transport are listed in Table 1.1; how they interact to maintain sodium balance will be discussed in Chapter 2.

Proximal Tubule

The proximal tubule has two major reabsorptive functions: It reabsorbs 50% to 55% of the filtered sodium and water, and it reabsorbs almost all of the filtered glucose, phosphate, amino acids, and other organic solutes by linking their transport to sodium.

Filtered sodium enters the proximal tubular cell via a series of transporters that also transport other solutes. Thus, there are specific sodium–glucose, sodium–phosphate, sodium–citrate, and several different sodium–amino acid cotransporters. Binding of the cotransported solute appears to lead to a conformational change in the carrier protein that results in an opening of the gate for transmembrane sodium movement.

Reabsorption via these transporters represents a form of *secondary active transport*. Although the cotransport process itself is passive, the energy is indirectly supplied by the Na^+–K^+-ATPase pump, which, as described above, creates the favorable electrochemical gradient that allows sodium to passively diffuse into the cell.

From a quantitative viewpoint, however, sodium–hydrogen exchange is of greatest importance. This transporter results in sodium reabsorption and hydrogen secretion; much of the secreted hydrogen then combines with filtered bicarbonate, leading to the reabsorption of approximately 90% of the filtered bicarbonate (see Chapter 5 for a detailed discussion of the role of the kidney in acid–base homeostasis).

The removal of solutes from the lumen initially lowers the tubular fluid osmolality, thereby creating an osmotic gradient that promotes an equivalent degree of water reabsorption. Osmotic water transport can occur because the apical and basolateral membranes are highly permeable to water due to the presence of transmembrane water channels (aquaporins). Water reabsorption can also occur between the cells across the relatively "leaky" tight junction that is present in the proximal tubule.

The net effect of this permeable epithelium is that concentration or osmotic gradients cannot be maintained in this segment. As a result, the sodium concentration and osmolality of the fluid leaving the proximal tubule are the same as that in plasma. This is also true of the concentration of solutes whose reabsorption is passively linked to that of sodium, such as urea, potassium, and calcium. Sodium-induced water reabsorption raises the tubular fluid concentration of these solutes, thereby allowing them to be passively reabsorbed down a favorable concentration gradient.

In comparison, the tight junctions are relatively impermeable in the more distal segments. As a result, concentration and osmotic gradients that can exceed 50:1 for sodium (urine sodium concentration ≤3 mEq/L with volume depletion) and almost 1000:1 for hydrogen (urine pH <5.0 with acid load) can be created and maintained.

 When patients become volume depleted, as with vomiting or diarrhea, the renin–angiotensin and sympathetic nervous systems are activated (see Chapter 2). Angiotensin II and norepinephrine enhance proximal sodium reabsorption by increasing the activity of the Na^+–H^+ exchanger; this response is appropriate since it limits urinary sodium losses that would exacerbate the volume deficit. What will happen to proximal urea reabsorption in this setting?

Loop of Henle

Thirty-five to forty percent of the filtered sodium and chloride is reabsorbed in the ascending limb of the loop of Henle. Reabsorption of sodium in the loop occurs in excess of that of water, since the apical membrane of the ascending limb is impermeable to water, lacking the aquaporins (water channels) present in the proximal tubule. This separation between sodium and water movement is an essential part of the countercurrent mechanism.

The major mechanism of active sodium chloride transport in the thick ascending limb is shown in Figure 1.3. Filtered sodium and chloride enter the cell via an electroneutral Na^+–K^+–$2Cl^-$ cotransporter in the apical membrane. The energy for Na^+–K^+–$2Cl^-$ cotransport is again derived from the favorable inward gradient for sodium (low intracellular Na^+ concentration due to constitutive activity of the basolateral Na^+–K^+-ATPase pump). However, the concentration of potassium in the lumen, and in the extracellular fluid, is much lower than that of sodium and chloride. Thus, continued sodium chloride reabsorption requires that the potassium entering the cell be recycled back into the tubular lumen through selective potassium channels in the apical membrane. This movement of potassium is electrogenic, making the lumen *electropositive*. Chloride exits the cell through a selective basolateral channel. The affinity of the Na^+–K^+–$2Cl^-$ cotransporter for sodium and potassium is very high, while it is the delivery of chloride to the active site that is rate limiting for transporter activity. The loop diuretics (furosemide) inhibit sodium chloride reabsorption by competing for the Cl^- binding site on the carrier.

The lumen positivity generated by potassium recycling is able to drive the passive reabsorption of cations (sodium, calcium, magnesium)

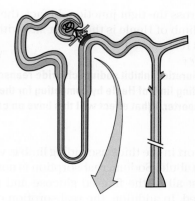

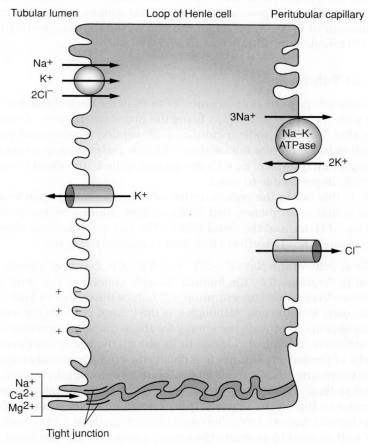

FIGURE 1.3. Schematic model of ion transport in the thick ascending limb of the loop of Henle. The lumen-positive potential generated by the recycling of potassium promotes the passive reabsorption of sodium, calcium, and magnesium between the cells across the tight junction.

between the cells across the tight junction. In fact, the cortical aspect of the thick ascending limb of Henle is the major site within the nephron at which magnesium is reabsorbed.

 Loop diuretics inhibit sodium chloride reabsorption in the thick ascending limb of Henle by competing for the chloride site on the $Na^+–K^+–2Cl^-$ cotransporter. What effect will this have on calcium reabsorption in this segment?

Note that transport in the thick ascending limb is very different from that in the proximal tubule. Sodium reabsorption is not linked to organic solutes, since almost all of the filtered glucose and amino acids have already been removed. In addition, the reabsorption of sodium without water progressively lowers the tubular fluid sodium concentration to a minimum of 50 to 75 mEq/L at the end of the thick ascending limb (vs. 140 mEq/L in the filtrate and proximal tubule).

Distal Tubule

The distal tubule normally reabsorbs 5% to 8% of the filtered sodium chloride, with $Na^+–Cl^-$ cotransport being the major mechanism of sodium entry (Fig. 1.4). This sodium chloride reabsorption is associated with a reduction in the tubular fluid sodium chloride concentration to approximately 40 mEq/L since, as with the ascending limb, the distal tubule is relatively impermeable to water.

It is this fall in the concentration of chloride, rather than sodium or the action of hormones, that limits sodium chloride reabsorption in the loop of Henle and the distal tubule. The fall in the luminal chloride concentration has two effects that limit continued transport:

- The activity of the $Na^+–K^+–2Cl^-$ and $Na^+–Cl^-$ cotransporters is primarily determined by the luminal chloride concentration; thus, a reduction in chloride concentration will reduce the rate of sodium chloride entry into the cell. Although it is the inward gradient for sodium that appears to provide the energy for these transport processes, the attachment of luminal chloride to its site on the transporter appears to be of primary importance in inducing the conformational change in the transporter that is required for solute movement into the cell.
- The sodium chloride concentration in the peritubular interstitium is similar to that in the plasma. Thus, the falling concentration within the lumen creates a favorable concentration gradient for the backflux of sodium and chloride into the lumen across the tight junctions.

Reabsorption ceases when the rate of sodium entry into the cell equals the rate of backflux.

The net effect is that transport in the loop of Henle and the distal tubule is *flow dependent*. If, for example, more fluid is delivered to the

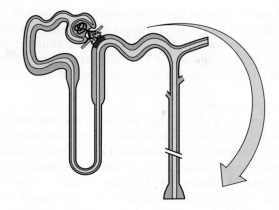

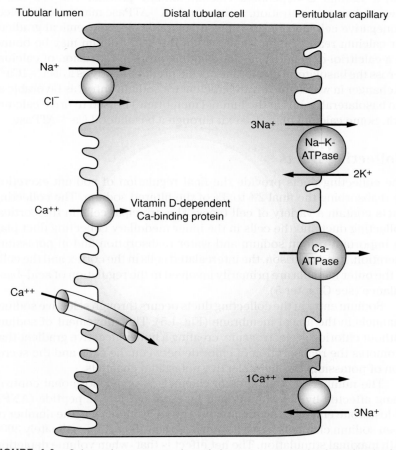

FIGURE 1.4. Schematic representation of the transport mechanisms involved in sodium chloride and calcium reabsorption in the distal tubule.

distal tubule because of the administration of a loop diuretic, then more sodium chloride can be reabsorbed. This distal response reduces the degree to which a loop diuretic can increase sodium excretion. However, inhibiting distal tubule Na^+–Cl^- transport (thiazide diuretics) potently augments sodium excretion in the presence of a loop diuretic.

Calcium Transport

The distal tubule and adjacent segments are the major sites at which urinary calcium excretion is actively regulated under the influence of parathyroid hormone and calcitriol (1,25 dihydroxyvitamin D, the active metabolite of vitamin D). A model for distal calcium reabsorption is shown in Figure 1.4. Calcium is able to enter the cell down a favorable electrochemical gradient through apical calcium channels and a vitamin D–dependent calcium-binding protein. The cell has a low calcium concentration, and the Na^+–K^+-ATPase maintains the electronegative cell interior providing a favorable electrochemical gradient for calcium reabsorption. Once within the cell, calcium may be bound to a calcitriol-dependent calcium-binding protein. Extrusion of calcium across the basolateral membrane occurs predominantly as a $3Na^+$–$1Ca^{2+}$ exchanger in which the inward gradient for sodium entry (as favorable at the basolateral as it is at the luminal membrane) is used to drive calcium exit. Some calcium may also exit through a basolateral Ca^{2+}-ATPase.

Collecting Ducts

The collecting ducts provide the final regulation of sodium excretion by reabsorbing the final 2% to 3% of the filtered sodium. The collecting ducts contain a variety of cell types. The principal cells in the cortical collecting duct and the cells in the inner medullary collecting duct play an important role in sodium and water reabsorption and in potassium secretion. In comparison, the intercalated cells in the cortex and the cells in the outer medulla are primarily involved in the regulation of acid–base balance (see Chapter 5).

Sodium entry in the collecting ducts occurs through selective sodium channels in the apical membrane (Fig. 1.5). This movement of sodium without chloride is electrogenic, creating a lumen-negative gradient that promotes the reabsorption of chloride between the cells and the secretion of potassium through selective potassium channels.

The number of open sodium channels is under hormonal control, being affected by aldosterone and by atrial natriuretic peptide (ANP). Aldosterone enhances sodium reabsorption by increasing the number of open sodium channels per cell from less than 100 to approximately 3000 with maximal stimulation. The net effect is that, when volume depletion activates the renin–angiotensin–aldosterone system, the urine sodium concentration can be reduced to less than 1 mEq/L by collecting duct reabsorption.

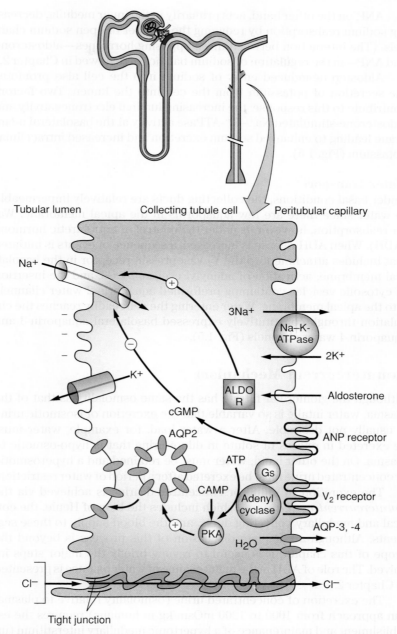

FIGURE 1.5. Schematic model of the transport pathways and hormonal factors—aldosterone, atrial natriuretic peptide (ANP), and antidiuretic hormone (ADH)—involved in sodium, potassium, and water handling in the collecting ducts. Different cells, such as the intercalated cells in the cortical collecting duct, are involved in the regulation of acid–base balance (see Chapter 5).

ANP, on the other hand, acts primarily in the inner medulla, decreasing sodium reabsorption by reducing the number of open sodium channels. (The interaction between these opposing hormones—aldosterone and ANP—in the regulation of sodium balance is reviewed in Chapter 2.)

Aldosterone-induced entry of sodium into the cell also promotes the secretion of potassium from the cell into the lumen. Two factors contribute to this response: the increasing luminal electronegativity and aldosterone-stimulated Na^+–K^+-ATPase activity at the basolateral membrane leading to enhanced sodium excretion and increased intracellular potassium (Fig. 1.5).

Water Transport
Under basal conditions, the collecting ducts are relatively impermeable to water since there are few aquaporins in the apical membrane. Water reabsorption, however, is under the control of antidiuretic hormone (ADH). When ADH release is increased, a sequence of events is initiated that includes attachment to the V_2 vasopressin receptor in the basolateral membrane, activation of adenylyl cyclase by Gs, and the insertion of cytosolic vesicles containing preformed aquaporin-2 water channels into the apical membrane. Water entering the cell readily reaches the circulation through constitutively expressed basolateral aquaporin-3 and aquaporin-4 water channels (Fig. 1.5).

Countercurrent Mechanism

Although the glomerular filtrate has the same osmolality as that of the plasma, water intake is so variable that the excretion of isosmotic urine is usually not desirable. After a water load, for example, water must be excreted in excess of solute in dilute urine that is hypo-osmotic to plasma. On the other hand, water must be retained and a hyperosmotic or concentrated urine must be excreted after a period of water restriction.

The excretion of dilute or concentrated urine is achieved via the *countercurrent mechanism*, which includes the loop of Henle, the cortical and medullary collecting ducts, and the blood supply to these segments. Although a complete discussion of this process is beyond the scope of this chapter, it is useful to review briefly the major steps involved. The role of ADH in the maintenance of water balance is presented in Chapter 2.

The excretion of concentrated urine (osmolality relative to plasma; can approach from 1000 to 1200 mOsm/kg in humans) requires the establishment and maintenance of a hypertonic medullary interstitium (up to 1200 mOsm/kg). The hairpin configuration of the loop of Henle *and* the unique microcirculation of the vasa recta that parallels the loop are essential for this process (Fig. 1.6). The factors resulting in countercurrent multiplication (countercurrent refers to the opposite direction of

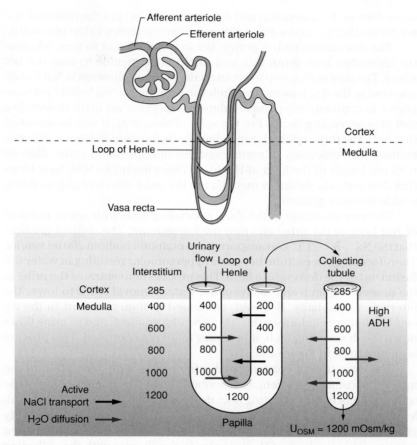

FIGURE 1.6. Relationship of vasa recta to tubule segments and depiction of the events in the renal medulla involved in the excretion of concentrated urine. The transport of sodium chloride without water from the ascending limb of the loop of Henle makes the tubular fluid dilute and the medullary interstitium and descending limb of the loop of Henle concentrated. The key points are as follows: (1) The descending limb is freely permeable to water and therefore able to equilibrate osmotically with the interstitium. (2) Active sodium chloride transport in the ascending limb maintains a gradient of approximately 200 mOsm/kg at each level. As urine flows down the descending limb, the urine concentrates and the interstitium maintains this 200 mOsm/kg gradient. The fluid leaving the medulla in the ascending limb has an osmolality of 200 mOsm/kg (less than plasma due to the active NaCl transport). In the presence of antidiuretic hormone (ADH), water is then reabsorbed in the cortical collecting duct by osmotic equilibration with the cortical interstitium, which has an osmolality similar to plasma (285 mOsm/kg). As a result, the fluid returning to the medulla in the medullary collecting duct is isosmotic to plasma. However, the osmolality of urine gradually rises in the collecting duct (in the presence of ADH) as the tubular fluid equilibrates with the medullary interstitium.

urine flow in the ascending and descending limbs) are the different water permeabilities and solute transport characteristics in the two limbs.

The descending limb is permeable to water but not to ions, whereas the ascending limb (both thin and thick) is permeable to ions but not water. The only *active* step in countercurrent multiplication is NaCl reabsorption in the thick ascending limb through the Na^+–K^+–$2Cl^-$ cotransporter. In contrast, only passive solute transport occurs in the descending and *thin* ascending limbs. For the sake of simplicity, it will be assumed that both the thin and thick ascending limbs function in a homogeneous manner. The efficiency of countercurrent multiplication varies directly with the length of the loop of Henle, so those nephrons with long loops that descend into the inner medulla are the most effective at generating a wide osmolar gradient.

The process starts in the thick ascending limb with active removal of NaCl out of the urine and into the interstitium. The sodium gradient that the Na^+–K^+–$2Cl^-$ cotransporter can maintain is about 200 mOsm/kg. Therefore, the interstitium becomes hypersomolar resulting in water diffusion *out* of the *descending* limb. This process concentrates the urine in the descending limb and the resulting water removal tends to lower the intersitital osmolality. However, continued sodium transport in the ascending limb reestablishes the 200 mOsm/kg gradient, and as urine flows down the descending limb, it becomes more concentrated. This process is summarized in Figure 1.6.

The excretion of concentrated urine begins with generation of the interstitial osmotic gradient as described above. The configuration of the tubule results in the collecting duct descending into the medulla in parallel with the loop of Henle (Fig. 1.6). As a result, the increasing osmolality gradient through the cortex and medulla generated by the countercurrent mechanism in the loop of Henle is also in equilibrium with the collecting duct. Unlike any other nephron segment, the collecting duct is dramatically responsive to ADH permitting it to be highly permeable to water in the presence of ADH, but impermeable in the absence of ADH. ADH activation of the V_2 receptor stimulates $G\alpha s$ and adenylyl cyclase leading to insertion of aquaporin-2 water channels from preformed vesicles into the apical membrane (Fig. 1.5). In the presence of ADH, urinary concentration within the collecting duct can reach levels approaching the interstitial concentrations at the papilla (bottom of the loop of Henle). The increase in urine osmolality varies with the circulating concentration of ADH. The role of the cortical collecting duct is essential to the production of concentrated urine. If the only processes were sodium chloride reabsorption without water in the medullary ascending limb and water reabsorption without sodium chloride in the medullary collecting duct, the excreted urine would essentially be isosmotic to plasma. This does not occur because most of the water is removed in the cortex. This marked reduction in water delivery to the medullary collecting duct allows osmotic water reabsorption to take place in the medulla without substantial washout of the interstitial osmotic gradient.

In the absence of ADH, the collecting duct is not permeable to water, allowing excretion of dilute urine without affecting medullary osmolality. After a maximum water load, for example, the urine osmolality in normal subjects can be reduced to as low as 30 to 60 mOsm/kg (as compared to a plasma osmolality of 280 to 290 mOsm/kg).

In addition to these basic steps, the hairpin (or loop) configuration of the vasa recta capillaries plays an important contributory role by minimizing removal of the excess medullary interstitial solute. The descending vasa recta enters the medulla at the corticomedullary junction and flows down to the tip of the papilla; it then turns around and becomes the ascending limb, which returns to the cortex. If the vasa recta continued straight through the medulla, then osmotic equilibration with the hyperosmotic medulla—by osmotic water movement out of the capillary into the interstitium and by interstitial solute movement into the capillary—would dissipate the countercurrent gradient and decrease concentrating ability. Although this does occur in the descending limb of the vasa recta, these processes are reversed as the direction of flow is reversed in the ascending limb. The net effect is that the fluid leaving the medulla is only slightly hyperosmotic to plasma and medullary tonicity is maintained.

SUMMARY

Although the preceding discussion has considered each nephron segment separately, it is important to appreciate that the different segments act in concert to maintain fluid and electrolyte balance. This can be illustrated by two examples that will be discussed in detail in Chapter 2. First, if the extracellular volume is reduced because of fluid losses (as with diarrhea or vomiting), the kidney attempts to compensate by minimizing sodium excretion to prevent a further fall in volume. Neurohumoral and hemodynamic mechanisms are activated that can increase sodium reabsorption in almost every segment: Angiotensin II and norepinephrine act in the proximal tubule; a volume depletion–induced fall in blood pressure acts in the loop of Henle via the phenomenon of pressure natriuresis; and aldosterone acts in the collecting ducts.

These compensatory mechanisms also come into play if urinary fluid loss is induced by administration of a loop diuretic, which diminishes sodium chloride reabsorption in the thick ascending limb of the loop of Henle (see Chapter 4). This fluid loss again activates the renin–angiotensin–aldosterone and sympathetic nervous systems. As a result, the net increase in sodium excretion resulting from decreased loop reabsorption is at first minimized and eventually abolished by enhanced sodium reabsorption in other tubule segments.

Glomerular Filtration Rate

Estimation of GFR is an essential part of the assessment of patients with kidney disease. The total kidney GFR is equal to the sum of the filtration rates in all of the functioning nephrons and there are approximately one million nephrons per kidney; as a result, *total GFR is an index of the functioning renal mass*. Thus, estimation of GFR can be used to evaluate the severity and the course of renal disease. For example, a fall in GFR means that the disease is progressing, whereas a rise in GFR is indicative of at least partial recovery.

Determinants of Glomerular Filtration

As with other capillaries, fluid movement across the glomerulus is governed by Starling's law, being determined by the net permeability of the glomerular capillary wall and the hydraulic and oncotic pressure gradients,

$$GFR = LpS\,(\Delta\,hydraulic\,pressure - \Delta\,oncotic\,pressure)$$
$$= LpS\,[(P_{gc} - P_{bs}) - s\,(\Pi_p - \Pi_{bs})]$$

where Lp is the unit permeability (or porosity) of the capillary wall, S is the surface area available for filtration, P_{gc} and P_{bs} are the hydraulic pressures in the glomerular capillary and Bowman's space, Π_p and Π_{bs} are the oncotic pressures in the plasma entering the glomerulus and Bowman's space, and s represents the reflection coefficient of proteins across the capillary wall (with values ranging from 0 if completely permeable to 1 if completely impermeable). Since the filtrate is essentially protein free, Π_{bs} is 0 and s is 1. Thus,

$$GFR = LpS\,(P_{gc} - P_{bs} - \Pi_p) \qquad \text{(Eq. 1)}$$

A reduction in GFR in disease states is most often due to a decrease in net permeability resulting from a loss of filtration surface area induced by some form of glomerular injury. In normal subjects, however, GFR is primarily regulated by alterations in P_{gc} that are mediated by changes in glomerular arteriolar resistance. The P_{gc} also plays a role in renal disease. For example, the initial fall in glomerular permeability in glomerular disease does not necessarily lead to reduction in GFR. In this setting, changes in arteriolar resistance can increase the P_{gc}, thereby raising the gradient favoring filtration and at least in part overcoming the effect of decreased permeability.

Arteriolar Resistance and Glomerular Filtration Rate

The glomerular capillaries are interposed between two arterioles: the afferent or precapillary arteriole and the efferent or postcapillary arteriole. As a result, the P_{gc} is governed by the interplay between three factors:

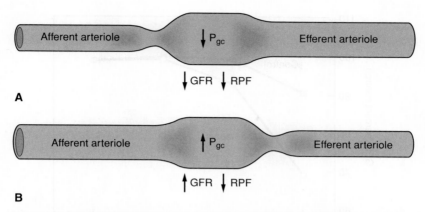

FIGURE 1.7. Relationship between glomerular arteriolar resistance, glomerular filtration rate (GFR), and renal plasma flow (RPF). Constriction of the afferent arteriole increases renal vascular resistance (thereby reducing RPF) and decreases the intraglomerular pressure and GFR, since less of the arterial pressure is transmitted to the glomerulus (**A**). Constriction of the efferent arteriole also lowers RPF but tends to elevate the intraglomerular pressure and GFR (**B**). Arteriolar dilation has the opposite effects.

the aortic pressure perfusing the kidney; the afferent resistance, which determines the degree to which the renal arterial pressure is transmitted to the glomerulus; and the efferent resistance (Fig. 1.7). If, for example, the P_{gc} must rise to counteract a reduction in glomerular permeability, this can be achieved by afferent dilation and/or efferent constriction.

Arteriolar resistance is partially under intrinsic myogenic control, but can also be influenced by other factors, including tubuloglomerular feedback, angiotensin II, norepinephrine, and other hormones (Chapter 2).

Autoregulation. In view of the importance of P_{gc}, it might be assumed that small variations in arterial pressure could produce large changes in glomerular filtration. However, GFR (and renal plasma flow) are almost constant over a relatively wide range of renal arterial pressures (Fig. 1.8). This phenomenon, which is also present in other capillaries, is called autoregulation.

Autoregulation in most capillaries is mediated by changes in precapillary resistance. In the kidney, for example, an increase in afferent arteriolar tone can, when perfusion pressure rises, prevent the elevation in pressure from being transmitted to the glomerulus, thereby preventing any significant change in P_{gc} and GFR. Conversely, GFR can be preserved by afferent dilation when renal perfusion pressure falls.

However, the mechanism of autoregulation of GFR is more complex. Angiotensin II makes an important contribution when renal perfusion pressure falls, a situation in which the renin–angiotensin system is

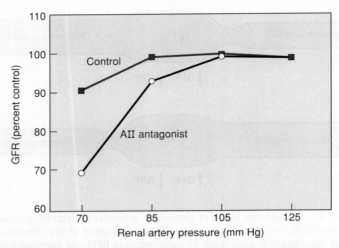

FIGURE 1.8. Autoregulation of glomerular filtration rate (GFR), expressed as a percentage of control values, as the renal artery pressure is reduced from a baseline level of 125 mm Hg in dogs. The *squares* represent control animals in which GFR was maintained until renal perfusion pressure was markedly reduced. The *circles* represent animals given an intrarenal infusion of an angiotensin II antagonist. In this setting, GFR is less well maintained. Although not shown, autoregulation also applies when renal artery pressure is initially raised.

activated. Angiotensin II preferentially increases the resistance at the efferent arteriole, thereby preventing the P_{gc} from declining in the presence of hypotension.

The contribution of angiotensin II to autoregulation can be seen in Figure 1.8. In normal animals, GFR begins to fall only when there is a marked reduction in renal perfusion pressure; this limitation presumably is due in part to maximal dilation of the afferent arteriole. In comparison, GFR begins to fall at a higher perfusion pressure in animals pretreated with an angiotensin II antagonist. Even in this situation, however, the ability to autoregulate is maintained with the initial reduction in renal perfusion pressure. This autoregulation at mild reductions in perfusion pressure is mediated by tubuloglomerular feedback (see next section) and the stretch receptors.

QUESTION 3   Narrowing of the renal arteries (renal artery stenosis) is a relatively common cause of severe or refractory hypertension, and is usually due to atherosclerotic lesions in older patients. What should happen to GFR in a stenotic kidney as BP is lowered with antihypertensive agents that act independently of angiotensin II? Would the response be different if any angiotensin-converting enzyme inhibitor, which decreases the formation of angiotensin II, were given?

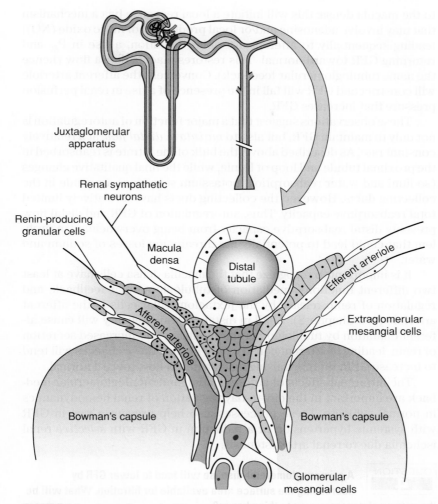

FIGURE 1.9. Juxtaglomerular apparatus and macula densa in tubuloglomerular feedback. The juxtaglomerular apparatus and macula densa cells at the beginning of the distal tubule are in close proximity. Chloride delivery is sensed by the $Na^+–K^+–2Cl^-$ cotransporter in the thick ascending limb and feedback regulates GFR. Renin release is also regulated at this site (see Chapter 2).

Tubuloglomerular Feedback. GFR is in part autoregulated by the rate of fluid delivery to the specialized cells in the *macula densa*, which begins at the end of the cortical thick ascending limb of the loop of Henle. These cells sense changes in the delivery and subsequent reabsorption of chloride, a process mediated by the $Na^+–K^+–2Cl^-$ cotransporter in the apical membrane (Figs. 1.3 and 1.9). If, for example, a reduction in renal perfusion pressure initially lowers GFR, less chloride will be delivered to the macula densa; this will initiate a local response [via a mechanism that may involve adenosine and/or local production of nitric oxide (NO)] leading sequentially to afferent arteriolar dilatation, a rise in P_{gc} and returning GFR toward normal. This restores macula densa flow (hence the name tubuloglomerular feedback). Conversely, the afferent arteriole will constrict and GFR will fall in the presence of a rise in renal perfusion pressure that increases GFR.

These observations suggest that a major function of autoregulation is not only to maintain GFR, but also to *maintain distal flow* at a relatively constant rate. As described above, the bulk of the filtrate is reabsorbed in the proximal tubule and loop of Henle, while the final qualitative changes (sodium and water reabsorption, potassium secretion) are made in the collecting ducts. However, the collecting ducts have a relatively limited total reabsorptive capacity. Thus, autoregulation of GFR and distal flow prevents distal reabsorptive capacity from being overwhelmed, a problem that could lead to potentially life-threatening losses of sodium and water.

It is important to recognize that the macula densa cells have at least two different functions: mediation of tubuloglomerular feedback, and regulation of renin release by the juxtaglomerular cells in the afferent arteriole (see Chapter 2). A fall in distal chloride delivery will cause afferent dilatation by tubuloglomerular feedback *and* increased secretion of renin, leading to efferent constriction. Both of these changes will tend to increase GFR, thereby raising macula densa flow toward normal.

The intrarenal effects of autoregulation and tubuloglomerular feedback are important in the day-to-day regulation of renal hemodynamics in normal subjects. These processes also help prevent a rise in GFR with systemic hypertension or a reduction in GFR with *selective* renal ischemia due to renal artery stenosis.

 A primary glomerular disease will tend to lower GFR by decreasing the surface area available for filtration. What will be the autoregulatory response to this change?

Neurohumoral Influences. A reduction in renal perfusion pressure in patients is most often due to effective circulating volume depletion (as with gastrointestinal fluid losses or congestive heart failure; see Chapter 2), rather than to selective renal ischemia. In these disorders, systemic hypoperfusion leads to increased release of the vasoconstrictors angiotensin II and norepinephrine. The former increases resistance at the efferent arteriole more than at the afferent arteriole, whereas norepinephrine affects both arterioles to a similar degree. The net effect is renal vasoconstriction (not vasodilatation as with pure autoregulation), a potentially marked reduction in renal plasma flow, and a slight fall or even no change in GFR due to the effect of efferent constriction. This is a physiologically appropriate adaptation since it preferentially shunts blood to the critical coronary and cerebral circulations, while maintaining GFR and therefore excretory capacity.

These vasoconstrictive effects are antagonized by renal vasodilator prostaglandins. Angiotensin II and norepinephrine stimulate glomerular prostaglandin production. The ensuing prostaglandin-induced decrease in arteriolar tone prevents excessive renal ischemia. This adaptation is important clinically because of the widespread use of nonsteroidal anti-inflammatory drugs to treat arthritis and other conditions. These drugs inhibit prostaglandin production and can produce an acute decline in GFR (acute renal failure) in susceptible subjects who are volume depleted and who therefore have relatively high levels of angiotensin II and norepinephrine. On the other hand, normal subjects are at little risk since, in the absence of high levels of vasoconstrictors, the rate of renal prostaglandin production is relatively low.

Clinical Estimation of Glomerular Filtration Rate

As described above, estimation of GFR is used clinically to assess the severity and course of renal disease. Measurement of GFR relies on the concept of clearance. Consider a compound such as the polysaccharide inulin (not insulin) or a radioisotope, such as iothalamate, with the following properties:

1 Able to achieve a stable plasma concentration
2 Freely filtered at the glomerulus
3 Not reabsorbed, secreted, synthesized, or metabolized by the kidney

With these characteristics,

Filtered inulin = excreted inulin

The filtered inulin is equal to the GFR times the plasma inulin concentration (P_{in}), and the excreted inulin is equal to the product of the urine inulin concentration (U_{in}) and the urine flow rate (V, in milliliters per minute or liters per day). Therefore,

$$GFR \times P_{in} = U_{in} \times V$$
$$GFR = [U_{in} \times V]/P_{in} \qquad \text{(Eq. 2)}$$

The term ($U_{in} \times V$)/P_{in} is called the clearance of inulin and is an accurate estimate of GFR. The inulin clearance, in mL/min, refers to *that volume of plasma cleared of inulin by renal excretion* in one minute. If, for example, 1.2 mg of inulin is excreted per minute ($U_{in} \times V$) and the P_{in} is 1.0 mg/dL (or to keep the units consistent, 0.01 mg/mL), then the clearance of inulin is 120 mL/min; that is, 120 mL of plasma has been cleared by urinary excretion of the 1.2 mg of inulin that it contained.

Creatinine Clearance

Although accurate, performance of the inulin or radioisotopic clearance is too cumbersome and expensive for routine clinical use. The most common method used to estimate GFR is the endogenous *creatinine clearance*:

$$Creatinine\ clearance = [U_{cr} \times V]/P_{cr} \qquad \text{(Eq. 3)}$$

Creatinine is derived from the metabolism of creatine in skeletal muscle. Like an inulin infusion, it has a relatively stable plasma concentration, it is freely filtered at the glomerulus, and it is not reabsorbed, synthesized, or metabolized by the kidney. However, a variable quantity of creatinine is secreted into the urine in the proximal tubule. As a result, creatinine excretion exceeds creatinine filtration by 10% to 20% in normal subjects; thus, creatinine clearance will tend to overestimate GFR by the same 10% to 20%. Creatinine clearance is usually determined by using venous blood for the plasma creatinine concentration and a 24-hour urine specimen for the urine volume and urine creatinine concentration. The normal values for creatinine clearance in adults are 95 ± 20 mL/min in women and 120 ± 25 mL/min in men.

Limitations. Two errors can occur with creatinine clearance. The first is underestimation of the true GFR due to an incomplete urine collection by the patient. The relative constancy of creatinine production and therefore of creatinine excretion in the steady state can be used to assess patient compliance. Creatinine production varies directly with muscle mass (which falls with age) and to a lesser degree with meat intake (which is a source of creatinine). In adults under the age of 50, daily creatinine excretion should be from 20 to 25 mg/kg (177 to 221 μmol/kg) of lean body weight in men and from 15 to 20 mg/kg (133 to 177 μmol/kg) of lean body weight in women. From the ages of 50 to 90, there is a progressive decline in creatinine excretion, due primarily to a fall in muscle mass. Values much below expected levels suggest an incomplete collection or severe malnutrition leading to a loss of muscle mass.

QUESTION
5

A 43-year-old woman weighing 65 kg is being evaluated for possible renal disease. Plasma creatinine concentration is 1.2 mg/dL, urine volume in the 24-hour urine collection is 1080 mL and the urine creatinine concentration is 72 mg/dL. Calculate the creatinine clearance in mL/min. Does the rate of creatinine excretion suggest that this is a complete urine collection?

As mentioned, a second frequent error is overestimation of GFR due to creatinine secretion. Although creatinine secretion accounts for only about 15% of urinary creatinine when GFR is normal, the secretory pump is not yet saturated. As a result, the rise in plasma creatinine concentration that accompanies a fall in GFR leads to more creatinine secretion, which can ultimately account for as much as 35% of urinary creatinine in advanced disease. In this situation, creatinine clearance can markedly overestimate the true GFR, masking the severity and perhaps even the presence of a decline in renal function. In one study, for example, creatinine clearance was normal (>90 mL/min) in one-half of patients with a true GFR of 61 to 70 mL/min and in one-quarter of patients with a true GFR as low as 51 to 60 mL/min.

It has been suggested that, in patients with moderate to advanced disease, a more accurate estimate of GFR can be obtained by averaging creatinine and urea clearances. Urea, an end product of protein metabolism, is filtered and then about 50% is reabsorbed. Thus, urea clearance will underestimate GFR, a change that will counteract overestimation by creatinine clearance when the two values are averaged.

Plasma Creatinine Concentration and Glomerular Filtration Rate

Exact knowledge of GFR is not required in most clinical conditions. Plasma levels of some drugs normally excreted by the kidneys can be monitored for potentially toxic effects (such as digoxin or an aminoglycoside antibiotic). In patients with renal disease, on the other hand, it is important to know roughly how much function has been lost and whether GFR is changing; this can usually be determined from measurement of plasma creatinine concentration alone, a much simpler test than creatinine clearance.

In a subject in the steady state in whom plasma creatinine concentration is stable,

$$Creatinine\ excretion = Creatinine\ production$$

Creatinine excretion is approximately equal to the amount of creatinine filtered—GFR × plasma creatinine concentration (P_{cr})—whereas the rate of creatinine production is relatively constant. If these substitutions are made in the above equation, then

$$GFR \times P_{cr} = Constant$$
$$P_{cr} = Constant/GFR$$

Thus, *plasma creatinine concentration varies inversely with GFR.* If, for example, GFR falls by 50%, creatinine filtration and subsequent excretion also will be diminished. As a result, newly produced creatinine will accumulate in the plasma until the filtered load again equals the rate of production. This will occur when plasma creatinine concentration has increased twofold, excluding the contribution from creatinine secretion:

$$GFR/2 \times 2P_{cr} = GFR \times P_{cr} = Constant$$

In adults, the range for normal plasma creatinine concentration is from 0.8 to 1.3 mg/dL in men and from 0.6 to 1.0 mg/dL (women have a smaller muscle mass and therefore a lower rate of creatinine production). Creatinine production can also be influenced by the intake of meat, which contains creatine, the precursor of creatinine. For example, plasma creatinine concentration can fall by as much as 15% by switching to a meat-free diet, without any change in GFR.

The idealized reciprocal relationship between GFR and plasma creatinine concentration is shown by the solid curve in Figure 1.10. There are three points to note about this relationship:

1 The relationship is valid only in the steady state when plasma creatinine concentration is stable. If, for example, GFR suddenly ceases,

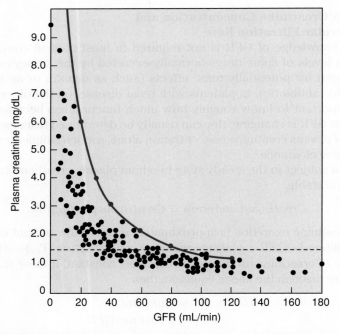

FIGURE 1.10. Relationship between true GFR (as measured by inulin clearance) and plasma creatinine concentration in 171 patients with glomerular disease. The *red circles* joined by the *solid line* represent the relationship that would exist if creatinine were excreted solely by glomerular filtration; the *dotted line* represents the upper limit of "normal" for plasma creatinine concentration of 1.4 mg/dL. In the patients (*dark circles*), however, variations in GFR between 120 and 60 mL/min were often associated with a plasma creatinine concentration that remained well within the normal range due to increased creatinine secretion. The latter becomes saturated at a plasma creatinine concentration above 1.5 to 2 mg/dL; as a result, plasma creatinine concentration rises as expected with further reductions in GFR.

plasma creatinine concentration will still be normal for the first few hours because there has not been time for nonexcreted creatinine to accumulate.

2 The shape of the curve is important, since there is a variable relation between a change in plasma creatinine concentration and the degree of change in GFR. An apparently minor elevation in plasma creatinine concentration from 1.0 up to 1.5 mg/dL reflects a major fall in GFR from 120 down to 80 mL/min. In comparison, a more prominent increase in plasma creatinine concentration from 5 up to 10 mg/dL in a patient with advanced renal failure represents a relatively small absolute decline in GFR from 24 down to 12 mL/min.

3 The shape of the curve is also dependent upon the rate of creatinine production, which is mostly determined by muscle mass. The horizontal dashed line in Figure 1.10 shows that a plasma creatinine concentration of 1.0 mg/dL represents a range of creatinine clearances from 30 to 130 mL/min. This extreme range reveals the necessity of interpreting the plasma creatinine in the context of the age and weight of the patient. A serum creatinine of 1.0 mg/dL may reflect a GFR of 120 mL/min in a young muscular man, whereas, an older frail women who has much less muscle may have a much lower GFR at the same plasma creatinine concentration. The following formula has been used to account for the effects of body weight and age on muscle mass and therefore on the relationship between plasma creatinine concentration and GFR:

$$Creatinine \; clearance \cong \frac{(140 - age) \times lean \; body \; weight \, (in \; kg)}{P_{cr} \, (in \; mg/dL) \times 72} \qquad \text{(Eq. 4)}$$

This value should be multiplied by 0.85 in women in whom a lesser fraction of body weight is composed of muscle.

Using this formula, which correlates fairly closely with a simultaneously measured creatinine clearance, we can see that a seemingly normal plasma creatinine concentration of 1.0 mg/dL represents a creatinine clearance of only 36 mL/min in a 50-kg, 80-year-old woman. Similar findings can be demonstrated in malnourished patients, such as those with advanced hepatic cirrhosis.

More recently, the MDRD (Modification of Diet in Renal Disease) study equation has been adopted by most clinical laboratories to express an estimated GFR (eGFR) along with serum creatinine. The original equation that was correlated with iothalamate GFR contained six variables has been simplified to

$$GFR \; (in \; mL/min/1.73 \; m^2) = 175 \times S_{cr} \, (exp[-1.154])$$
$$\times Age(exp[-0.203]) \times (0.742 \; if \; female)$$
$$\times (1.21 \; if \; African \; American) \qquad \text{(Eq. 5)}$$

Web sites are available to aid in the calculation of the GFR through these formulas. These include www.kidney.org/professionals/KDOQI/gfr_calculator.cfm

However, this equation was derived from white patients with nondiabetic kidney disease and is less precise in obese patients, patients with normal or near-normal GFR, and other ethnic populations.

QUESTION 6   **A 76-year-old man who weighs 70 kg has been unable to urinate for several days due to obstruction of the urethra by an enlarged prostate. Back pressure up the nephron will raise the intratubular pressure and cause GFR to fall to very low levels. A catheter is placed in the bladder to relieve the obstruction. Over the next 24 hours, plasma creatinine concentration falls from 6 mg/dL to the previous baseline of 1.3 mg/dL. What accounts for this reduction in plasma creatinine concentration?**

Limitations. Significant disease progression can occur with little or no elevation in plasma creatinine concentration, particularly in patients with a GFR above 60 mL/min. Three factors can contribute to this problem, two of which prevent or minimize any reduction in GFR and one of which minimizes the rise in plasma creatinine concentration when GFR does fall:

■ As discussed in Question 4, glomerular diseases can cause a substantial decline in glomerular permeability by decreasing the surface area available for filtration. Nevertheless, GFR is initially maintained at normal or near-normal levels by a compensatory elevation in intraglomerular pressure that may be mediated by tubuloglomerular feedback.

■ Nephron loss of any cause leads to a compensatory elevation in GFR above normal in the remaining nephrons with more normal function. As many as 25% to 30% of nephrons can be lost with little or no reduction in GFR because of this adaptation. Even the loss of one kidney leads to a fall in total GFR of only 20% to 25%. This means that the filtration rate in each glomerulus in the remaining kidney must increase by an average of 50%.

■ Once GFR does fall, the rise in plasma creatinine concentration will, as described above, be minimized by increased creatinine secretion.

The potential effect of enhanced creatinine secretion is illustrated in Figure 1.10. Although a fall in GFR from 120 to 60 mL/min should ideally induce a doubling of plasma creatinine concentration, many patients have only a small increase (as little as 0.1 to 0.2 mg/dL) in plasma creatinine concentration. Thus, a stable value within the normal or high-normal range does not necessarily reflect stable disease. However, plasma creatinine concentration rises as expected with reductions in GFR in more advanced disease (plasma creatinine concentration greater than 1.5 to 2 mg/dL), presumably due to saturation of the secretory mechanism.

Blood Urea Nitrogen and Glomerular Filtration Rate

Changes in GFR can also be detected by alterations in the concentration of urea in the blood, measured as blood urea nitrogen (BUN). Like plasma creatinine concentration, BUN is excreted by glomerular filtration and tends to vary inversely with GFR.

However, this relationship is less predictable, since two factors can affect BUN without a change in GFR (or plasma creatinine concentration). First, urea production is not constant. Urea is formed from the hepatic metabolism of amino acids that are not utilized for protein synthesis. Amino acid deamination leads to the generation of ammonia (NH_3), which is then converted into urea in a reaction that can be summarized by the following reaction:

$$2NH_3 + CO_2 \rightarrow H_2O + H_2N - CO - NH_2 \; (urea)$$

Thus, urea production and BUN increase with a high-protein diet or enhanced tissue breakdown; conversely, a low-protein diet or liver disease will lower urea production and BUN.

Second, approximately 50% of the filtered urea is reabsorbed, much of which occurs in the proximal tubule as urea movement passively follows the reabsorption of sodium and water. Thus, increased proximal reabsorption as appropriately occurs in hypovolemic states will raise BUN out of proportion to any change in GFR or plasma creatinine concentration (see Chapter 11 for a discussion of how this relationship can be useful in the differential diagnosis of acute renal failure).

ANSWERS TO QUESTIONS

1 Increased reabsorption of sodium and water will raise the tubular fluid urea concentration, resulting in enhanced passive urea reabsorption. This will reduce urea excretion, thereby increasing the BUN concentration. This selective elevation in BUN is, in the appropriate clinical setting, suggestive of volume depletion and decreased renal perfusion as the cause of renal dysfunction, rather than intrinsic renal disease (see Chapter 11).

2 Calcium reabsorption will fall because the decrease in $Na^+–K^+–2Cl^-$ cotransport will result in less potassium recycling and therefore a diminution in the lumen-positive electrical gradient that drives passive

calcium transport in this segment. This ability to increase calcium excretion makes a loop diuretic a key component of therapy for hypercalcemia.

3 The intrarenal pressure distal to the stenosis should be lower than the arterial pressure. As a result, lowering systemic blood pressure will further reduce intrarenal pressure to below normal. Nevertheless, autoregulation will maintain GFR unless the stenosis is so severe or the systemic pressure is lowered so much that intraglomerular pressure falls below the autoregulatory range. The administration of an angiotensin-converting enzyme inhibitor will tend to lower GFR by blocking angiotensin II–mediated regulation at the efferent arteriole. Therefore, the combination of reduced afferent flow distal to the stenosis and inhibition of normal efferent regulatory mechanisms by angiotensin-converting enzyme inhibitor can lead to acute renal failure (if bilateral renal artery stenoses or unilateral stenosis in a solitary kidney).

4 The fall in GFR will lead sequentially to decreased fluid delivery to the macula densa, activation of tubuloglomerular feedback, afferent arteriolar dilatation, and a rise in intraglomerular pressure that will return GFR and macula densa flow toward normal. Thus, estimation of GFR will underestimate the severity of glomerular disease, since substantial damage can occur without any significant fall in GFR. In addition, the compensatory elevation in intraglomerular pressure may be maladaptive over the long term, since intraglomerular hypertension can produce progressive glomerular injury independent of the activity of the underlying disease (see Chapter 12).

5 Creatinine clearance is 45 mL/min: Total urine creatinine is 1080 mL/24 h × 72 mg/dL = 777 mg/24 h,

$$\text{Creatinine clearance} = \frac{777 \text{ mg/24 h}}{1.2 \text{ mg/dL}} \equiv 647.5 \text{ dL/24 h}$$

$$\equiv 64{,}750 \text{ mL/1440 min} \equiv 45 \text{ mL/min}$$

which is about one-half the expected value. Total creatinine excretion of 777 mg is well below the expected 15 to 20 mg/kg (975 to 1300 mg) suggesting an incomplete collection.

6 The very low GFR during the period of almost complete urinary tract obstruction caused creatinine to accumulate in the plasma. Relief of the obstruction allowed GFR to return to near-normal levels. However, a normal GFR at a plasma creatinine concentration that is more than four times greater than normal (6 vs. 1.3 mg/dL) means that the filtered creatinine load is also initially more than four times normal, and therefore more than four times the rate of creatinine production. As a result, plasma creatinine concentration will fall toward normal.

SUGGESTED READINGS

Nielsen S, Agre P. The aquaporin family of water channels in kidney. Kidney Int 1995;48:1057–1068.

Poggio ED, Wang X, Greene T, et al. Performance of the modification of diet in renal disease and Cockcroft–Gault equations in the estimation of GFR in health and in chronic kidney disease. J Am Soc Nephrol 2005;16:459.

Rose BD. Diuretics. Kidney Int 1991;39:336.

Rose BD, Post TW. Clinical Physiology of Acid–Base and Electrolyte Disorders, 5th Ed. New York: McGraw-Hill, 2001, Chapters 2–5.

Shemesh O, Golbetz H, Kriss JP, et al. Limitations of a creatinine as a filtration marker in glomerulopathic patients. Kidney Int 1985;28:830.

2

REGULATION OF SALT AND WATER BALANCE

CASE PRESENTATION A 63-year-old woman is noted to have mild essential hypertension on a routine office visit. She is started on a salt-restricted diet, but little antihypertensive effect is noted. As a result, 25 mg of hydrochlorothiazide—a thiazide-type diuretic that inhibits sodium chloride reabsorption in the distal tubule—is added. Five days later, she is noted to be lethargic and feeling very weak.

Physical examination reveals a tired woman in no acute distress. Her blood pressure is now 130/85 and her weight is 2.5 kg below her baseline value. The remainder of the examination is unremarkable; there are no focal neurologic findings.

Initial laboratory data reveal the following:

BUN	$= 42$ mg/dL (9–25)
Creatinine	$= 1.2$ mg/dL (0.8–1.4)
Na	$= 134$ mEq/L (136–142)
K	$= 3.4$ mEq/L (3.5–5)
Cl	$= 90$ mEq/L (98–108)
Total CO_2	$= 32$ mEq/L (21–30)

Urine Na   = 84 mEq/L (variable)
K   = 59 mEq/L (variable)
Osmolality   = 553 mOsm/kg (variable)

OBJECTIVES

By the end of this section, you should have an understanding of each of the following issues:

- The relationship between water balance and the regulation of the plasma osmolality, which is primarily determined by the plasma sodium concentration.
- The important differences between osmoregulation and volume regulation, with emphasis on the role of alterations in water and sodium excretion.
- The role of osmotic pressure in determining the distribution of water between the cells and the extracellular fluid.
- The roles of the renin–angiotensin–aldosterone system, atrial natriuretic peptide, and antidiuretic hormone in the regulation of sodium and water balance.
- The concepts of the steady state (as it applies to fluid and electrolyte balance) and of the effective circulating volume.

Introduction

Water and sodium balance are regulated *independently* by specific pathways that are designed to prevent large changes in the plasma osmolality (which is primarily determined by the plasma sodium *concentration*) and the effective circulating volume. The differences between these pathways can be appreciated by considering the clinical manifestations of impaired regulation:

- Too much water—hyponatremia (low plasma sodium concentration)
- Too little water—hypernatremia (high plasma sodium concentration)
- Too much sodium—edema
- Too little sodium—volume depletion

Although these disorders will be reviewed in the following chapters, one point is central to this chapter: The plasma sodium concentration is regulated by changes in water balance, not by changes in sodium or volume balance.

Physiologic Role of Osmotic Pressure

An approach to the regulation of water balance begins with the processes of osmosis and osmotic pressure, which can be easily understood from the simple experiment in Figure 2.1. Distilled water in a beaker is separated into two compartments by a membrane that is freely permeable to water but not to sodium chloride (NaCl). Water molecules exhibit random motion and can diffuse across a membrane by a mechanism that is similar to that for diffusion of solutes. When a solute such as NaCl is added to one compartment, the intermolecular cohesive forces reduce the random movement (or activity) of the water molecules in that compartment. Since water will move from an area of high activity to one of low activity, water will flow into the solute-containing compartment.

This increase in volume in the solute-containing compartment will raise the pressure within this compartment; this hydrostatic pressure can be measured by the height of the fluid column above the compartment. Equilibrium will be reached when the hydrostatic pressure, which tends to push water back into the solute-free compartment, is equal to the osmotic forces generated by the addition of NaCl, which tends to cause water movement in the opposite direction. This equilibrium pressure is called the *osmotic pressure.*

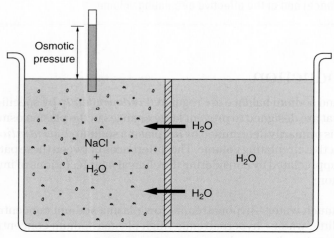

Semipermeable membrane

FIGURE 2.1.   Effect of adding sodium chloride on fluid distribution in a rigid beaker separated into two compartments by a semipermeable membrane, which is permeable to water but not to sodium chloride. The addition of solute decreases the random movement of water, resulting in water diffusion into the solute-containing compartment at a faster rate than diffusion in the opposite direction. In a rigid compartment as in this experiment, the net force promoting water movement can be measured as the osmotic pressure.

The osmotic pressure generated by a solute is proportional to the number of solute particles, not to the size, weight, or valence of the particles. Since 1 mol of any nondissociable substance has the same number of particles (6.02×10^{23}), the osmotic pressure is determined by the molar concentrations of the solutes that are present.

The unit of measurement of osmotic pressure is osmole (Osm). One osmole is defined as one gram molecular weight (or 1 mol) of any nondissociable substance. In relatively dilute physiologic fluids, however, it is more appropriate to use units of millimoles (mmol) and milliosmoles (mOsm) (one-thousandth of a mol). For example, glucose has a molecular weight of 180; thus, 180 mg is equal to 1 mmol and can potentially generate 1 mOsm of osmotic pressure. In comparison, 1 mmol of NaCl will generate approximately 2 mOsm due to its dissociation into sodium and chloride ions.

Solutes generate an osmotic pressure by their inability to cross membranes. Some solutes like urea are lipid soluble and can freely cross membranes. As a result, the addition of urea to one compartment will lead to a new equilibrium that is reached by urea entry into the solute-free compartment, rather than by water movement in the opposite direction. Thus, no osmotic pressure is generated at equilibrium and urea is called an *ineffective* osmole. The same principles apply to other lipid-soluble solutes such as ethanol. Plasma ethanol levels can reach relatively high levels in a patient who is drunk, but there will be little change in the effective plasma osmotic pressure or therefore in water distribution.

Osmotic Pressure and Distribution of Body Water

Osmotic pressure is important physiologically because it determines the distribution of the body water between the different fluid compartments. In normal adults, water comprises 55% to 60% of *lean* body weight in men and 45% to 50% in women. Adipose tissue contains no water and is not included in this calculation. The body water is primarily contained in two compartments that are separated by the cell membrane: inside the cells (the intracellular fluid) and in the extracellular space (the extracellular fluid). The extracellular fluid is further divided into two compartments: the interstitial fluid that bathes the cells and the intravascular compartment of circulating plasma water. These extracellular fluid spaces are separated by the capillary wall.

Since virtually all cell membranes and peripheral capillaries are permeable to water, the distribution of water between these compartments is entirely determined by osmotic pressure. Each compartment has one solute that is primarily limited to that compartment and therefore acts to pull water into that compartment: potassium salts in the cells; sodium salts in the interstitial fluid; and proteins (particularly albumin) in the plasma (Fig. 2.2). The distribution of potassium and sodium is

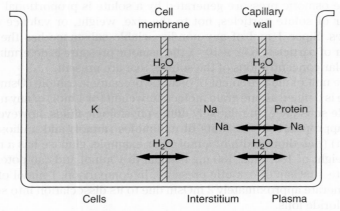

FIGURE 2.2. Schematic representation of the osmotic factors that determine the distribution of the body water among its three major compartments: potassium salts in the intracellular fluid; sodium salts in the interstitial fluid; and proteins in the plasma water.

primarily determined by the Na^+–K^+-ATPase pumps in the cell membranes that actively transport sodium out of and potassium into cells (see Chapter 1).

In comparison, sodium is freely able to cross the capillary wall and therefore acts as an ineffective osmole at the site separating the interstitial from intravascular compartments. The much larger plasma proteins, however, cannot easily diffuse across the capillary. As a result, these macromolecules are the primary effective solutes in the plasma; the pressure they generate to hold water within the vascular space is called the *plasma oncotic pressure*. It might be suspected that water would continually move from the interstitium into the vascular space down this favorable osmotic gradient. However, this does not occur because the plasma oncotic pressure is counterbalanced by the capillary hydraulic pressure (generated by cardiac contraction) that tends to cause water movement in the opposite direction. This relationship is described in detail in Chapter 4 and Figure 4.1.

Relation between Plasma Osmolality and Sodium Concentration

Since the osmolality in all the fluid compartments is essentially equal, we can estimate the osmolality of the body water simply by measuring the plasma osmolality. The latter can be estimated from the following formula:

$$Plasma\ osmolality \cong 2 \times PNa + \frac{[glucose]}{18} + \frac{BUN}{2.8} \qquad \textbf{(Eq. 1)}$$

Since sodium is the major extracellular cation, the plasma sodium concentration (PNa) is multiplied by 2 to account for the osmotic contribution of accompanying anions—primarily chloride and bicarbonate. The concentrations of glucose (molecular weight 180 g/mol) and blood urea nitrogen (BUN; 28 g/mol) are divided by 18 and 2.8, respectively, to convert from the frequently measured units of mg/dL into mmol/L. The normal plasma sodium concentration is between 139 and 143 mmol/L (or mEq/L, since the valence of sodium is 1) and the normal osmolality of the body water is between 280 and 290 mOsm/kg.

In normal subjects, the effective plasma osmolality can be simplified to

$$Effective\ Posm \cong 2 \times PNa \qquad \text{(Eq. 2)}$$

Glucose can be ignored, since it is present in a much lower concentration (less than 6 mmol/L) than sodium salts, and urea can be ignored, since it is present in low concentrations and is an ineffective osmole.

These observations illustrate an important difference between *osmolality*, which is measured in the laboratory and reflects the total number of particles in solution, and the *osmotic pressure*, which determines fluid distribution and reflects the number of osmotically active particles in each compartment. It is important to note the following:

■ Urea contributes to the plasma osmolality but not to osmotic pressure.
■ Sodium contributes to the plasma osmolality and to the osmotic pressure at the cell membrane but not at the capillary wall (Fig. 2.2).
■ Plasma proteins, particularly albumin, are the main determinant of the plasma oncotic pressure (since they are essentially the only effective osmoles in the plasma). However, albumin (mol wt 69,000) does not contribute to the plasma osmolality since a normal plasma albumin concentration of 4 g/dL or 40 g/L represents less than 1 mmol/L or 1 mOsm/kg.

Osmoregulation and Volume Regulation

The relationship between plasma osmolality and plasma sodium concentration is often thought to reflect the importance of sodium balance in osmoregulation. However, these are separate processes since the plasma osmolality is regulated by changes in *water intake* and *water excretion*, while sodium balance is regulated by changes in *sodium excretion*.

The different characteristics of osmoregulation and sodium regulation can be illustrated by evaluating the effects of adding NaCl alone (as with eating salted potato chips), water alone (as with drinking but not excreting water), or isotonic salt and water (as with an infusion of isotonic

TABLE 2.1

How Adding Sodium Chloride, Water, and an Isotonic Sodium Chloride Solution to the Extracellular Fluid Affects the Plasma Sodium Concentration, the Extracellular Fluid (ECF) Volume, Urinary Sodium Excretion, and the Intracellular Fluid (ICF) Volume

	NaCl	H$_2$O	Isotonic Saline
Plasma Na	↑	↓	0
ECF volume	↑	↑	↑
Urine Na	↑	↑	↑
ICF volume	↓	↑	0

saline, which has a sodium concentration similar to that in the plasma water). The results of these experiments are summarized in Table 2.1:

■ When sodium is ingested without water, the excess sodium will remain in the extracellular space, where it will raise the plasma sodium concentration and the plasma osmolality. The increase in osmolality will, as in Figure 2.1, result in the osmotic movement of water out of the cells into the extracellular space until the osmolality is the same in the two compartments. The net effect is hypernatremia (a high plasma sodium concentration), an elevation in plasma osmolality, an increase in the extracellular fluid volume, and an equivalent reduction in the intracellular fluid volume that results in a similar increase in intracellular osmolality. Note that the osmotic effect of the added sodium is distributed through the total body water even though the sodium is restricted to the extracellular fluid. The increased extracellular fluid volume inhibits renin–angiotensin–aldosterone and stimulates atrial natriuretic peptide (see next section) to increase urinary sodium excretion.

■ The retention of water without sodium lowers both the plasma sodium concentration and the plasma osmolality. As a result, some of the excess water will move into the cells until osmotic equilibrium is achieved. The net result is hyponatremia (a low plasma sodium concentration), hypo-osmolality, and an increase in both the extracellular (also leading to increased urinary sodium excretion) and intracellular fluid volumes.

■ The administration of isotonic saline will not affect water movement between the cells and the extracellular fluid, since there is no change in osmolality. All of the excess salt and water will remain in the extracellular fluid, producing extracellular volume expansion but no alteration in the plasma sodium concentration.

A number of important observations can be appreciated when we summarize these experiments (Table 2.1):

- The plasma sodium concentration is determined by the *ratio* between the amounts of solute and water that are present, whereas the extracellular fluid volume is determined by the *absolute amounts* of solute and water that are present.
- The plasma sodium concentration and the plasma osmolality vary *in parallel* as predicted from Eq. 2.
- There is *no predictable relationship between the plasma sodium concentration and the extracellular fluid volume*: The latter is increased in all three experiments, whereas the plasma sodium concentration rises, falls, and is unchanged.
- There is *no predictable relationship between the plasma sodium concentration and urinary sodium excretion.* As will be reviewed below, the extracellular fluid volume is regulated by changes in sodium excretion. Since volume expansion occurred in all three experiments, there will be an appropriate increase in sodium excretion (in an attempt to lower the extracellular fluid volume toward normal), even though the plasma sodium concentration may vary widely.
- Alterations in plasma osmolality lead to changes in intracellular fluid volume: Hyponatremia and hypo-osmolality induce fluid movement into the cells, whereas hypernatremia and hyperosmolality induce fluid movement out of the cells. These changes in volume within the brain are largely responsible for the symptoms associated with hyponatremia and hypernatremia (see Chapter 3).

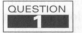 **Suppose that you exercised on a hot day, leading to the loss of sweat, which is a relatively dilute fluid containing low concentrations of sodium and potassium. What will happen to the plasma sodium concentration, extracellular fluid volume, and urinary sodium excretion?**

Hormonal Role in Water and Sodium Balance

The lack of predictable relationship between the plasma sodium concentration and extracellular fluid volume means that these parameters must be regulated independently. Table 2.2 lists the major neurohumoral factors involved in the regulation of osmolality and volume; note that these are separate pathways with almost no overlap (except for the

TABLE 2.2

	Osmoregulation	Volume Regulation
Major Sensors and Effectors of the Osmoregulatory and Volume Regulatory Pathways		
What is sensed	Plasma osmolality	Effective tissue perfusion
Sensors	Hypothalamic osmoreceptors	Macula densa Afferent arteriole Atria Carotid sinus
Effectors	Antidiuretic hormone Thirst	Renin–angiotensin–aldosterone Atrial natriuretic peptide (ANP) ANP-related peptides Norepinephrine Antidiuretic hormone
What is affected	Urine osmolality Water intake	Urinary sodium Thirst

hypovolemic stimulus to the secretion of antidiuretic hormone, which occurs only when tissue perfusion is substantially reduced).

Osmoregulation

Plasma osmolality is regulated by osmoreceptors in the hypothalamus that influence the release of antidiuretic hormone (ADH) and thirst. ADH reduces water excretion while thirst increases water intake. The combined effects result in water retention, which will tend to lower plasma osmolality and plasma sodium concentration by dilution. Thus, regulation of the plasma sodium concentration is mediated almost entirely by *changes in water balance*, not in the handling of sodium.

Volume Regulation

Multiple receptors and effectors are involved in volume regulation. These include the juxtaglomerular cells of the afferent arteriole (Fig. 1.9), which release renin—leading to the subsequent generation of the sodium-retaining hormones angiotensin II and aldosterone; the atria, which release natriuretic peptides that promote sodium excretion; and the carotid sinus, which regulates the activity of the sympathetic nervous system and mediates the hypovolemic stimulus to ADH. As will be described below, these systems affect urinary sodium excretion and, via angiotensin II and norepinephrine, systemic vascular resistance.

Can you think of a physiologic reason why it is beneficial to have multiple receptors for volume regulation, while only one receptor in the hypothalamus is sufficient for osmoregulation?

Before discussing the basic aspects of these humoral pathways, it is useful to review the changes that will occur in the three experimental conditions summarized in Table 2.1:

■ The administration of isotonic saline causes volume expansion without affecting the plasma osmolality. Thus, only the volume regulatory pathway will be activated: Renin release will be suppressed, while atrial natriuretic peptide (ANP) secretion will be enhanced. This increase in pronatriuretic forces will appropriately enhance sodium excretion in an attempt to excrete the volume load.

■ The ingestion of free water will initially lower the plasma osmolality, thereby suppressing the release of ADH. The ensuing fall in water reabsorption will allow the excess water to be excreted rapidly in dilute urine.

■ The ingestion of salt without water causes both hyperosmolality and extracellular fluid volume expansion, thereby activating both pathways. The rise in plasma osmolality will enhance both ADH release and thirst, thereby reducing water excretion and increasing water intake in an attempt to lower the plasma osmolality toward normal. Volume expansion, on the other hand, will suppress the secretion of renin and increase that of ANP. The net effect will be enhanced excretion of sodium in a relatively small volume of urine, a composition that is similar to intake.

 In the above example of unreplaced sweat losses in Question 1, what will happen to the osmoregulatory and volume regulatory pathways?

Antidiuretic Hormone, Thirst, and Maintenance of Water Balance

The following review of ADH, the renin–angiotensin–aldosterone system, and ANP will primarily emphasize those hormonal effects related to the regulation of water and sodium balance.

ADH (the human form is called arginine vasopressin; AVP) is a polypeptide synthesized in the supraoptic and paraventricular nuclei in the hypothalamus (Fig. 2.3). Secretory granules containing AVP migrate down the axons of the supraopticohypophysial tract into the posterior lobe of the pituitary, where they are stored and subsequently released after appropriate stimuli.

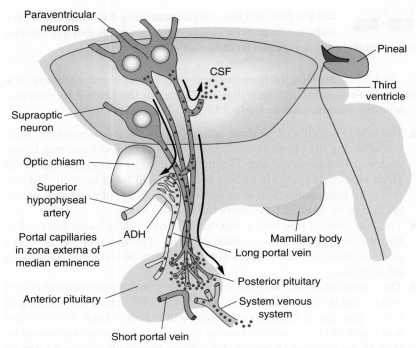

FIGURE 2.3.   Schematic representation of the mammalian hypothalamus and pituitary gland showing pathways for the secretion of antidiuretic hormone (ADH). ADH is synthesized in the supraoptic and paraventricular nuclei, transported in granules along their axons, and then secreted at three sites: the posterior pituitary gland, the portal capillaries of the median eminence, and the cerebrospinal fluid (CSF). *Black arrows* indicate transport pathways to secretory sites.

Actions

The absence or presence of ADH is the major physiologic determinant of urinary free water excretion or retention. ADH acts on the collecting ducts, to allow water reabsorption *independent* of sodium down the osmotic gradients created by the countercurrent system (see Chapter 1).

The ADH-induced increase in collecting duct water permeability occurs primarily in the principal cells, as the adjacent intercalated cells are mostly involved in acid or bicarbonate secretion (see Chapter 5). There are three major receptors for ADH: the V_{1a}, V_{1b} (also called V_3), and V_2 receptors. Activation of the V_1 receptors induces vasoconstriction and enhancement of prostaglandin release while the V_2 receptors mediate the antidiuretic response. The V_{1b} (V_3) receptor appears to mediate the effect of ADH on the pituitary, facilitating the release of ACTH.

Activation of adenylylcyclase by ADH via the V_2 receptor on the basolateral membrane initiates a sequence of events in which a protein kinase is activated (see Chapter 1 and Fig. 1.5). This leads to apical membrane insertion of aquaporin-2 water channels from preformed cytoplasmic vesicles that contain aquaporin-2 water channels. Once the water channels span the luminal membrane, water is reabsorbed into the cells, and then rapidly returned to the systemic circulation across aquaporin-3 and aquaporin-4 water channels in the basolateral membrane. These channels are water permeable (even in the absence of ADH) and the basolateral membrane has a much greater surface area than the luminal membrane. When the ADH effect has worn off, the water channels aggregate within clathrin-coated pits and they are removed from the luminal membrane by endocytosis.

The net effect is that the urine osmolality may be as high as 1000 to 1200 mOsm/kg in the presence of ADH, a concentration that is four times that of the plasma. In contrast, the urine osmolality can fall to as low as 30 to 50 mOsm/kg in the complete absence of ADH, a situation in which there is minimal water reabsorption in the collecting ducts.

A defect in any step in this pathway, such as attachment of ADH to its receptor or the function of the water channel, can cause resistance to the action of ADH and an increase in urine output. This disorder is called nephrogenic diabetes insipidus. Nephrogenic diabetes insipidus can occur through inherited defects in the V_2 receptor or the aquaporin-2 gene, or can be acquired most commonly as a side effect of lithium therapy or hypercalcemia.

Vascular Resistance

The antidiuretic effects of ADH are mediated by the V_2 receptors and adenylylcyclase stimulation, while the V_1 receptors stimulate phospholipase C and primarily act to increase vascular resistance (hence the name vasopressin). Thus, ADH may contribute to the regulation of vascular resistance, although it is clear that the renin–angiotensin and sympathetic nervous systems are of much greater importance.

Renal Prostaglandins

ADH stimulates the production of prostaglandins (particularly prostaglandin E_2 and prostacyclin) in a variety of cells within the kidney, including those in the thick ascending limb, collecting ducts, medullary interstitium, and glomerular mesangium. The prostaglandins that are produced then impair both the antidiuretic and vascular actions of ADH. The antidiuretic effect is due to a reduction in ADH-induced generation of cyclic AMP in the collecting ducts through activation of the inhibitory G protein, G_i, and protein kinase C stimulation.

These findings have suggested that a short *negative feedback loop* may be present in which ADH enhances local prostaglandin production, thereby preventing an excessive antidiuretic response. However, the effect of ADH on prostaglandin synthesis is mediated by the V_1, not the antidiuretic V_2, receptors. Thus, the major function of the ADH–prostaglandin relationship may be to maintain renal perfusion as ADH-induced vasoconstriction is minimized by the vasodilator prostaglandins.

Control of Antidiuretic Hormone Secretion

Two major stimuli to ADH secretion are hyperosmolality and volume depletion (Fig. 2.4). These responses are physiologically appropriate, since the water retention induced by ADH will lower the plasma osmolality and raise the extracellular volume toward normal. Conversely, lowering the plasma osmolality by water loading will diminish ADH release. The ensuing reduction in collecting duct water reabsorption will decrease the urine osmolality, thereby allowing the excess water to be excreted. Since the half-life of ADH in the circulation is several minutes, the maximum diuresis after a water load is delayed for 90 to 120 minutes—the time required for the metabolism of the previously circulating ADH.

Osmoreceptors

The location of the osmoreceptors governing ADH release was initially demonstrated by experiments utilizing local infusions of hypertonic saline, which raised the local but not the systemic plasma osmolality.

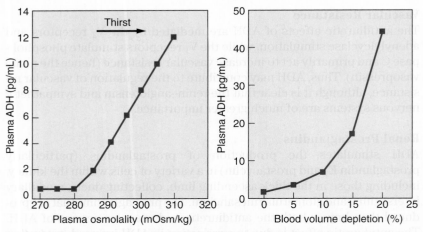

FIGURE 2.4. Relationship of the plasma ADH concentration to plasma osmolality in normal humans (in whom the plasma osmolality was varied by changing the state of hydration) and to isosmotic blood volume depletion in the rat. Although volume depletion produces a more pronounced increase in ADH levels, a relatively large fall in blood volume is required for this to occur.

ADH secretion was enhanced and the urine output fell following infusion into the carotid artery, but not the femoral artery. These findings indicated that the osmoreceptors were located in the brain (hypothalamus), and not in the periphery (Fig. 2.3).

The signal sensed by the hypothalamic osmoreceptors is an effective osmotic gradient between the plasma and the receptor cell, leading to water movement out of or into the cell. The ensuing change in the intracellular osmotic pressure stimulates both ADH secretion and synthesis.

The plasma sodium concentration is the major osmotic determinant of ADH release, since sodium salts are the primary effective extracellular solutes. In contrast, alterations in the BUN do not affect ADH release, because urea is an ineffective osmole that readily crosses cell membranes.

The osmoreceptors are extremely sensitive, responding to alterations in the plasma osmolality of as little as 1%. In humans, the osmotic threshold for ADH release is between 280 and 290 mOsm/kg (Fig. 2.4). There is little circulating ADH below this level, a setting in which the urine should be maximally dilute with an osmolality below 100 mOsm/kg. Above the osmotic threshold, there is a progressive and relatively linear rise in ADH secretion.

This system is so efficient that the plasma osmolality usually does not vary by more than 1% to 2%, despite wide fluctuations in water intake. For example, a large water load will lower the plasma osmolality and essentially shut off the release of ADH. The net effect is the excretion of the excess water within 4 hours. The range of maximum water excretion is so much above intake that normal subjects rarely can retain water and become hyponatremic. Thus, the development of hyponatremia in almost all cases implies an inability to excrete water, which, in the absence of advanced renal failure, implies an *inability to suppress ADH release*. This issue will be reviewed in detail in Chapter 3.

Thirst

The response to a rise in the effective plasma osmolality, as can occur with water loss due to exercise-induced sweating on a hot day, leads to increased thirst, as well as ADH release (Fig. 2.4). The combination of increased water intake and reduced water excretion will then return the plasma osmolality to normal.

Even though thirst is regulated centrally, it is sensed peripherally as the sensation of a dry mouth. Even small increases in plasma osmolality (2 to 3 mOsm/kg) will lead to increased thirst (Fig. 2.4) and the sensation of thirst is so powerful that *normal subjects cannot become hypernatremic* as long as they have access to water. This is true even in patients with central diabetes insipidus who make little or no ADH. Although these patients excrete a large volume of dilute urine, this water loss is matched by increased intake so that the plasma sodium concentration remains in the normal or high-normal range. In theory, shutting off thirst should be an equally powerful protection against the development of hyponatremia, since the plasma sodium concentration cannot fall if there is no water intake. However, most of the fluid we drink is for cultural or social reasons and is not regulated by the osmoreceptors.

Volume Receptors

Patients with effective circulating volume depletion (which is defined below) may secrete ADH even in the presence of a low plasma osmolality (Fig. 2.4). These findings indicate the existence of nonosmolal, volume-sensitive receptors for ADH release.

Parasympathetic afferents primarily located in the carotid sinus baroreceptors play a major role in this response. Changes in the rate of afferent discharge from these neurons affect the activity of the vasomotor center in the medulla and subsequently the rate of ADH secretion by the cells in the paraventricular nuclei. The supraoptic nuclei, in comparison, are important for osmoregulation but do not appear to participate in this volume-sensitive response.

The sensitivity of the volume receptors is different from that of the osmoreceptors. The latter respond to alterations in plasma osmolality of as little as 1%. In comparison, small, acute reductions in volume that are sufficient to increase the secretion of renin and norepinephrine have little effect on the release of ADH. Acutely, ADH is secreted nonosmotically in humans only if there is a large enough change in the effective volume to produce a reduction in the systemic blood pressure. Once hypotension occurs, there may be a marked rise in ADH secretion, resulting in circulating hormone levels that can easily exceed that induced by hyperosmolality (compare the *left* and *right* panels in Fig. 2.4 and note the different *y*-axis scales).

Thirst is also stimulated by volume depletion. Hypovolemia stimulates angiotensin II production (discussed below), and angiotensin II is a highly potent stimulus of thirst.

Interactions of Osmotic and Volume Stimuli

The hormone-producing cells in the supraoptic and paraventricular nuclei receive input from both the osmotic and volume receptors, resulting in positive or negative interactions. For example, volume depletion potentiates the ADH response to hyperosmolality, and volume depletion can prevent the inhibition of ADH release normally induced by a fall in the plasma osmolality.

The hypovolemic stimulus to ADH release and thirst is beneficial from the viewpoint of volume regulation. Water retention will expand the extracellular fluid volume, and the vasopressor activity of ADH may contribute to an elevation in the systemic blood pressure. However, these changes often occur at the expense of osmoregulation. The persistent nonosmotic stimulation of ADH release impairs water excretion, potentially leading to water retention and hyponatremia. As an example, hyponatremia is commonly present in patients with persistent marked effective volume depletion, as with congestive heart failure and hepatic cirrhosis (see Chapter 3).

Hormonal Regulation of Sodium Excretion

As listed in Table 2.2, the factors involved in the regulation of sodium excretion are different from those involved in water excretion. The only important area of overlap is the hypovolemic stimulus to ADH release and thirst.

The presence of multiple receptors for the hormonal control of sodium excretion illustrates an important difference between the regulation of volume and that of osmolality. Maintenance of concentration can often be achieved with only a single sensor (such as the hypothalamic osmoreceptors), since all tissues are perfused by the same arterial blood. In comparison, there may be marked variability in regional perfusion, necessitating the presence of local volume sensors. A simple example is changing from the sitting to the standing position, which, by gravity, results in hyperperfusion of (and fluid accumulation in) the lower extremities, and in hypoperfusion of the brain. In this setting, activation of the carotid sinus baroreceptors with a subsequent increase in sympathetic activity helps to preserve cerebral perfusion by maintaining the systemic blood pressure.

Definition of Effective Circulating Volume

Before discussing the major hormones that affect sodium excretion, it is important to first define what is being regulated. The *effective circulating volume* is an unmeasurable parameter that refers to that part of the extracellular fluid that is in the arterial system and is therefore effectively perfusing the tissues. Although a 70kg man would have approximately 42 liters of water there is less than 1 liter (approximately 700ml) actually perfusing tissues through the arterial limb. A detailed breakdown of the approximate distribution of water (both in % body weight and volume (liters)) is shown in Figure 2.5. The effective circulating volume varies directly with the extracellular fluid volume in normal subjects, being largely determined by total body sodium stores, since sodium salts are the primary extracellular solutes that act to hold water within the extracellular space. As a result, maintenance of the effective circulating volume and regulation of sodium balance (by alterations in urinary sodium excretion) are closely related functions. Sodium loading will tend to produce volume expansion, whereas sodium loss will lead to volume depletion.

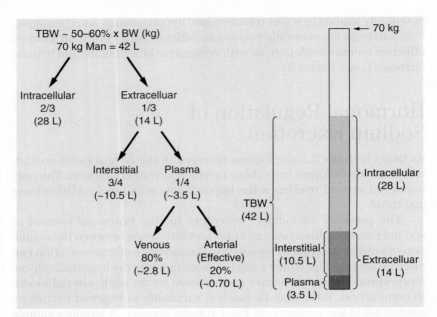

FIGURE 2.5. Approximate relationships of body water compartments to total body weight that can be used to estimate amounts of water in specific body compartments. Note that plasma volume is only about 3.5 liters of total 42 liters of total body water (TBW). These relationships will be useful for calculating disorders of water balance (Chapter 3).

Although the effective circulating volume varies with the extracellular fluid volume in normal subjects, it may be *independent of the extracellular fluid volume, the plasma volume, or even the cardiac output in a variety of disease states* (Table 2.3). Patients with congestive heart failure, for example, have a reduced effective circulating volume due to the primary decrease in cardiac output. However, the ensuing activation of sodium-retaining hormones (in an attempt to increase perfusion toward normal) leads to edema formation and increases in the plasma volume and total extracellular fluid volume (see Chapter 4). Thus, these parameters may be dissociated from the rate of tissue perfusion.

The effective circulating volume may, in some cases, also be independent of the total cardiac output. In addition to a reduction in cardiac output, effective volume depletion can also result from hypotension induced by a fall in systemic vascular resistance (peripheral vasodilatation). In the presence of a low-resistance arteriovenous fistula, for example, the cardiac output is elevated by an amount equal to the flow through the fistula. However, this fluid is circulating *ineffectively*, since it bypasses the capillary circulation. Thus, the patient is normovolemic, despite the presence of a cardiac output that may be substantially elevated.

The potential dissociation between the effective circulating volume and the cardiac output can also be illustrated by the hemodynamic

TABLE 2.3

Potential Independence of Effective Circulating Volume from Other Hemodynamic Parameters—Extracellular Fluid Volume, Plasma Volume, and Cardiac Output

	Effective Circulating Volume	Extracellular Fluid Volume	Plasma Volume	Cardiac Output
Hypovolemia due to vomiting	↓	↓	↓	↓
Heart failure	↓	↑	↑	↓
Arteriovenous fistula	Normal	↑	↑	↑
Severe hepatic cirrhosis	↓	↑	↑	Normal – ↑

changes seen in advanced hepatic cirrhosis and ascites (which refers to fluid accumulation in the peritoneum). The extracellular fluid volume is expanded in this disorder primarily by the ascites; the plasma volume is increased due in part to fluid accumulation in the markedly dilated but slowly circulating splanchnic venous circulation (induced by portal hypertension); and the cardiac output is often elevated because of multiple arteriovenous fistulas throughout the body such as the spider angiomas on the skin.

Despite all of these signs of volume expansion, most of the excess fluid is hemodynamically ineffective and these patients *behave as if they are volume depleted*. The cause of the effective circulating volume depletion is a reduction in systemic vascular resistance resulting from the low-resistance shunting by the arteriovenous fistulas and from vasodilatation within the splanchnic circulation. The presence of decreased effective tissue perfusion is manifested clinically by relatively low blood pressures, a low rate of urinary sodium excretion (often below 10 mEq/day in advanced cases) and by a progressive increase in the secretion of the hormones typically released in response to hypovolemia: renin, norepinephrine, and ADH.

Assuming there is no defect in renal sodium handling (most often due to blocking tubular sodium transport with diuretic agents), one of the major clinical hallmarks of effective circulating volume depletion of any cause is a low level of sodium excretion, usually manifested by a urine sodium concentration below 25 mEq/L. Sodium intake on a regular diet in the United States usually ranges from 80 to 250 mEq/day (approximately 1.8 to 5.8 g/day). However, the urine sodium *concentration* is variable, since it is also determined by the rate of water intake and excretion. The only common clinical setting in which a low rate of sodium excretion does not reflect systemic hypoperfusion is *selective* renal ischemia. This most commonly occurs with bilateral renal arterial narrowing, usually due to atherosclerotic lesions in older patients.

Renin–Angiotensin System

The renin–angiotensin system plays an important role in the regulation of the systemic blood pressure, urinary sodium excretion, and renal hemodynamics. Renin is a proteolytic enzyme secreted by specialized cells—the juxtaglomerular cells—in the afferent arteriole of each glomerulus. In addition, more proximal cells in the interlobular artery can be recruited for renin release when the stimulus is prolonged.

Renin initiates a sequence of steps (Fig. 2.6) that begins with cleavage of angiotensinogen (renin substrate) to a decapeptide, angiotensin I.

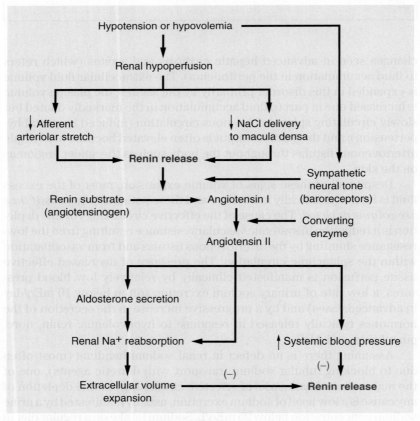

FIGURE 2.6.   Pathway of angiotensin production.

Angiotensin I is then converted into an octapeptide, angiotensin II, in a reaction catalyzed by angiotensin-converting enzyme (ACE). Initial studies suggested that renin released from the kidneys acted on angiotensinogen produced in the liver; the angiotensin I formed by this reaction was then converted into angiotensin II primarily in the pulmonary circulation, since the lung has the highest concentration of ACE.

It is now clear, however, that angiotensin II can be synthesized at a variety of sites, including the kidney, vascular endothelium, adrenal gland, and brain. Within the kidney, for example, locally generated angiotensin II can participate in the regulation of the glomerular filtration rate and sodium excretion without requiring activation of the systemic renin–angiotensin system. The observation that the concentration of angiotensin II in the renal peritubular capillary and proximal tubule is roughly 1000 times higher than that in the systemic circulation is consistent with this local effect.

Actions

Angiotensin II has two major systemic effects, which are mediated by binding to specific angiotensin II receptors in the cell membrane. Both of these actions, vasoconstriction and sodium retention, will tend to reverse the hypovolemia or hypotension usually responsible for the stimulation of renin secretion.

First, angiotensin II produces arteriolar vasoconstriction, thereby raising the systemic blood pressure. This represents an appropriate response in hypovolemic subjects, but can contribute to the development of hypertension if there is an abnormality in renin regulation. The importance of angiotensin II in hypertension in humans can be illustrated by the fall in blood pressure that often follows the administration of an ACE inhibitor or angiotensin receptor blocker (ARB). Second, angiotensin II leads to enhanced renal tubular sodium reabsorption, thereby expanding the extracellular fluid volume. At least two factors contribute to this response: direct stimulation of transport in the early proximal tubule by angiotensin II, and increased release of aldosterone, resulting in enhanced collecting duct sodium reabsorption (see Fig. 2.6 and Chapter 1 for a review of sodium transport). Since water reabsorption in the proximal tubule passively follows that of sodium, angiotensin II enhances the reabsorption of *both* sodium and water. Thus, the *extracellular fluid volume will be expanded but there will be no change in the plasma sodium concentration*, which as described previously is primarily regulated by ADH.

Regulation of Glomerular Filtration Rate.

Angiotensin II also plays an important role in the regulation of the glomerular filtration rate (GFR). Angiotensin II constricts the efferent and, to a lesser degree, the afferent arteriole. The efferent constriction tends to raise the intraglomerular pressure, a change that will increase the GFR. This is particularly important when renal perfusion pressure is reduced, as with any of the causes of volume depletion. In this setting, the decline in perfusion pressure can be counterbalanced by the efferent constriction, resulting in initial maintenance of the intraglomerular pressure and the GFR (see Chapter 1 and Fig. 1.8 for a review of the role of angiotensin II and the consequences of angiotensin II blockade in this process of autoregulation).

Control of Renin Secretion.   The main determinant of renin secretion in normal subjects is salt intake. A high salt intake expands the extracellular fluid volume and decreases renin release; these changes are reversed with a low salt intake (or with fluid loss from any site; see Figure 2.6). The associated alterations in angiotensin II and aldosterone then allow sodium to be excreted with volume expansion or retained with volume depletion.

The net effect for renin (and for all the regulatory hormones discussed in this chapter) is that there is *no fixed normal value* for the plasma renin activity or the plasma concentration of angiotensin II or aldosterone. The levels observed must be correlated with the patient's volume status, as partially determined clinically from the rate of urinary sodium excretion. Sodium excretion in a normovolemic subject is roughly equal to intake, which ranges from 80 to 250 mEq/day in a typical American diet.

These changes in volume or pressure that affect renin release and synthesis are sensed at one or more of three sites: the *afferent arteriole*, the *cardiopulmonary baroreceptors*, and the *macula densa cells* in the early distal tubule:

■ The baroreceptors in the wall of the afferent arteriole are stimulated by a reduction in renal perfusion pressure. The ensuing increase in renin release appears to be mediated in part by the local production of prostaglandins, particularly prostacyclin.

■ The cardiopulmonary baroreceptors are also affected by a fall in perfusion pressure, leading to increased activity of the sympathetic nervous system. The ensuing stimulation of β_1 receptors in the juxtaglomerular apparatus results in enhanced release of renin.

■ The macula densa cells, in comparison, respond to changes in the luminal delivery of chloride. As with the thick ascending limb of the loop of Henle, NaCl entry into these cells is mediated by a Na^+–K^+–$2Cl^-$ cotransporter in the luminal membrane (see Chapter 1 and Fig. 1.9). The activity of this transporter is primarily regulated by the luminal chloride concentration. With volume expansion, for example, more NaCl is delivered to and *reabsorbed* in the macula densa (due to diminished proximal reabsorption), leading to suppression of renin release. The mechanism by which the chloride signal is translated into alterations in renin secretion appears to be mediated by PGE-2 and PGI-2.

Loop diuretics are commonly used in the treatment of edema. They increase NaCl excretion by inhibiting the luminal Na^+-K^+ $-2Cl^-$ carrier in the loop of Henle and macula densa. What effect should this have on renin release (independent of any changes in extracellular volume)?

In many clinical conditions, these three sites act in concert to regulate renin release. Consider the systemic and local responses to volume depletion, which initially lead to a small reduction in systemic blood pressure. This will decrease the stretch in both the afferent arteriolar and cardiopulmonary baroreceptors; distal chloride delivery will also be diminished due in part to enhanced proximal reabsorption. Each of these changes will promote the secretion of renin.

Aldosterone

Aldosterone is synthesized in the adrenal zona glomerulosa (the outermost layer of the adrenal cortex), while cortisol and androgens are produced in the zona fasciculata (middle layer) and reticularis (inner layer) of the cortex, respectively. The zona glomerulosa is well adapted for the production of aldosterone. It has a low concentration of 17α-hydroxylase, the enzyme necessary for cortisol and androgen synthesis (Fig. 2.7). More importantly, the final step in the conversion of corticosterone to aldosterone, oxidation of a hydroxyl group at the 18-carbon

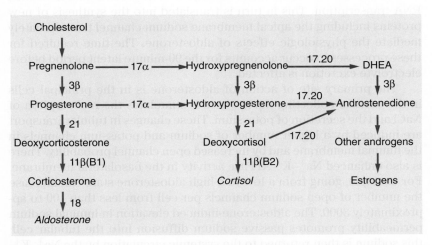

FIGURE 2.7. Pathways of adrenal steroid synthesis. DHEA is dehydroepiandrostenedione, and the numbers at the *arrows* refer to specific enzymes: 17α refers to 17α-hydroxylase; 3β refers to 3β-hydroxysteroid dehydrogenase; 21 refers to 21-hydroxylase; 11β refers to 11β-hydroxylase; 18 refers to a two-step process resulting in the oxidation of a hydroxyl group to an aldehyde at the 18-carbon position.

position to an aldehyde, occurs only in the zona glomerulosa. The enzymes that catalyze this reaction, known as aldosterone synthase, are normally suppressed in the zona fasciculata. This suppression is important because it prevents aldosterone secretion from being inappropriately regulated by ACTH.

A rare form of familial hyperaldosteronism resulting in glucocorticoid sensitive hypertension results in ACTH-sensitive aldosterone production occurring in the zona fasciculata. 11β hydroxylase has two isoforms, one in the cortisol pathway (β2) and the other in the aldosterone pathway (β1) (Fig. 2.7). The mutation in patients with GRA (glucocorticoid-remedial aldosteronism) is fusion of the 11β-hydroxylase promoter from the cortisol isoform (β2) to the coding sequence of the β1 isoform in the aldosterone pathway. This results in ACTH-dependent activation of aldosterone synthase leading to high levels of unique biochemical end products, 18-oxocortisol and 18-hydroxycortisol, that have mineralocorticoid activity similar to aldosterone.

Actions

The major effects of aldosterone occur in the distal nephron, the site at which the final composition of the urine is determined. As with other steroid hormones, aldosterone acts by diffusing into the tubular cell and then attaching to a specific cytosolic receptor (Fig. 1.5). The hormone–receptor complex migrates to the nucleus, where it interacts with specific sites on the nuclear chromatin to enhance messenger RNA and ribosomal RNA transcription. This in turn is translated into the synthesis of new proteins including the apical membrane sodium channel that ultimately mediate the physiologic effects of aldosterone. The time required for these processes to occur accounts for the 90-minute latent period before electrolyte excretion is affected.

The primary site of action of aldosterone is in the principal cells in the cortical collecting duct, where it stimulates the reabsorption of NaCl and the secretion of potassium. These changes in tubular transport are induced by a higher number of sodium and potassium channels in the luminal membrane and by increased open channel probability. There is also enhanced $Na^+–K^+$-ATPase activity in the basolateral membrane. For example, going from a low to a high aldosterone state can increase the number of open sodium channels per cell from less than 100 to approximately 3000. The aldosterone-induced elevation in luminal sodium permeability promotes passive sodium diffusion into the tubular cell; this sodium is then returned to the systemic circulation by the $Na^+–K^+$-ATPase pump. The movement of cationic sodium through its channel is *electrogenic* in that the loss of cationic sodium from the lumen creates a lumen-negative potential difference. Electroneutrality is maintained in this setting either by passive chloride reabsorption via the paracellular pathway between the cells or by potassium secretion from the cell into the lumen. This effect on potassium handling is clinically important, since collecting duct potassium secretion is the primary determinant of urinary potassium excretion (see Chapter 7).

QUESTION	Deoxycorticosterone is an ACTH-dependent steroid that has
5	aldosterone-like (mineralocorticoid) activity. Children with one

of the forms of congenital adrenal hyperplasia have impaired activity of one of the enzymes in Figure 2.7. Remembering that cortisol deficiency stimulates ACTH secretion, what effect will decreased activity of each of these enzymes have on aldosterone production, total mineralocorticoid activity (aldosterone plus deoxycorticosterone), and renal sodium and potassium handling?

In addition to its role in sodium and potassium handling, aldosterone also can affect acid handling in part by increasing the activity of the H^+-ATPase secretory pumps in the intercalated cells in the cortical collecting duct. The factors involved in the regulation of acid excretion are reviewed in Chapter 5.

Control of Aldosterone Secretion

Aldosterone plays an important role in volume and potassium balance via its renal effects. It is therefore appropriate that volume depletion (acting via angiotensin II) and an elevation in the plasma potassium concentration are the primary stimuli to aldosterone secretion. Angiotensin II and potassium act on the zona glomerulosa, promoting the conversion of cholesterol to pregnenolone and, more importantly, the conversion of corticosterone to aldosterone (Fig. 2.7).

The volume stimulus to aldosterone secretion is primarily mediated by the renin–angiotensin system. In normal subjects, both renin and aldosterone release rise with a low-salt diet and fall with a high-salt diet. These changes contribute to the maintenance of sodium balance. With salt restriction, for example, the increments in renin, angiotensin II, and aldosterone enhance proximal and collecting duct sodium reabsorption, thereby minimizing further sodium excretion.

The stimulatory effect of potassium increases linearly as the plasma potassium concentration rises above 3.5 mEq/L, with increments in the plasma potassium concentration of as little as 0.1 to 0.2 mEq/L increasing aldosterone release. The ensuing elevation in potassium excretion returns the plasma potassium concentration toward normal.

Although potassium acts directly on the adrenal gland, the ensuing elevation in aldosterone secretion may be mediated in part by a local *intra-adrenal* renin–angiotensin system. In isolated zona glomerulosa cells, for example, a rise in the extracellular potassium concentration increases renin release. Furthermore, the associated elevation in aldosterone release in this setting is impaired by the presence of an ACE inhibitor that reduces the local generation of angiotensin II.

Maintenance of Sodium and Potassium Balance

Since aldosterone simultaneously affects both sodium and potassium handling, it might be expected that the regulation of sodium excretion would interfere with that of potassium. However, this potential maladaptive response does not occur because the secretion of potassium is also strongly affected by the delivery of sodium and water to the distal secretory site (see Chapter 7). Thus, the hyperaldosteronism induced by volume depletion is also associated with decreased distal delivery due in part to enhanced proximal reabsorption. These two effects tend to balance out and potassium secretion remains relatively constant. These responses are reversed by volume expansion: reduced aldosterone counteracted by increased distal delivery.

 Aldosterone increases and ANP decreases the reabsorption of sodium in the collecting ducts. Although these changes are important for the regulation of sodium balance, they do not produce alterations in the plasma sodium concentration or plasma osmolality. Why? Consider this question carefully, since it is essential to understanding the difference between volume regulation and osmoregulation.

Atrial Natriuretic Peptide

ANP is released from myocardial cells in the atria and, in heart failure, from the ventricles as well. It circulates primarily as a 28-amino acid polypeptide. Most of its actions are mediated by attachment to specific receptors on the cell membrane of target cells. The interior domain of these receptors has guanylate cyclase activity, leading to the formation of the second messenger cyclic GMP.

Actions

ANP has two major actions that may contribute to volume regulation: It is a direct vasodilator that lowers the systemic blood pressure, and it increases urinary sodium and water excretion. The natriuretic effect may be mediated both by an increase in GFR (due to combined afferent arteriolar vasodilatation and efferent arteriolar vasoconstriction) and by a reduction in tubular sodium reabsorption. The inner medullary collecting duct has been the best-documented tubular site of action. ANP acts in this segment by directly closing the luminal membrane sodium channels through which luminal sodium normally enters the cell. ANP may also indirectly diminish sodium transport at this site by suppressing the release of both renin from the kidney and aldosterone from the adrenal gland.

The relative roles of increased filtration and decreased reabsorption in the natriuresis induced by ANP are uncertain. The decline in collecting duct sodium reabsorption may be the initial response, since the hormone concentration required to achieve this effect is significantly lower than that to affect glomerular hemodynamics. The increment in GFR may contribute to the natriuresis with more marked volume expansion and higher ANP levels.

Control of Atrial Natriuretic Peptide Secretion

ANP is primarily released from the atria in response to volume expansion, which is sensed as an increase in atrial stretch. The right atrium may be more important than the left in normal subjects. With chronic cardiac overload in congestive heart failure, however, there is recruitment of hormone production by myocardial cells in the ventricles and, at least in animals, by the lungs.

The release of ANP is increased in any condition associated with an elevation in cardiac filling pressures. Examples include a high-salt diet, congestive heart failure, and salt retention in renal failure. The rise in ANP secretion in these settings can be reversed by removal of the excess fluid.

Physiologic Role of Atrial Natriuretic Peptide

Despite the multiple sites at which ANP can affect sodium excretion and its appropriate release in response to changes in volume, the physiologic role of ANP as a natriuretic hormone remains uncertain. For example, infusion of ANP into normal humans generally induces only a modest diuresis.

The vasodilatation and subsequent fall in systemic and renal perfusion pressure induced by ANP may be responsible for its seemingly limited natriuretic activity. It is possible, for example, that hypotension acts by diminishing the quantity of sodium delivered to the ANP-sensitive site in the inner medullary collecting duct. A clinical example of this phenomenon may occur in congestive heart failure, a disorder in which cardiac output and renal perfusion are reduced. These patients have high ANP levels but avidly retain sodium.

The importance of reducing renal perfusion pressure on the natriuretic effect of ANP has been demonstrated experimentally in transgenic mice given an extra ANP gene. These animals have a 10-fold elevation in plasma ANP levels, normal sodium balance, and a lower blood pressure than control animals. If, however, the blood pressure is elevated by volume expansion, the natriuretic effect of ANP is unmasked, resulting in a marked increase in sodium excretion. Similarly, the apparent resistance to ANP in congestive heart failure can be largely reversed in animals by restoring renal perfusion to normal.

Other Atrial Natriuretic Peptide–like Hormones

It is possible that the major physiologic role of ANP is on circulatory hemodynamics and that other ANP-like hormones are more important regulators of sodium excretion. For example, a separate ANP-like hormone (ANP plus four additional N-terminal amino acids) has been identified in human urine and called *urodilatin*. Distal nephron cells have been shown to secrete an ANP prohormone that could be the precursor to urodilatin. Urodilatin excretion appropriately increases in response to volume expansion, and it can contribute to the ensuing natriuresis by binding to the renal ANP receptors with the same activity as ANP itself. However, the mechanism by which urodilatin production is regulated is not known, and it is possible that the receptors controlling the secretion of ANP also regulate secretion of ANP-like peptides in the kidney.

Brain natriuretic peptide (BNP) is an additional natriuretic hormone that is moderately homologous to ANP. It was initially identified in the brain but is also present in the heart, particularly the ventricles, not the atria. The circulating concentration of BNP is less than 20% of that of ANP in normal subjects, but can equal or exceed that of ANP in patients with congestive heart failure. BNP levels are routinely available and are elevated in patients with congestive heart failure. However, BNP levels are also elevated in numerous other clinical conditions and in patients with renal failure limiting its sensitivity.

C-type natriuretic peptide (CNP) is structurally similar to the other natriuretic peptides. It activates cyclic GMP via a different receptor from ANP and BNP. CNP is produced by vascular endothelial cells and in the kidney. Initial studies suggested that its major function may involve regulation of local blood flow. However, the rate of urinary excretion (but not the plasma CNP concentration) is increased in congestive heart failure (CHF), raising the possibility of a paracrine or autocrine role in sodium excretion.

SUMMARY

From the viewpoint of the hormonal regulation of volume balance, ANP (or related hormones) and the renin–angiotensin–aldosterone system appear to function as counterbalancing systems. Renin release is stimulated (and that of ANP reduced) by volume depletion or a low-salt diet. The subsequent generation of angiotensin II and aldosterone results in appropriate sodium retention (in the proximal tubule and collecting duct) and systemic vasoconstriction (to prevent a fall in the systemic blood pressure). In comparison, the release of ANP is enhanced by volume expansion (as with a high-salt diet) and results in increased sodium excretion and systemic vasodilatation.

Although it is useful for the student to view sodium regulation in terms of these two hormonal systems, there are a number of other hormones that also may play a contributory role in certain settings. These include sodium-retaining hormones such as norepinephrine (which is released in response to volume depletion and increases proximal reabsorption) and natriuretic hormones such as dopamine (which is produced in the kidney from circulating L-dopa and which reduces proximal reabsorption in part by diminishing the activity of Na^+–K^+-ATPase pump). A putative endogenous digitalis-like hormone, which may be identical to ouabain, also may increase sodium excretion by impairing Na^+–K^+-ATPase activity.

In the aggregate, the hormonal regulation of sodium excretion allows sodium balance to be maintained in the face of varying sodium intake without any significant alteration in the systemic blood pressure. If, however, one or more of these regulatory systems are impaired, the reduced efficiency of sodium regulation will lead to initial changes in the plasma volume and systemic blood pressure. In this setting, the renal perfusion pressure becomes an important determinant of sodium excretion.

Pressure Natriuresis

An essential "backup" feature of the volume regulatory system that can compensate for an abnormality in the humoral control of Na^+ excretion is the phenomenon of *pressure natriuresis*. In normal subjects, a small elevation in blood pressure results in a relatively large increase in the urinary excretion of Na^+ and water. In contrast to the other mediators of tubular Na^+ transport, this pressure natriuresis phenomenon does not require neurally or humorally mediated sensor mechanisms, since changes in volume directly affect the cardiac output and therefore the systemic blood pressure. The mechanisms mediating these events are unclear but may involve prostaglandins and nitric oxide.

The potential importance of pressure natriuresis can be illustrated by the phenomenon of *aldosterone escape*. Normal animals or humans given aldosterone and a high-salt diet initially retain sodium, leading to volume expansion and a mild rise in blood pressure; hypokalemia also occurs due to the stimulation of potassium secretion. Within a few days, however, there is a spontaneous natriuresis that lowers the plasma volume toward normal. Thereafter, sodium intake and excretion remain equal, although mild hypertension and hypokalemia persist.

ANP and pressure natriuresis have been thought to contribute to this response by decreasing tubular reabsorption at sites other than the aldosterone-sensitive cortical collecting duct. To evaluate experimentally the effect of pressure natriuresis, a clamp was placed around the suprarenal aorta to prevent the increase in systemic pressure from being transmitted to the kidneys. As shown in Figure 2.8, there is now no escape phenomenon as sodium excretion remains at low levels. The continuing sodium retention in this setting leads to ever-increasing plasma

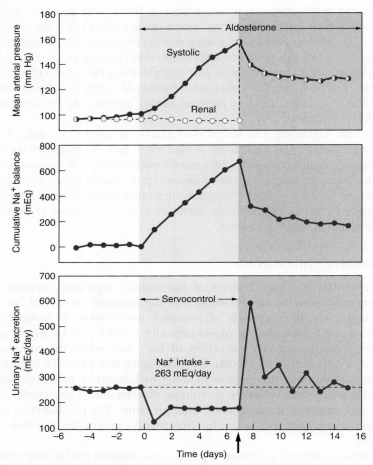

FIGURE 2.8. Effect of the administration of aldosterone and a high-sodium diet on mean arterial pressure, cumulative sodium balance, and urinary sodium excretion in dogs in which renal perfusion pressure is initially held constant (*red circles*) by a suprarenal aortic clamp (servocontrol). In this setting, the administration of aldosterone leads to a persistent fall in sodium excretion, producing progressive sodium retention and hypertension. When the clamp is released on day 7 (*arrow*), the increase in systemic pressure is now transmitted to the kidneys, resulting in a spontaneous diuresis, a reduction in the degree of sodium retention, and much less severe hypertension.

volume expansion (as evidenced from the positive sodium balance) and hypertension.

When, however, the clamp is released on day 7, the renal perfusion pressure rises and aldosterone escape can now occur. The new steady state in which sodium intake and excretion are again equal on days 10 to 14 is similar to that seen in dogs given aldosterone but no aortic clamp: mild hypertension but no edema, since only a small amount of sodium has been retained.

QUESTION 7 Patients with marked narrowing of one or both renal arteries develop hypertension due primarily to increased renin release by the ischemic kidney(s) and subsequent angiotensin II generation. One of the interesting observations in this disorder (renovascular hypertension) is that it occurs in fewer than 1% of patients with mild hypertension but in up to 40% with severe or refractory hypertension. Can you devise a hypothesis that would explain this propensity to produce only severe disease, even in patients with unilateral renal artery narrowing?

Steady State

Regulation of solute and water balance can occur via one of two mechanisms: (1) a *set-point*, in which the aim is to maintain solute concentration or volume at a specific level; or (2) a *steady state*, in which intake and output are maintained at an equal level. Although they produce a similar end result, these two mechanisms are somewhat different in that the plasma concentration or volume varies with the steady state model to provide the signal that allows intake and output to remain equal.

Fluid and electrolyte balance is primarily achieved by maintenance of the steady state. Figure 2.9, for example, illustrates the expected humoral responses—falling renin and aldosterone, rising ANP—to increasing sodium intake from 10 up to 350 mEq/day (sodium intake in a regular

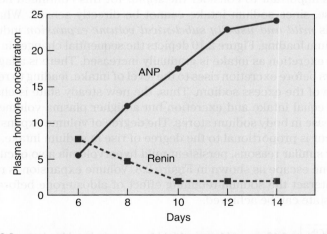

FIGURE 2.9. Effect of gradually increasing sodium intake in normal subjects from a low value of 10 up to 350 mEq/day. Decreased activity of the renin–angiotensin–aldosterone system and increased ANP release are required for the excess sodium to be excreted.

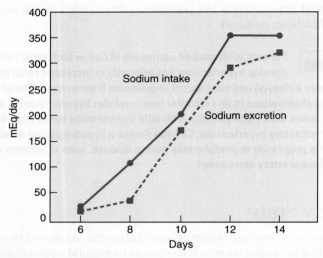

FIGURE 2.10. Effect of gradually increasing sodium intake (*top curve*) in normal subjects from a low value of 10 up to 350 mEq/day on urinary sodium excretion (*bottom curve*). There is a lag of several days before sodium excretion reaches the level of intake; it is this volume expansion that is the continuing signal for high ANP and low renin levels as seen in Figure 2.9. These changes would be reversed with the institution of a low-sodium diet.

American diet is usually between 80 and 250 mEq/day). These appropriate hormonal changes will persist as long as the high-sodium diet is continued.

It is important to consider the *signal* for this continued hormonal response, since sodium intake cannot be directly sensed. What is required is *mild and usually subclinical volume expansion* induced by the sodium loading. Figure 2.10 depicts the sequential changes in urinary sodium excretion as intake is gradually increased. There is a lag of several days before excretion rises to the level of intake, leading to retention of some of the excess sodium. Thus, the new steady state is characterized by equal intake and excretion but a higher plasma volume due to an increase in body sodium stores. The degree of volume expansion that will occur is proportional to the degree of rise in sodium intake.

For similar reasons, persistent mild hypervolemia also occurs in aldosterone escape as shown in Figure 2.8. Volume expansion is required to counteract the sodium-retaining effect of aldosterone before a new steady state can be achieved.

A 43-year-old man with kidney stones is told to increase his water intake, since lowering the concentrations of calcium and oxalate and raising the urine flow rate will tend to diminish the likelihood of

stone formation and growth. Describe the hormonal change that will occur to allow the excess water to be excreted. What will be the ongoing signal for this hormonal change to persist?

Role of Impaired Renal Excretion in Electrolyte Disorders

The concept of the steady state has a number of important clinical implications, two of which will be considered here. First, the central role of the kidney in excreting ingested fluid and electrolytes implies that developing an electrolyte disorder characterized by retention of a substance will be markedly facilitated if there is an *impairment in its renal excretion*.

As an example, Figure 2.11 shows the sequential changes in potassium balance after intake is increased from a relatively normal level of 100 mEq/day up to 400 mEq/day. By the second or third day, the steady state is restored as excretion has risen to match intake. This is associated with elevations in the two major factors that enhance potassium excretion: aldosterone and the plasma potassium concentration itself (see Chapter 7). At day 20, intake and output are still equal but aldosterone levels have returned almost to baseline and the plasma potassium concentration is now 4.3 mEq/L, higher than the initial level of 3.8 mEq/L

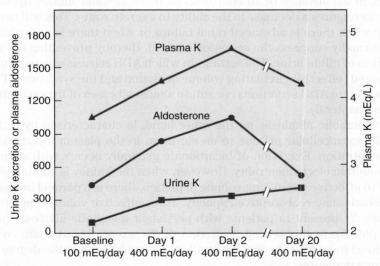

FIGURE 2.11. Effect of increasing potassium intake from 100 up to 400 mEq/day on urinary potassium excretion and the plasma aldosterone and potassium concentrations in normal subjects. Urinary excretion rises to equal intake by day 2 and persists through the study until day 20. Both a mild elevation in the plasma potassium concentration and an initial elevation in aldosterone release contribute to the reattainment of the steady state.

but lower than the peak level of 4.8 mEq/L. The increased efficiency of potassium excretion at this time has been called *potassium adaptation* and probably reflects a selective rise in Na^+–K^+-ATPase activity in the potassium-secreting principal cells in the cortical collecting duct.

This experiment demonstrates the ability to markedly increase the rate of potassium excretion without much of an elevation in the plasma potassium concentration. The clinical lesson that can be drawn from this observation is that persistent hyperkalemia (plasma potassium concentration above 5.3 mEq/L) *cannot occur in the absence of impaired renal potassium excretion.* Thus, the differential diagnosis of this problem can be derived simply by knowing the factors that normally regulate potassium excretion other than the plasma potassium concentration: aldosterone and the distal delivery of sodium and water. One or both of these factors must be reduced if there is to be a defect in potassium excretion. Thus, one of the forms of hypoaldosteronism or decreased distal delivery (due to advanced renal failure or to marked volume depletion as in severe CHF) constitutes most of the differential diagnosis of persistent hyperkalemia. Enhanced potassium intake may contribute but cannot alone lead to potassium retention.

Similar considerations apply to hyponatremia and metabolic alkalosis. Hyponatremia is essentially always due to the retention of ingested water. Normal subjects can excrete more than 10 L of water per day; thus, in the absence of an enormous increase in water intake, hyponatremia requires a decrease in the ability to excrete water. This will occur only when there is advanced renal failure or when there is an inability to normally suppress the secretion of ADH, thereby preventing the excretion of dilute urine. The settings in which ADH release is persistently elevated (effective circulating volume depletion and the syndrome of inappropriate ADH secretion) constitute almost all cases of hyponatremia (see Chapter 3).

Metabolic alkalosis, on the other hand, is characterized by a rise in the extracellular pH due to an elevation in the plasma bicarbonate concentration. Excretion of bicarbonate generally occurs with sodium to maintain electroneutrality. However, when the kidney is sodium avid due to effective circulating volume depletion, there is a parallel increase in bicarbonate reabsorptive capacity. Thus, effective volume depletion is usually present in patients with persistent metabolic alkalosis (see Chapter 5). In this setting, excretion of the excess bicarbonate (with sodium) to correct the metabolic alkalosis would worsen the degree of volume depletion.

QUESTION 9 **The patient described at the beginning of this chapter was put on a low-salt diet in an attempt to lower blood pressure. What changes in hormone secretion and volume will be present in the new steady state?**

The patient did not respond to salt restriction and a thiazide diuretic was added. Although her blood pressure fell to the normal range, she complained of lethargy and weakness. What do you think accounted for these symptoms? What protects such a patient from excessive diuretic-induced sodium loss?

Time Course of Diuretic Action

The steady state also has important implications for the use of diuretics. These drugs are used to increase NaCl excretion in hypertension and edematous states (see Chapter 4). The initial salt and water loss induced by the diuretic will activate counterregulatory systems that will serve to limit further losses. The hormonal changes that may occur include activation of the renin–angiotensin–aldosterone and sympathetic nervous systems and decreased release of ANP.

From a balance viewpoint, the natriuretic effect of the diuretic is gradually counteracted by increased activity of antinatriuretic forces. The latter will gradually rise until a new steady state is reached in which sodium intake and output are again equal.

This relationship leads to two important rules concerning diuretic use, which apply as long as diuretic dose, dietary intake, and the severity of the underlying problem requiring administration of the diuretic are relatively constant:

■ Assuming that there is not a problem with drug absorption, the *maximum natriuretic response to a diuretic will be seen with the first dose.* As soon as the initial fluid loss occurs, the hypovolemia-induced activation of the counterregulatory systems will diminish the response to the second dose.
■ The attainment of the new steady state is generally achieved within 1 to 2 weeks. Thus, all of the fluid and electrolyte disturbances that can occur (volume depletion, hypokalemia, hyponatremia, and metabolic alkalosis) will develop within this time. Whatever the values are at the end of this period, they represent the new steady state for that patient. Repeated blood samples do not need to be obtained at every visit unless there are new clinical circumstances affecting overall balance (such as gastrointestinal losses, acute renal failure).

SUMMARY

This chapter has reviewed the basic principles involved in two largely separate pathways: osmoregulation (which maintains the plasma sodium concentration by affecting water excretion and water intake) and volume regulation (which maintains tissue perfusion by affecting sodium excretion). The disorders of water and sodium balance will be reviewed in Chapters 3 and 4. As will be seen, the approach to these disorders is markedly simplified by an understanding of normal physiology.

What factors protect against the development of hypernatremia (a high plasma sodium concentration)? Patients with central diabetes insipidus have a variable decrease in ADH production, leading to a potentially marked increase in urine output. Nevertheless, the plasma sodium concentration is usually normal or high normal in this setting. Why?

CASE DISCUSSION

The patient presented at the beginning of the chapter has clearly become volume depleted following the institution of diuretic therapy. Her weight has fallen by 2.5 kg, her blood pressure has fallen to a level that, although normal, might have occurred too quickly for her to adjust to, and her BUN is elevated out of proportion to the plasma creatinine concentration (see Chapter 11). In this setting, we might expect these symptoms in addition to high levels of angiotensin II and aldosterone, low levels of ANP, and a urine sodium concentration below 25 mEq/L. The urine sodium concentration, however, is high (84 mEq/L) because persistent diuretic effect masks the hormonal tendency to sodium retention.

Hypovolemia is also a stimulus to the release of ADH, and the relatively high urine osmolality of 553 mOsm/kg suggests that ADH is present. Although the persistently concentrated urine would also predispose to retention of ingested water and the development of hyponatremia (see Chapter 3), the plasma sodium concentration is in the low-normal range. The absence of a more prominent reduction in the plasma sodium concentration probably reflects a lack of water intake due to the patient's general malaise.

ANSWERS TO QUESTIONS

1 The loss of a dilute fluid such as sweat will lead to a rise in the plasma sodium concentration and a reduction in the extracellular fluid volume; the latter will lead to an appropriate reduction in urinary sodium excretion in an attempt to minimize further losses.

2 Only one receptor is required to regulate concentration or osmolality, since all tissues are perfused by the same arterial blood. In comparison, tissues are often perfused at different rates, requiring local regulation. A simple example occurs with standing, as gravity results in increased flow to the lower extremities and decreased perfusion of the brain.

3 Sweat loss will lead to increased thirst and ADH release in an attempt to replace the water losses and lower the plasma sodium concentration toward normal. On the other hand, the associated volume depletion

will activate the renin–angiotensin–aldosterone system and lower ANP release, thereby limiting further sodium losses.

4 Loop diuretics inhibit NaCl uptake both in the loop of Henle and in the macula densa. Thus, the cells within the macula densa cells perceive decreased NaCl delivery, leading to increased renin release.

5 Deficiency in aldosterone synthase will lead to a selective decrease in aldosterone production, a change that will tend to induce hyperkalemia and a modest tendency to sodium wasting. An abnormality in any of the other adrenal enzymes will diminish cortisol and aldosterone production, with the former enhancing the release of ACTH. The net mineralocorticoid effect will depend upon what happens to the production of deoxycorticosterone. Deficiency of 21-hydroxylase (which is the most common) or deficiency of 3β-hydroxysteroid dehydrogenase will impair deoxycorticosterone synthesis, producing findings similar to isolated hypoaldosteronism. In comparison, deoxycorticosterone release will be enhanced with 17α-hydroxylase or 11β-hydroxylase deficiency, leading to findings of mineralocorticoid excess: hypokalemia due to urinary potassium wasting and mild volume expansion and hypertension. Edema will not occur due to the phenomenon of aldosterone escape.

6 Although aldosterone and ANP affect sodium reabsorption, they produce parallel changes in water handling so that the plasma sodium concentration is not affected. Aldosterone, for example, increases sodium reabsorption in the cortical collecting duct. Water will follow (if ADH is present) down the osmotic gradient that has been created by loss of sodium from the tubular lumen. In the absence of ADH, aldosterone will initially increase the plasma sodium concentration; this change, however, will stimulate both ADH release and thirst, leading to water retention and a return to normonatremia. These steps are reversed with ANP. If, for example, ADH is present, then the decline in sodium reabsorption will induce an equivalent reduction in water transport. These simple examples again illustrate the central role of ADH and thirst, not the volume regulatory hormones, in osmoregulation.

7 Bilateral renal artery narrowing (also called stenosis) prevents the increase in systemic pressure from being transmitted to the kidneys, thereby impairing pressure natriuresis and predisposing to relatively severe hypertension as in Figure 2.8. With unilateral renal artery stenosis, the increased release of renin and angiotensin II from the stenotic kidney will produce contralateral vasoconstriction that will tend to impair pressure natriuresis on that side even in the absence of a stenotic lesion.

8 Increased water intake requires a reduction in ADH release to allow the excess water to be excreted. Retention of a small amount of this water on day 1 to lower the plasma sodium concentration (usually by no more than

1 mEq/L) and plasma osmolality constitutes the ongoing signal to maintain relatively low levels of ADH.

9 Dietary sodium restriction will increase the activity of the renin–angiotensin–aldosterone and sympathetic nervous systems and lower ANP release. Mild volume depletion due to the sodium deficit sustained on the first few days before the steady state was reestablished constitutes the signal for the hormonal changes to persist and for sodium excretion to remain at a low level.

10 The symptoms in this patient were probably due to excess fluid loss (2.5 kg in 5 days) induced by the diuretic. The hormonal changes described in the answer to Question 9 act to minimize diuretic-induced sodium losses. A patient such as this with symptomatic volume depletion also may have a hypovolemic stimulus to ADH release (Fig. 2.4), a change that can lead to the retention of ingested water and a fall in the plasma sodium concentration.

11 ADH release and thirst normally protect against the development of hypernatremia, since they induce water retention that will lower the plasma sodium concentration toward normal. Even in the relative absence of ADH, stimulation of thirst is sufficient to prevent hypernatremia. Thus, patients with central diabetes insipidus complain of polydipsia (increased thirst) as well as polyuria (increased urine output). The thirst stimulus is so strong that hypernatremia is primarily seen in patients with impaired mental status or in infants who cannot express their desire to drink. The presence of hypernatremia in an alert adult is virtually diagnostic of a hypothalamic disorder affecting the thirst center.

SUGGESTED READINGS

deZeeuw D, Janssen WMT, de Jong PE. Atrial natriuretic factor: its (patho)physiological significance in humans. Kidney Int 1992;41:1115.

Gonzalez-Campoy JM, Romero JC, Knox FG. Escape from the sodium-retaining effects of mineralocorticoids: role of ANF and intrarenal hormone systems. Kidney Int 1989;35:767.

Guyton AC. Blood pressure control—special role of the kidneys and body fluids. Science 1991;252:1813.

Hall JE, Granger JP, Smith MJ Jr, et al. Role of renal hemodynamics and arterial pressure in aldosterone "escape." Hypertension 1984;6(Suppl. 1):I183.

Lifton RP, Gharavi AG, Geller DS. Molecular mechanisms of human hypertension. Cell 2001;104:545–556.

Rabelink TJ, Koomans HA, Hené RJ, et al. Early and late adjustment to potassium loading in humans. Kidney Int 1990;38:942.

Rose BD, Post TW. Clinical Physiology of Acid–Base and Electrolyte Disorders, 5th Ed. New York: McGraw-Hill, 2001.

Wagner C, Jensen BL, Kramer BK, et al. Control of the renal renin system by local factors. Kidney Int 1998;54(Suppl. 67):S78.

3

DISORDERS OF WATER BALANCE

Hyponatremia, Hypernatremia, and Polyuria

CASE PRESENTATION

A 53-year-old man has been feeling tired and weak for several weeks and now presents with several days of vomiting. He has a 60-pack-year history of smoking.

Physical examination shows an ill-appearing man in no acute distress. Vital signs reveal a blood pressure of 120/80 with a 10 mm Hg decline after assumption of the upright posture. The skin turgor is moderately reduced and the estimated jugular venous pressure is less than 5 cm H_2O. These findings plus the orthostatic fall in blood pressure are compatible with volume depletion, presumably induced by the vomiting.

A left lower lobe mass is noted on chest x-ray. Further evaluation shows the mass to be an oat cell carcinoma.

Initial blood and urine tests reveal the following:

BUN   = 42 mg/dL (9–25)
Creatinine = 1.2 mg/dL (0.8–1.4)
Na   = 107 mEq/L (136–142)

K	$= 3.9$ mEq/L (3.5–5)
Cl	$= 75$ mEq/L (98–108)
Total CO_2	$= 22$ mEq/L (21–30)
Urine Na	$= 8$ mEq/L (variable)
Osmolality	$= 553$ mOsm/kg (variable)

OBJECTIVES

By the end of this section, you should have an understanding of each of the following issues:

■ The factors that determine the plasma sodium concentration, including the role of potassium.
■ The central role of impaired water regulation, not sodium regulation, in the genesis of hyponatremia (low plasma sodium concentration) and hypernatremia (high plasma sodium concentration).
■ The role of alterations in brain volume in the symptoms induced by changes in the plasma osmolality.
■ The mechanisms by which hyponatremia and hypernatremia occur and the basic principles involved in the differential diagnosis and treatment of these disorders.
■ A general approach to the patient complaining of polyuria, which may be arbitrarily defined as a urine output above 3 L/day (normal output ranges from 800 to 2500 mL/day).

Chapter 2 reviewed the basic principles involved in the regulation of sodium and water balance. One of the central concepts in Chapter 2 is that regulation of the plasma osmolality and its main determinant, the plasma sodium concentration, is achieved by alterations in water intake and excretion. It is not surprising, therefore, that alterations in the plasma sodium concentration (hyponatremia and hypernatremia) generally require an abnormality in one or both of the factors that affect water balance: ADH release and thirst.

Before discussing the pathogenesis and approach to these disorders, it is helpful to review briefly the factors that determine the plasma sodium concentration and why maintenance of a relatively constant plasma sodium concentration is clinically important.

Determinants of Plasma Sodium Concentration

The main determinants of the plasma sodium concentration can be appreciated from a few simple calculations related to the plasma osmolality.

The plasma osmolality can be estimated from two times the plasma sodium concentration (PNa), because sodium salts comprise most of the extracellular osmoles (see Chapter 2):

$$Plasma\ osmolality \cong 2 \times PNa \qquad \text{(Eq. 1)}$$

The plasma osmolality is also equal to the osmolality of the total body water since the osmolality of almost all the body water compartments is the same. The osmolality of the total body water is equal to the ratio of total body solutes to total body water (TBW):

$$Plasma\ osmolality = Total\ body\ water\ osmolality = \frac{Total\ body\ solutes}{Total\ body\ water}$$
$$\text{(Eq. 2)}$$

Total body solutes are comprised of extracellular (primarily sodium salts) and intracellular solutes (primarily potassium salts). Thus,

$$Plasma\ osmolality \equiv Extracellular + Intracellular\ solutes/TBW$$

or

$$Plasma\ osmolality \cong (2 \times Na_e + 2 \times K_e)/TBW \qquad \text{(Eq. 3)}$$

where 2 refers to the anions accompanying sodium and potassium and the subscript (e) refers to the exchangeable (or osmotically active) quantities, since some of the body sodium and potassium are bound in bone and in the cells where they are osmotically inactive. If Eqs. 1 and 3 are combined,

$$Plasma\ Na \cong (Na_e + K_e)/TBW \qquad \text{(Eq. 4)}$$

The relationship described by Eq. 4 indicates that the plasma sodium concentration varies directly with Na_e and K_e and inversely with TBW. This prediction is confirmed experimentally in Figure 3.1 where a linear correlation is found between plasma sodium concentration and the sum of exchangeable sodium plus potassium divided by TBW. An important implication of Eq. 4 and Figure 3.1 is that changes in concentrations of solutes that do not affect water movement (i.e., urea) will not impact the plasma sodium concentration. Adding sodium without water will raise the plasma sodium concentration, while adding water without sodium will lower the plasma sodium concentration. The effect of potassium is less direct, involving a transcellular cation exchange. For example, the loss of potassium from the extracellular fluid (as with diarrhea or vomiting) will lead to the movement of potassium out of the cells in an attempt to replete extracellular stores. The major intracellular anions are proteins and inorganic phosphates that are too large to leave the cells. Thus, the loss of potassium must be balanced by the movement of a cation into the cell (sodium or hydrogen) in order to maintain electroneutrality. The entry of sodium into the cells will tend to lower the plasma sodium concentration.

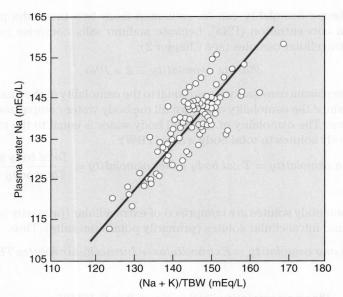

FIGURE 3.1. Direct relationship between the sodium concentration in the plasma water and the ratio of total body exchangeable sodium plus potassium to the total body water.

One setting in which this relationship is often clinically important is the administration of intravenous fluids to replete a patient who has become volume depleted. For example, lowering the plasma sodium concentration toward normal in a patient who is hypernatremic requires the administration of a dilute solution, such as dextrose in water or one-half isotonic saline. The latter solution has a sodium concentration of 77 mEq/L, roughly one-half that of the plasma. In some cases, potassium is added to the replacement fluid since the patient has also become potassium depleted. However, potassium is as active osmotically as sodium and the addition of 40 mEq/L of potassium will make the fluid less dilute, being now equal to approximately three-quarters isotonic saline. Thus, it may be desirable to lower the sodium content (using one-quarter isotonic saline, which contains 38 mEq/L of sodium) to maintain the dilute nature of the replacement fluid.

| QUESTION 1 | The patient described at the beginning of this chapter develops severe diarrhea due to viral gastroenteritis. The diarrheal fluid is |

isosmotic to plasma and has a sodium plus potassium concentration of 85 mEq/L. What effect will loss of this fluid have on the plasma sodium concentration?

Clinical Importance of Osmoregulation

In view of the ability of water to diffuse freely across virtually all cell membranes, maintenance of a relatively constant plasma sodium concentration and plasma osmolality is essential for the maintenance of cell volume, particularly in the brain. As shown in Figure 3.2, acute reduction in the plasma osmolality and plasma sodium concentration (from 140 down to 119 mEq/L) over 2 hours creates an osmotic gradient that promotes the movement of water from the extracellular fluid into the brain (and other cells). The ensuing cerebral edema led to severe neurologic symptoms and all of the animals died.

The outcome was very different when the plasma sodium concentration was slowly reduced. In this setting, there was a lesser increase in brain water and the animals were asymptomatic (Fig. 3.2). Similar findings occur in humans as chronic hyponatremia typically produces no symptoms.

Osmolytes and Cell Volume Regulation

The only way for the brain cell volume to fall toward normal with persistent hyponatremia is for the cells to lose solutes, which will be followed by osmotic water loss. Both ions (sodium and potassium salts)

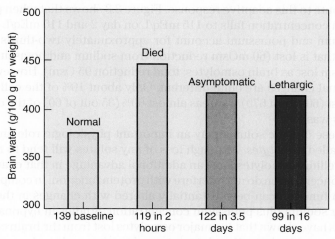

FIGURE 3.2. Brain water content in normal rabbits and three groups of rabbits with varying degrees of hyponatremia developing over a variable period of time. Cerebral edema and death occurred with acute hyponatremia (*second panel*), but more chronic reductions in the plasma sodium concentration produced a lesser degree of cerebral edema and few, if any, neurologic symptoms. A similar pattern, although in the opposite direction, occurs with hypernatremia.

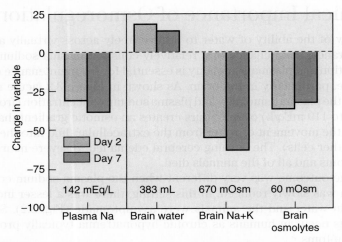

FIGURE 3.3. Changes in brain water, sodium plus potassium content, and three brain osmolytes—inositol, glutamine, and taurine—after onset of hyponatremia. The changes in values reported on the y-axis are in the same units that are listed along the bottom of each group. The numbers at the bottom represent the baseline values before the onset of hyponatremia. The return of brain water toward normal at day 7 even as hyponatremia worsened is due to increased loss of sodium, potassium, and osmolytes.

and organic solutes (inositol and the amino acids glutamine and taurine) contribute to this adaptive response. Figure 3.3 shows that when plasma sodium concentration falls to 115 mEq/L on day 2 and 110 mEq/L on day 7, sodium and potassium account for approximately two-thirds of the solute that is lost (60 mOsm reduction from sodium and potassium and 35 mOsm lost as brain osmolytes; total reduction 95 Osm). However, the fractional changes are quite different. Only about 10% of the cell cation was lost (60 out of 670) whereas almost 60% (35 out of 60) of the organic solutes was lost.

These organic solutes play an important physiologic role and have been called *osmolytes*. Although loss of any solutes will tend to reverse cell swelling, osmolytes have an additional advantage in that changes in their concentration do not interfere with protein function. In comparison, protein function can be substantially altered with changes in the intracellular sodium plus potassium concentration. Studies in hyponatremic animals have shown that the major osmolytes lost from the brain cells are the amino acids glutamine, glutamate, and taurine, and to a lesser degree the carbohydrate myoinositol. In humans with chronic hyponatremia, myoinositol and choline compounds were the primary organic solutes lost, with a smaller change occurring in glutamine and glutamate.

Similar considerations apply to hypernatremia, although water and solutes move in the opposite direction. The initial rise in the plasma sodium concentration produces osmotic water movement out of the cells and cerebral shrinkage. Beginning on the first day, however, the cell solute concentration increases, resulting in water movement into the cells and the restoration of brain cell volume toward normal. Osmolytes account for approximately one-third of this response. Enhanced my-oinositol uptake from the extracellular fluid is mediated by an increased number of myoinositol transporters in the cell membrane.

Implications for Symptoms and Treatment

The sequential water fluxes induced by changes in the plasma sodium concentration and osmolality have important implications both for the possible development of neurologic symptoms and for therapy. In general, *only acute hyponatremia or hypernatremia produces neurologic symptoms* (lethargy, seizures, coma) due to cerebral edema and cerebral shrinkage, respectively. The subsequent adaptations that restore brain volume toward normal are so effective that, unless very severe, few if any symptoms are seen in patients with chronic (induced over more than a few days) changes in the plasma sodium concentration (Fig. 3.2).

These adaptations are also important considerations for the rate of correction. If, for example, the cerebral edema induced by hyponatremia developed rapidly (over hours as is sometimes seen in hyponatremia of marathon runners who overhydrate), then rapid correction of the plasma sodium concentration to normal leads to a rapid efflux of water from the brain and safely lowers the brain volume back to the previous baseline.

The outcome, however, is different when the cerebral edema has been partially corrected by the loss of cell solutes. In this setting, rapid correction can reduce the brain volume below normal and produce an osmotic demyelination syndrome that may include findings of central pontine myelinolysis. This disorder, which may lead to irreversible severe neurologic damage, is characterized by paraparesis or quadriparesis, dysarthria (difficulty in speaking), dysphagia (difficulty in swallowing), and coma.

Studies in animals and observations in humans suggest that this is most likely to occur when the plasma sodium concentration is raised in a patient with severe hyponatremia at a rate exceeding 0.5 mEq/L/hour or, more importantly, 12 mEq/L over the course of the day (Fig. 3.4). Similar recommendations apply to chronic hypernatremia, as overly rapid reduction in the plasma sodium concentration can lead to cerebral edema and seizures.

The aim of therapy is different in patients with symptomatic hyponatremia or hypernatremia. In these settings, initially rapid correction is safe and may be lifesaving. The plasma sodium concentration can at first be returned toward normal at 1.5 to 2 mEq/L/hour until the symptoms resolve, followed by slower correction toward normal, again trying to keep the maximal daily change in the plasma sodium concentration from

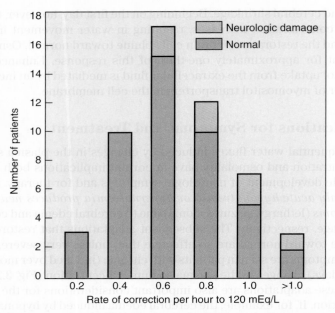

FIGURE 3.4. Incidence of delayed neurologic complications (*gray bars*) in patients with severe hyponatremia (plasma sodium concentration less than 111 mEq/L) according to rate of correction (expressed as mEq/L per hour) to a plasma sodium concentration of 120 mEq/L. Neurologic deterioration occurred only in patients corrected faster than 0.5 mEq/L/hour.

exceeding 12 mEq/L. How the rate of correction can be controlled will be discussed below.

Hyponatremia

Hyponatremia (plasma sodium concentration below 135 mEq/L) is one of the most common electrolyte disorders. From Eq. 4, hyponatremia can be induced in only two ways: the loss of sodium plus potassium, or the retention of ingested or infused water. However, solute loss (as with vomiting or diarrhea) almost always occurs in an isosmotic fluid that has a sodium plus potassium concentration less than that of the plasma. Loss of these fluids cannot directly lower the plasma sodium concentration.

Thus, water retention leading to an *excess of water in relation to solute* is the common denominator in almost all hyponatremic states. The ingestion of water in normal subjects reduces the plasma osmolality and rapidly lowers ADH release, thereby allowing the excess water to be excreted in dilute urine. In the absence of ADH, the urine osmolality can fall to a level between 40 and 100 mOsm/kg (below one-third that in the plasma) with a maximum water excretory capacity that can exceed 10 L in subjects on a regular diet. This enormous capacity for water excretion is much greater than the normal level of water intake, which is usually below 2.5 L/day.

The net effect is that water retention resulting in hyponatremia generally occurs *only when there is a defect in renal water excretion.* An exception to this rule occurs in patients (often schizophrenic) with primary polydipsia who drink such large volumes of fluid that they can overwhelm even the normal excretory capacity.

Etiology

In the absence of advanced renal failure, a defect in water excretion that promotes the development of hyponatremia is almost always associated with an *inability to suppress the secretion of ADH.* Persistent ADH release is usually due to one of four conditions: effective circulating volume depletion, the syndrome of inappropriate antidiuretic hormone (SIADH) secretion, cortisol deficiency, or hypothyroidism (Table 3.1).

TABLE 3.1

Major Causes of Hyponatremia and Hypo-osmolality

I. Disorders in which water excretion is impaired
  A. Effective circulation volume depletion
    1. Gastrointestinal losses: Vomiting, diarrhea, nasogastric tube drainage, bleeding
    2. Renal losses: Diuretics, salt-wasting kidney diseases
    3. Skin losses in which relatively dilute fluids are replaced with free water
    4. Congestive heart failure
    5. Hepatic cirrhosis
    6. Thiazide diuretics (which may act in part by inducing volume depletion)
  B. Syndrome of inappropriate antidiuretic hormone secretion
    1. Virtually any neuropsychiatric disorder or severe pain with or without narcotic administration
    2. Drugs: Such as the oral hypoglycemic agent chlorpropamide
    3. Ectopic production by tumors: Most often oat cell carcinoma of lung
    4. Postoperative patient, a response mediated by pain afferents
    5. Pulmonary diseases
  C. Advanced renal failure
  D. Hormonal changes
    1. Hypothyroidism
    2. Cortisol deficiency
    3. Pregnancy

II. Primary polydipsia

III. Reset osmostat (see text)

The degree of water retention that will occur is related both to the level of water intake and to the severity of the diluting defect. Suppose that a patient with high ADH levels excretes 600 mOsm of solute (primarily sodium and potassium salts and urea) and has a net water intake (intake minus insensible losses from the skin) of 2000 mL. The urine osmolality will average 300 mOsm/kg (600 mOsm in 2 L) if all the ingested water can be excreted. If, however, the minimum urine osmolality were 400 mOsm/kg due to the persistent secretion of ADH, then the 600 mOsm of solute will be excreted in only 1500 mL (600 mOsm/400 mOsm per kg), resulting in the retention of 500 mL of water and a gradual fall in the plasma sodium concentration. Water balance could be maintained in this setting only if water intake were lowered to 1500 mL/day.

 Although water handling is impaired in SIADH, the volume regulatory pathways are intact (such as the renin–angiotensin–aldosterone system). What effect will the initial water retention have on volume regulation and urinary sodium excretion?

An examination of all of the causes of hyponatremia is beyond the scope of this book. Nevertheless, it is instructive to review the underlying mechanisms responsible for the development of hyponatremia in three of these disorders: congestive heart failure and SIADH (the two most common), and a reset osmostat.

Congestive Heart Failure

Increasing cardiac dysfunction is associated with a progressive fall in cardiac output that promotes the development of hyponatremia in two major ways (each of which also may apply to the other hypovolemic states in Table 3.1):

- The low cardiac output leads to enhanced secretion of the three "hypovolemic hormones": renin, norepinephrine, and ADH (see Chapter 2). ADH directly enhances water retention, whereas angiotensin II and norepinephrine induce renal vasoconstriction and lower renal blood flow, another factor that can impair water excretion.
- The hypovolemic stimulus to ADH release also increases thirst. The ensuing elevation in water intake will further enhance the tendency to water retention.

Each of these problems increases in parallel with the severity of the cardiac disease. Thus, hyponatremia alone is an important prognostic finding in the absence of some other cause for a low plasma sodium concentration. Patients with advanced congestive heart failure who have a plasma sodium concentration below 137 mEq/L have a mean survival that is only one-half that of normonatremic patients with clinically equivalent cardiac dysfunction. A plasma sodium concentration below 125 mEq/L is indicative of almost end-stage heart disease. Similar considerations apply to hepatic cirrhosis. (See Chapter 2 for a discussion of the mechanism of effective volume depletion in hepatic cirrhosis.)

 Assume that increased ADH release plays an important role in diuretic-induced hyponatremia. Why would a loop diuretic that inhibits NaCl transport in the thick ascending limb of the loop of Henle be less likely than a thiazide to cause hyponatremia? Consider the physiology of the countercurrent mechanism (see Chapter 1).

Syndrome of Inappropriate Antidiuretic Hormone

SIADH is most often seen with neurologic disease, malignancy, and after major surgery (Table 3.1). The persistent secretion of ADH in this disorder occurs either in the hypothalamus or ectopically in patients with tumor-induced disease. There is typically a gradual reduction in the plasma sodium concentration (unless water intake is very high) and most patients are asymptomatic.

As mentioned above, the degree of hyponatremia is proportional both to the severity of the diluting defect and to the level of water intake. It is important to emphasize that ADH alone cannot cause hyponatremia in the absence of water intake. For example, patients with tumor-induced disease may present to the hospital with a relatively normal plasma sodium concentration because decreased appetite limited the amount of fluid intake. Once admitted, however, intravenous fluid administration is begun and hyponatremia develops.

 Sodium handling is intact in SIADH where the only defect is in water excretion. Assume that a patient with this disorder has a plasma sodium concentration of 115 mEq/L and a urine osmolality that is relatively fixed at 616 mOsm/kg. In this setting, what will happen to the plasma sodium concentration in the steady state after the administration of 1 L of isotonic saline (containing 154 mEq/L each of sodium and chloride or 308 mOsm)? Consider that isotonic saline is composed of sodium and chloride mixed in water.

Reset Osmostat

A subset of patients with mild hyponatremia and SIADH have a reset osmostat. The characteristics of this disorder are determined by the almost normal functioning of the osmoreceptors and therefore of ADH release:

■ The urine can be appropriately diluted after a water load, as ADH secretion is shut off.

■ The urine can be appropriately concentrated if the plasma osmolality is raised by water restriction, as ADH secretion is increased.

■ The plasma sodium concentration is *stable*.

Thus, these patients behave similarly to normal subjects except that the *threshold for ADH release is reduced*, occurring at a plasma sodium concentration of 125 mEq/L rather than at the normal level of 138 to 140 mEq/L.

The main clue suggesting that a patient has a reset osmostat rather than relatively unregulated ADH release as in SIADH is that the plasma sodium concentration varies within a narrow range of only a few milliequivalents per liter over many days of observation.

Establishing the diagnosis is clinically important because the *hyponatremia cannot and should not be treated*. These patients are asymptomatic and are not at risk of more severe hyponatremia, since they can appropriately suppress ADH release and excrete excess water. Furthermore, attempting to raise the plasma sodium concentration will have the same effect as in normal subjects: intense stimulation of thirst and of ADH release that will prevent any elevation from persisting. Therapy should be directed, if possible, only at correcting the underlying disorder, such as severe malnutrition, hypothyroidism, or adrenal insufficiency.

Diagnosis

The history and physical examination often provide important clues suggesting the presence of one of the disorders in Table 3.1. Routine laboratory tests should include measurement of the plasma creatinine concentration (to rule out renal failure) and, if indicated, evaluation of adrenal and thyroid function. In addition, three simple tests can help to establish the correct diagnosis: plasma osmolality, urine osmolality, and urine sodium concentration.

Plasma Osmolality

Patients with any of the causes of true hyponatremia in Table 3.1 will have a proportionate reduction in the plasma osmolality. There are, however, some disorders in which the plasma osmolality is normal or even increased and in which treatment is not directed at the hyponatremia. Some of these disorders are characterized by the movement of water out of cells into the plasma volume. The most common is hyperglycemia in uncontrolled diabetes mellitus. In this setting, the rise in the plasma glucose concentration will increase the plasma osmolality, leading to osmotic water movement out of the cells and a dilutional reduction in the plasma sodium concentration. Correction of the hyperglycemia with insulin will reverse this process and raise the plasma sodium concentration toward normal. *Pseudohyponatremia* refers to those disorders in which marked elevations of substances, such as lipids and proteins, result in a reduction in the fraction of plasma that is water and an artificially low measured serum sodium concentration.

Urine Osmolality

Patients with primary polydipsia are able to appropriately suppress ADH release, leading to excretion of a maximally dilute urine with an osmolality below 100 mOsm/kg. Patients with a higher urine osmolality have an impairment in water excretion that is usually due to the presence of ADH.

Urine Sodium Concentration

Effective circulating volume depletion and (assuming that adrenal and thyroid disease have been excluded) SIADH are the two major causes of true hyponatremia with an inappropriately high urine osmolality. These disorders can generally be distinguished by measuring the urine sodium concentration. Patients with hypovolemia are sodium avid in an attempt to limit further losses; as a result, the urine sodium concentration is generally below 25 mEq/L. In comparison, patients with SIADH are normovolemic and sodium excretion in the steady state is equal to intake. Since normal sodium intake generally is greater than 80 mEq/day, the urine sodium concentration is typically above 40 mEq/L.

 In the case presented at the beginning of this chapter, the patient is initially hypovolemic (as evidenced by the low urine sodium concentration) but may have underlying SIADH due to the carcinoma of the lung. Therapy is begun with isotonic saline and the next morning the plasma sodium concentration has partially corrected up to 122 mEq/L. At this time, there are three possibilities: Hypovolemia alone was responsible for the hyponatremia and the patient is still volume depleted, since not enough saline was given; hypovolemia alone was responsible for the hyponatremia and the patient is now normovolemic; the patient is now normovolemic but also has underlying SIADH. How could you use the urine sodium concentration and urine osmolality to distinguish between these possibilities?

Basic Principles of Therapy

There are two basic mechanisms by which the plasma sodium concentration can be raised in a hyponatremic patient: the administration of sodium (or potassium if the patient is also hypokalemic), or restricting water intake to induce negative water balance. The choice of therapy depends in part upon the underlying disease:

■ Water restriction in an edematous patient with congestive heart failure, hepatic cirrhosis, or renal disease. These patients also have too much sodium (as manifested by the edema) and therefore should not be given sodium unless they have symptomatic hyponatremia.
■ Isotonic saline or oral salt in patients with true volume depletion due to gastrointestinal losses or bleeding. This regimen will correct the

hyponatremia by two mechanisms. First, the sodium concentration in the saline (154 mEq/L) is higher than that in the plasma. Second, saline will reverse the volume depletion, eventually removing the hypovolemic stimulus to ADH release and allowing the excess water to be excreted.

■ Water restriction in patients with primary polydipsia (in whom increased intake is the primary problem) and in most patients with SIADH. As shown in Question 4, isotonic saline should generally be avoided in SIADH: The administered salt will be excreted and some of the water will be retained, leading to a further reduction in the plasma sodium concentration. This adverse effect does not occur with volume depletion, since both the salt and the water will be retained.

■ Cortisol or thyroid hormone replacement in patients with adrenal insufficiency or hypothyroidism.

■ No therapy for a reset osmostat.

As described above, patients with chronic hyponatremia are typically asymptomatic and may suffer neurologic damage if the plasma sodium concentration is raised too rapidly (Fig. 3.5). In comparison, more rapid correction is indicated in symptomatic patients with acute hyponatremia. In this setting, hypertonic saline (which contains 513 mEq of sodium per

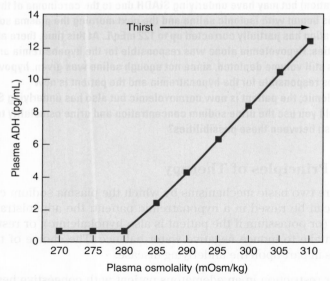

FIGURE 3.5. Relationship of the plasma ADH concentration to plasma osmolality in normal humans in whom the plasma osmolality was varied by changing the state of hydration. The threshold for ADH release is usually between 280 and 285 mOsm/kg; little or no ADH is released below this level, while ADH secretion rises progressively with higher plasma osmolalities. The threshold for thirst is thought to be 2 to 5 mOsm/kg higher than that for ADH release.

liter) is usually administered in an attempt to raise the plasma sodium concentration at an initial rate of 1.5 to 2 mEq/L/hour until the symptoms resolve. The amount of sodium required can be estimated from the following formula to estimate the plasma sodium deficit:

$$Sodium\ deficit = Volume\ of\ distribution \times sodium\ deficit\ per\ liter$$

The volume of distribution of the plasma sodium concentration is equal to the TBW, which is approximately 60% and 50% of lean body weight in men and women, respectively. Thus, to raise the plasma sodium concentration from 105 up to 120 mEq/L in a 50-kg lean woman,

$$Sodium\ required \cong 50 \times 0.5 \times (120 - 105)$$
$$\cong 375\ mEq$$

Since the aim is to correct the hyponatremia at an average rate of 0.5 mEq/L/hour in an asymptomatic patient, these 375 mEq should be given over 30 hours (or 12.5 mEq/hour) to produce a 15-mEq/L elevation in the plasma sodium concentration. This requires approximately 25 mL/hour of hypertonic saline, each milliliter of which contains roughly 0.5 mEq of sodium (513 mEq/L). Careful monitoring is required during this period to ascertain that the desired rate of correction is being achieved. It is important to emphasize that although therapy for correction of hyponatremia is often directed at sodium replacement, these clinical conditions are disorders of ADH and water regulation. Although water intake can be restricted, the options for increasing renal water excretion or blocking ADH actions in the collecting duct are limited. V_2 receptor antagonists promote an aquaresis and raise serum sodium concentration, but the only approved preparation for SIADH must be administered intravenously. Oral V_2 receptor antagonists are being tested in clinical trials for SIADH and congestive heart failure.

 Why is the TBW used as the volume of distribution even though the administered sodium will be limited to the extracellular space, which is only about 20% of the lean body weight?

Hypernatremia

Hypernatremia (plasma sodium concentration above 146 mEq/L) is associated with hyperosmolality, since sodium salts are the major extracellular solutes. In almost all cases, the elevation in the plasma sodium concentration is induced by unreplaced water losses, although a similar effect can result from the administration or ingestion of a hypertonic sodium solution in which the sodium concentration is higher than that in the plasma.

To appreciate the settings in which hypernatremia is most likely to occur, it is important to remember that the normal defense against an elevation in the plasma sodium concentration is the stimulation of ADH release and thirst (Fig. 3.5). The ensuing combination of decreased water excretion and increased water intake results in water retention and a reduction in the plasma sodium concentration toward normal.

Although ADH is clearly important, *it is thirst that provides the ultimate protection against hypernatremia.* For example, patients with severe central diabetes insipidus secrete little or no ADH, leading to diminished water reabsorption in the collecting duct and a marked increase in the urine output. Nevertheless, water balance is maintained and the plasma sodium concentration is normal or in the high-normal range because water intake is appropriately enhanced to match output.

Thus, hypernatremia due to water loss occurs primarily when thirst cannot be normally expressed: in adults with altered mental status, intubated patients in an intensive care unit (ICU), and in children who are unable to ask for water.

 An alert patient is asymptomatic but has a plasma sodium concentration that ranges between 150 and 160 mEq/L. What defect must be present and where would the anatomic location of such a lesion be?

Etiology

The major causes of hypernatremia are listed in Table 3.2, with unreplaced water losses being most common. For example, the osmolality of fluid lost from the skin and respiratory tract ranges from near zero (with evaporative losses) to less than 200 mOsm/kg (with sweat).

However, even isosmotic losses can cause hypernatremia if the water is not replaced. As described previously, the plasma sodium

TABLE 3.2

Major Causes of Hypernatremia

I. Increased water losses that are unreplaced due to impairment of thirst
    A. Insensible and sweat losses: Fever, respiratory infections
    B. Urinary losses: Central or nephrogenic diabetes insipidus, osmotic diuresis due to glucose or mannitol
    C. Gastrointestinal losses
    D. Hypothalamic lesion affecting the thirst center (very rare)

II. Administration of hypertonic sodium chloride or sodium bicarbonate concentration is determined by three factors: sodium, potassium, and water (see Eq. 3). As a result, when considering the osmotic effect of fluid that is lost, it is the sodium plus potassium concentration, not the total osmolality that is most important. This principle can be illustrated by considering the different forms of diarrhea in which the fluid lost is generally isosmotic to plasma. Secretory diarrheas such as cholera have a sodium plus potassium concentration similar to that in the plasma. Loss of this fluid will cause volume and potassium depletion but will have no direct effect on the plasma sodium concentration.

In comparison, the fluid lost with most other infectious diarrheas usually has a sodium plus potassium concentration between 40 and 100 mEq/L (vs. 145 to 150 mEq/L in the plasma) with urea and other organic solutes (that do not affect the plasma sodium concentration) accounting for most of the remaining solutes. The loss of fluid with a sodium plus potassium concentration below that of the plasma will directly raise the plasma sodium concentration. In this circumstance, the water losses are proportionally greater than the sodium and potassium losses resulting in hypernatremia. The concurrent presence of fever also may contribute by increasing insensible water losses.

Loss of water in excess of sodium plus potassium also occurs in uncontrolled diabetes mellitus. In this setting, the plasma glucose concentration is so high that the filtered glucose load exceeds glucose reabsorptive capacity in the proximal tubule. The ensuing presence of large amounts of nonreabsorbed glucose in the tubular lumen carries water with it (a process called an *osmotic diuresis*). The net effect is that the sodium plus potassium concentration in the urine is well below that of the plasma, thereby raising both the plasma sodium concentration and the plasma osmolality.

However, the plasma sodium concentration is often not elevated in patients who present with uncontrolled diabetes mellitus because of the counteracting hyponatremic effect of hyperglycemia. As described above, the elevation in plasma glucose concentration causes osmotic water movement out of the cells, thereby lowering the plasma sodium concentration by dilution. However, unlike hyponatremia that occurs with lower serum osomolality, this form of hyponatremia is associated with elevated serum osomolality resulting from the hyperglycemia. Treatment with insulin will correct this form of hyponatremia. The subsequent reduction in plasma osmolality will cause water to move back into the cells, unmasking the underlying hypernatremia induced in part by the osmotic diuresis.

The most common cause of hypernatremia is an infection (such as pneumonia or a urinary tract infection) in an elderly patient with diminished mental status. The infection will increase insensible water losses, while the dementia will limit the protecting effect of thirst.

Other causes of hypernatremia, such as central (diminished ADH release) or nephrogenic (renal resistance to ADH) diabetes insipidus, will be discussed in the section on polyuria.

Diagnosis

Assuming that the hypernatremia is not due to the administration of a hypertonic sodium solution or salt tablets, the differential diagnosis is aimed at identifying the source of the water loss. The history is helpful in many cases, as the examiner should ask about a possible recent infection, vomiting, diarrhea, or increased urinary losses (polyuria). Both the plasma glucose concentration and a test of the urine for glucose (with a dipstick or tablet) should be performed.

In some cases, the information that can be obtained is initially limited by neurologic abnormalities induced either by hypernatremia or much more commonly by the cerebral disease responsible for impairing the thirst mechanism. In this setting, the *urine osmolality* should be measured to assess the integrity of the ADH–renal axis (Table 3.3).

The normal response to hypernatremia is to increase ADH release (Fig. 3.5), resulting in a urine osmolality that can reach a maximum of 1000 to 1200 mOsm/kg in normal subjects (a level more than three times that in the plasma). Renal responsiveness to ADH is reduced in elderly subjects who are most at risk of developing hypernatremia, so that a urine osmolality above 500 mOsm/kg can be accepted as representing relatively intact ADH release and renal response in this group. The presence of concentrated urine suggests that the water loss responsible for the elevation in the plasma sodium concentration is, in the absence of on osmotic diuresis, coming from extrarenal sources.

TABLE 3.3

Diagnostic Utility of Urine Osmolality in Hypernatremia		
Urine Osmolality	**Cause**	**Response to Antidiuretic Hormone**
>500 mOsm/kg	Extrarenal water losses Osmotic diuresis	Little or none, since maximum endogenous release
<300 mOsm/kg	Central diabetes insipidus (complete or severe) Nephrogenic diabetes insipidus (severe)	More than 50% rise in urine osmolality Little or none

In comparison, a urine osmolality below that of the plasma (less than 300 mOsm/kg) is indicative of a major impairment either in ADH release (central) or response (nephrogenic). Although this distinction will be discussed below, the diagnosis can usually be established in the hypernatremic patient by administering DDAVP, an analog of ADH. The urine osmolality should rise by at least 50% in the first 2 hours (with a concomitant fall in urine volume) in patients with central diabetes insipidus who are ADH deficient. In contrast, patients with nephrogenic diabetes insipidus show little or no response since their defect is in the response to, rather than in the production of, ADH.

Values between 300 and 500 mOsm/kg are relatively nonspecific, and can be seen in almost any of the causes of hypernatremia, including partial central diabetes insipidus.

QUESTION 8 **Polyuria is one of the major clinical findings in either central or nephrogenic diabetes insipidus. However, the urine output may not be very high on admission when the patient is volume depleted due either to unreplaced urinary water loss or to concurrent extrarenal water loss. Remembering that ADH increases water reabsorption in the collecting duct by enhancing the water permeability of the luminal membrane, by what mechanisms might volume depletion lower the urine output when ADH release or renal responsiveness is reduced?**

Treatment

The basic concerns in the correction of hypernatremia are similar to those described for hyponatremia: A slowly developing elevation in the plasma sodium concentration is unlikely to produce many neurologic symptoms, and overly rapid correction may be dangerous. The development of hypernatremia causes water movement out of the brain; this is followed by the generation of osmolytes that return brain volume toward normal (Fig. 3.6). At this time, often when the patient is being evaluated by the physician, overly rapid reduction in the plasma sodium concentration can cause excessive water movement into the brain and potentially symptomatic cerebral edema.

To minimize this risk, it is recommended that the plasma sodium concentration be reduced at a maximum rate of 12 mEq/L/day, similar to the recommended rate in hyponatremia. This is usually achieved by the administration of water orally or intravenously (as dextrose in water). Sodium or potassium can be added if there are concurrent volume or potassium deficits.

Water Deficit

Attaining a proper rate of fluid replacement requires calculation of the estimated water deficit. The formula used in this setting can be derived

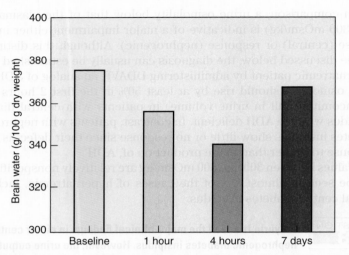

FIGURE 3.6. Effect of sustained elevation in plasma sodium concentration to a level between 170 and 180 mEq/L on brain water content in rabbits. The initial osmotic brain shrinkage begins to correct on the first day and brain volume is near normal by day 7.

in the following way. The quantity of osmoles in the body is equal to the osmolal space (the TBW) times the osmolality of the body fluids or plasma osmolality:

$$Total\ body\ osmoles = TBW \times plasma\ osmolality$$

Since the plasma osmolality is primarily determined by the plasma sodium (Na) concentration,

$$Total\ body\ osmoles \cong TBW \times plasma\ [Na] \qquad \textbf{(Eq. 5)}$$

If hypernatremia results only from water loss, then

$$Current\ body\ osmoles = Normal\ body\ osmoles$$

or, if the normal plasma Na^+ concentration is 140 mEq/L,

$$Current\ body\ water\ (CBW) \times plasma\ [Na]$$
$$= Normal\ body\ water\ (NBW) \times 140$$

By rearrangement,

$$NBW = CBW \times \frac{plasma\ [Na]}{140} \qquad \textbf{(Eq. 6)}$$

The water deficit can then be estimated from

$$Water\ deficit = NBW - CBW$$

or by substituting from Eq. 6:

$$Water\ deficit \cong \left(CBW \times \frac{plasma\ [Na]}{140} \right) - CBW$$

$$Water\ deficit \cong CBW \times \left(\frac{plasma\ [Na]}{140} - 1 \right) \qquad \text{(Eq. 7)}$$

The TBW is normally about 60% and 50% of lean body weight (LBW) in men and women, respectively. However, it is probably reasonable to use values about 10% lower in hypernatremic patients who are water depleted. Thus, in women, Eq. 7 becomes

$$Water\ deficit \cong 0.4 \times LBW \times \left(\frac{plasma\ [Na]}{140} - 1 \right) \qquad \text{(Eq. 8)}$$

This formula estimates the amount of positive water balance required to return the plasma Na^+ concentration to 140 mEq/L. It does not, however, include ongoing losses and any additional *isosmotic fluid deficit* that is frequently present when both Na^+ and water have been lost, as occurs with an osmotic diuresis or diarrhea.

| QUESTION 9 | A 60-kg man in a nursing home becomes confused and stops drinking after developing diarrhea due to viral enteritis. He is |

admitted to the hospital with a plasma sodium concentration of 168 mEq/L; the urine osmolality is 543 mOsm/kg. What factors contributed to the hypernatremia?

Calculate the water deficit required to raise the plasma sodium concentration from 140 to 168 mEq/L in this patient. Over what period of time should this quantity of free water be given to correct the hypernatremia at the recommended rate? Is this the total amount of water that must be given to correct the free water deficit? Would your orders change if, because of concurrent hypokalemia, 40 mEq of potassium were added to each liter of fluid?

One additional aspect of therapy is treatment of the underlying disease to minimize further free water losses. This is most important with a glucose-induced osmotic diuresis (which should be treated with insulin) and with central diabetes insipidus (which should be treated with DDAVP).

Concept of Free Water Clearance

To adequately replace free water loss in hypernatremia, regardless of the etiology, it is necessary to replace urinary free water losses. In the setting of nephrogenic diabetes insipidus, these ongoing losses can be many liters per day. To measure the amount of solute-free water that the kidney can excrete per unit time, one can calculate the free water clearance, C_{H_2O}. The total urine volume can be thought of as the volume necessary to excrete the solute load isosmotic to plasma plus the urinary free water clearance. The excretion of the solute load is obligatory (fixed) while the free water clearance can be negative or positive depending upon whether the urine is hyper- or hypo-osomolar with respect to the plasma:

$$Volume\ (V) = C_{osm} + C_{H_2O} \qquad \text{(Eq. 9)}$$

The C_{osm} can be calculated from the general formula for clearance,

$$C = UV/P$$

$$C_{osm} = (U_{osm} \times V)/P_{osm}$$

If Eq. 9 is now solved for the C_{H_2O}, then

$$C_{H_2O} = V - C_{osm}$$

$$C_{H_2O} = V - V(U_{osm}/P_{osm}) \qquad \text{(Eq. 10)}$$

However, in terms of plasma sodium concentration, only the exchangeable extracellular solutes (sodium and potassium) will contribute to plasma osmolality (see above). Therefore, it is the electrolyte free water clearance that is important for calculating losses. Substituting into Eq. 10, we get

$$C_{H_2O} = V - V(U_{Na+K}/P_{Na+K}) \qquad \text{(Eq. 11)}$$

Polyuria

Polyuria (an increase in urine output) is a relatively common clinical complaint that is arbitrarily defined as an output exceeding 3 L/day. We can derive most of the differential diagnosis by considering how water is reabsorbed in the different nephron segments: It passively follows the reabsorption of sodium in the proximal tubule and loop of Henle, and it is reabsorbed independent of sodium in the collecting duct under the influence of ADH (see Chapters 1 and 2). Urine volume is intrinsically linked to two factors: (1) the amount of solute to be excreted, and (2) the effects of ADH. Solutes generated from metabolism and oral intake are relatively constant and averages from 600 to 800 mOsm/day; ADH is regulated as described in Chapter 2. Figure 3.7 shows the linear increase in urine volume as solute excretion increases. However, this is dramatically affected by whether the urine is maximally dilute (no ADH; urine osmolality ~70 mOsm/kg) or maximally concentrated (maximum ADH; urine osmolality ~1400 mOsm/kg). Based upon this range of urine osmolality generated by healthy kidneys, the normal extremes in urinary volume per day can be appreciated; a minimum of approximately 500 mL (600 to 800 mOsm) in maximally concentrated (1400 mOsm/kg) urine to approximately 9 to 11 L (600 to 800 mOsm) in maximally dilute (70 mOsm/kg).

Thus, there are two major mechanisms that result in polyuria: those that decrease sodium reabsorption in the proximal nephron (filtration

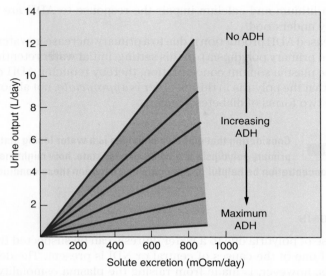

FIGURE 3.7. Effects of ADH and solute excretion on urine volume. It is assumed that the U_{osm} is 70 mOsm/kg in the absence of ADH and 1400 mOsm/kg with maximum ADH effect.

of osmotically active molecules such as glucose) resulting in an *osmotic diuresis* (>800 mOsm/day) and processes that affect ADH levels or renal responsiveness to ADH in the collecting duct (resulting in a *water diuresis*). Decreased sodium reabsorption is most often due to the glucose-induced osmotic diuresis in uncontrolled diabetes mellitus but can also be seen with any solute that is filtered but not reabsorbed (i.e., mannitol). In other cases, the diuresis reflects an appropriate response to volume expansion as might be seen with the excessive administration of intravenous saline.

Other than diabetes mellitus, most cases of polyuria represent a water diuresis in which the urine osmolality is less than that in the plasma due to decreased water reabsorption in the collecting ducts. The polyuria in this setting is due to diminished ADH effect, which can be induced in one of three ways:

■ Decreased ADH production in central diabetes insipidus (CDI). This disorder is often idiopathic, but also can be induced by a variety of diseases, the most common of which are trauma, pituitary surgery, and hypoxic encephalopathy.
■ Reduced renal response to ADH in nephrogenic diabetes insipidus (NDI). ADH resistance that is severe enough to produce polyuria in adults is rare in adults except for two settings: chronic lithium ingestion (for bipolar disease) and hypercalcemia. The mechanisms by

which lithium and calcium impair the response to ADH are incompletely understood.

■ Decreased ADH production is due to a primary increase in water intake (called primary polydipsia). In this setting, initial water retention lowers the plasma sodium concentration, thereby reducing ADH release. Note that the polyuria in this disorder is *appropriate*, not abnormal as in the two forms of diabetes insipidus.

 Considering that diabetes insipidus is a water losing state and primary polydipsia is a water excess state, how might the plasma sodium concentration be helpful in distinguishing between these conditions?

Diagnosis

The cause of polyuria due to a water diuresis can be suspected from the history if one of the causes of central or NDI is present. The definitive diagnosis, however, is made from raising the plasma osmolality, using either water restriction or the administration of hypertonic saline (Fig. 3.8). Plasma ADH levels or, more simply and cheaply, the urine osmolality and urine volume are then monitored along with the plasma osmolality. As shown in Figure 3.5, the normal response to this elevation in plasma osmolality is a progressive increase in ADH release, which should be associated with a rise in urine osmolality.

The test is continued until one of two points is reached: the urine osmolality reaches a level that represents clearly adequate concentrating ability (above 500 to 600 mOsm/kg), or the plasma osmolality exceeds 295 to 300 mOsm/kg, the level at which there is sufficient circulating ADH in normal subjects to induce a maximal increase in the urine osmolality. At this point, exogenous ADH is given and the urine osmolality and urine volume monitored for 2 hours (Fig. 3.8). Only patients in whom ADH release is impaired (i.e., with CDI) should respond with a further elevation in urine osmolality.

A maximum urine osmolality of 500 to 600 mOsm/kg is considered relatively normal in this setting, even though it is only one-half of that achievable in normal subjects. Both primary polydipsia and CDI are associated with a usually modest impairment in maximum concentrating ability, even though renal function and the tubular response to ADH are intact. This mild form of "nephrogenic" diabetes insipidus is induced by the chronic diuresis, which partially washes out the medullary interstitial gradient (see Chapter 1). Remember that the increase in collecting duct water permeability induced by ADH allows the fluid in the tubular lumen to equilibrate osmotically with the hypertonic medullary interstitium. A reduction in interstitial osmolality will therefore lead to a reduction in maximum urine osmolality that can be attained.

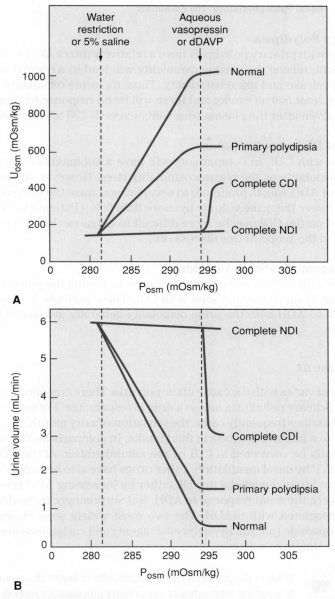

FIGURE 3.8. Effect of the induction of hyperosmolality, either by water restriction or the administration of hypertonic saline, and exogenous ADH (vasopressin or DDAVP) on (**A**) the urine osmolality and (**B**) the urine volume in normal subjects and patients with polyuria. Normal subjects show a maximum rise in urine osmolality as the plasma osmolality exceeds 295 mOsm/kg and do not respond to ADH at this time. Patients with primary polydipsia behave in a similar fashion to normal patients, except that the maximum urine osmolality is somewhat lower due to partial washout of the medullary gradient. Complete or severe CDI and NDI show little increase in urine osmolality or fall in urine volume as the plasma osmolality rises—only patients with CDI respond to ADH.

Primary Polydipsia

Patients with primary polydipsia have a relatively intact ADH–renal axis; as a result, raising the plasma osmolality will lead to a normal increase in ADH release and urine osmolality. Thus, the urine osmolality should rise to at least 500 mOsm/kg and there will be no response to exogenous ADH if given after the plasma osmolality exceeds 295 to 300 mOsm/kg.

Central Diabetes Insipidus

Patients with CDI, in comparison, will have a submaximal increase in urine osmolality as the plasma osmolality rises. However, the administration of ADH will, in moderate to severe cases, raise the urine osmolality and lower the urine volume by more than 50%. (Patients with milder forms of partial CDI may be more difficult to diagnose, but this problem is beyond the scope of this discussion.)

Nephrogenic Diabetes Insipidus

Patients with NDI show an initial response to raising the plasma osmolality that is similar to that seen with CDI. These patients, however, are resistant to ADH with the urine osmolality generally increasing by less than 10%.

Treatment

Treatment varies with the cause of the polyuria. There is generally no therapy for primary polydipsia unless a drug is responsible. For example, the phenothiazines frequently cause the sensation of a dry mouth, potentially leading to a marked increase in fluid intake. In comparison, the polyuria can usually be corrected in CDI by the administration of the ADH analog DDAVP by nasal insufflation. Other drugs have also been incidentally discovered to be beneficial in CDI, either by increasing ADH release or, more likely, the renal response to ADH. Not surprisingly, these drugs are often associated with SIADH. The two most widely studied drugs are chlorpropamide (an oral hypoglycemic agent) and carbamazepine (used in the treatment of seizures).

 QUESTION 11   **What is the potential risk of giving ADH to lower the urine output in a patient who actually has primary polydipsia, rather than CDI?**

ADH or drugs that depend upon ADH are typically ineffective in NDI. The major drug that has been useful in this setting is a thiazide diuretic. Although it seems paradoxical to give a diuretic to treat a diuresis, the thiazides act by inducing mild volume depletion. The ensuing activation of the renin–angiotensin–aldosterone and sympathetic nervous systems will increase proximal sodium and water reabsorption, limiting water delivery to the ADH-sensitive site in the collecting ducts. A 1 to 1.5 kg weight loss can lower the urine output by as much as two-thirds in a patient with NDI. This regimen is also effective as adjunctive therapy in CDI. Another potential treatment option for both central and NDI is the use of nonsteroidal anti-inflammatory drugs (NSAID). These drugs inhibit renal prostaglandin synthesis, and this has the effect of increasing concentrating ability, since prostaglandins normally antagonize the action of ADH. The net effect in patients with DI may be a 25% to 50% reduction in urine, a response that is partially additive to that of a thiazide diuretic.

Would a loop diuretic be likely to be as effective as a thiazide diuretic in these disorders?

CASE DISCUSSION   The patient presented at the beginning of this chapter has hyponatremia. The differential diagnosis includes disorders of ADH and water regulation, and volume depletion. In this case, the hyponatremia may be due to two causes: SIADH and vomiting-induced hypovolemia. The presence of an oat cell carcinoma makes SIADH likely. However, the decreased skin turgor, orthostatic hypotension, and low urine sodium concentration are indicative of volume depletion, which is also a stimulus to ADH release. The diagnosis can be unmasked by the administration of salt, as with hypertonic saline to raise the plasma sodium concentration slowly to a safe level. Reversal of the hypovolemia will cause rapid correction of the hyponatremia if only vomiting were responsible, since the stimulus to ADH secretion and water retention will be removed. If, however, there is also underlying SIADH, then volume repletion will lead to a rise in the urine sodium concentration above 40 mEq/L but hypersecretion of ADH will persist resulting in inappropriately elevated urine osmolality and some degree of hyponatremia.

ANSWERS TO QUESTIONS

1 From Eq. 4, the plasma sodium concentration is determined only by sodium, potassium, and water. Since the sodium plus potassium concentration in the diarrheal fluid is less than that in the plasma (85 vs. 111 mEq/L), the plasma sodium concentration will tend to rise since water is being lost in excess of an effective solute. Although the diarrheal fluid has the same total osmolality as the plasma, it contains urea and other organic solutes as well as sodium and potassium. However, the loss of these organic solutes has no effect on the plasma sodium concentration since they do not affect water movement across the cell membranes.

Urea, for example, can freely diffuse across cell membranes and is considered to be an ineffective osmole. The loss of urea will lower the plasma urea concentration (measured as the blood urea nitrogen or BUN). This will lead to urea diffusion out of the cells until the concentration is equal in the two compartments; there will, however, be no osmotic water movement and therefore no change in the plasma sodium concentration.

2 Volume expansion induced by water retention will decrease renin release and increase that of atrial natriuretic peptide. These changes will lead to enhanced sodium and water excretion that will tend to return the extracellular fluid volume toward normal. The net effect in terms of the hyponatremia is that the fall in plasma sodium concentration in SIADH is due both to an increase in TBW and to a decrease in total body sodium stores. However, sodium excretion will equal intake after the initial volume expansion, and the hyponatremia will persist from persistent ADH secretion.

3 The first step in countercurrent multiplication that creates the interstitial osmotic gradient is NaCl reabsorption in the thick ascending limb of the loop of Henle (see Chapter 1). Blocking this step with a loop diuretic will markedly diminish the interstitial gradient. Thus, even though the loop diuretic may lead to enhanced ADH release and increased collecting duct water permeability, there will be less net water reabsorption since the osmotic gradient that promotes water reabsorption at this site has been markedly diminished. A thiazide diuretic, in comparison, acts in the distal tubule, which is in the renal cortex and therefore does not interfere with generation of the countercurrent gradient.

4 It is tempting to assume that the plasma sodium concentration will rise, since the sodium concentration in the administered fluid is higher than that in the plasma. However, all of this sodium will be excreted as would occur in normal subjects. The excretion of the 308 mOsm in each liter will occur in only 500 mL of water because of the fixed urine osmolality (308 mOsm in 500 mL equals an osmolality of 616 mOsm/kg). Thus, approximately 500 mL of the water will be retained, leading to a further fall in the plasma sodium concentration.

5 Measurement of the urine sodium concentration and the urine osmolality can easily distinguish between these possibilities. If hypovolemia alone were present and the patient were still volume depleted, then the urine sodium concentration will remain below 15 mEq/L and the urine osmolality will remain elevated due to persistent secretion of ADH. If the patient is now normovolemic but also has underlying SIADH, then the urine sodium concentration will rise to above 20 mEq/L but the urine osmolality will still be inappropriately high. If hypovolemia alone were present and the patient is volume depleted, then sodium excretion will rise and there will *no longer be any hypovolemic stimulus to ADH*. As a result, the persistent

hyponatremia will suppress ADH release and the urine osmolality will fall to less than 100 mOsm/kg. Rapid excretion of the excess water in this setting will quickly correct the hyponatremia.

6 Although the administered sodium will be limited to the extracellular space, as seen in Eq. 4, plasma sodium concentration depends upon exchangeable sodium and potassium (the major intracellular cation). Therefore, the effect of sodium administration will be distributed through the TBW. The ensuing rise in the plasma sodium concentration will cause osmotic water movement out of the cells, since the cell membranes are freely permeable to water.

7 A plasma sodium concentration greater than 150 mEq/L is virtually never seen in an alert patient who has access to water. Thus, the patient must have a hypothalamic lesion affecting the thirst center, resulting in diminished sensation of thirst (hypodipsia).

8 Collecting duct water reabsorption is limited by the amount of water delivered to this segment. Hypovolemia may lower the glomerular filtration rate and increase proximal sodium and water reabsorption (mediated in part by angiotensin II and norepinephrine). The ensuing decline in water delivery to the collecting ducts will lower the urine output even though water permeability in this segment remains abnormally low.

9 Three factors contributed to the development of hypernatremia in this patient: impaired mental status, which limited the expression of thirst; increased insensible losses from the skin due to fever; and the loss of diarrheal fluid, which usually has a sodium plus potassium concentration below that of the plasma.

   From Eq. 8, the estimated water deficit is $[0.5 \times 60 \times (168/140) - 1]$, which is equal to 6 L. To correct at the rate of 12 mEq/L/day or 0.5 mEq/L/hour, the 6 L should be given over 56 hours; approximately 100 mL/hour. This is an underestimate of the amount of fluid required to correct the plasma sodium concentration since there will be ongoing dilute losses from the skin and respiratory tract averaging about 50 mL/hour. Thus, the total rate of free water administration should be 150 mL/hour to correct the water deficit. (If this patient had diabetes insipidus, then dilute urinary losses would also have to be replaced.)

   Adding 40 mEq/L to each liter of free water is roughly equivalent to one-quarter isotonic saline, since potassium is as osmotically active as sodium. Therefore, each liter is only three-quarters free water and the rate of fluid administration must be multiplied by 4/3, which results in a rate of 200 mL/hour.

10 The plasma sodium concentration tends to be in the high-normal range in diabetes insipidus (142 to 145 mEq/L) due to tendency toward water loss

and in the low normal range (136 to 139 mEq/L) in primary polydipsia due to the continuing excess water intake. Thus, a finding at either extreme is helpful diagnostically, whereas a plasma sodium concentration of 140 mEq/L is of little help.

11 Patients with primary polydipsia usually maintain a relatively normal plasma sodium concentration because they are able to excrete the excess water by suppressing the release of ADH. The administration of ADH to such a patient would rapidly lead to water retention and acute and possibly symptomatic hyponatremia. Thus, establishing the correct diagnosis is vital in this setting.

12 As described in the answer to Question 3, loop diuretics block the first step in the countercurrent mechanism (the reabsorption of sodium chloride without water in the thick ascending limb), thereby diminishing responsiveness to ADH. Thus, a loop diuretic should be less effective in lowering the urine output in diabetes insipidus, particularly when given as an adjunct to DDAVP in CDI.

SUGGESTED READINGS

Ayus JC, Wheeler JM, Arieff AI. Postoperative hyponatremic encephalopathy in menstruant women. Ann Intern Med 1992;117:891.

Gross P. Treatment of severe hyponatremia. Kidney Int 2001;60:2417.

McManus ML, Churchwell KB, Strange K. Mechanisms of disease: regulation of cell volume regulation in health and disease. N Engl J Med 1995;333:1260.

Rose BD, Post TW. Clinical Physiology of Acid–Base and Electrolyte Disorders, 5th Ed. New York: McGraw-Hill, 2001.

Schrier RW, Gross P, Gheorghiade M, et al. Tolvaptan, a selective oral vasopressin V_2-receptor antagonist, for hyponatremia. N Engl J Med 2006;355(20):2099–2112.

Strange K. Regulation of solute and water balance and cell volume in the central nervous system. J Am Soc Nephrol 1992;3:12.

4

EDEMATOUS STATES AND THE USE OF DIURETICS

CASE PRESENTATION

A 34-year-old woman noted the relatively sudden onset of weight gain, puffiness of the face, and swelling of her legs. She had been previously well and has no history of a systemic disease that might predispose her to edema formation.

Physical examination reveals a healthy-appearing young woman whose face appears slightly swollen. Her weight is 132 lb, 15 lb above her baseline level. Her blood pressure is 120/75; the estimated jugular venous pressure is 6 cm H_2O, and there is 4+ pitting edema two-thirds of the way up the calf. Examination of the heart, lungs, and abdomen are normal; there is no evidence of either ascites or pulmonary congestion.

Pertinent laboratory data show a normal BUN and plasma creatinine concentration, 4+ protein on dipstick of the urine, an otherwise normal urinalysis without cells or cellular casts, 24-hour protein excretion of 4.3 g/day (normal <150mg/day). The plasma albumin concentration is 2.1 mg/dL (normal = 3.5 to 4.5 mg/dL).

OBJECTIVES

By the end of this section, you should have an understanding of each of the following issues:

- The role of Starling's forces in governing the movement of water between the plasma water and the interstitial space.
- The central importance of renal sodium retention in the development of clinically detectable edema.
- The different factors that promote edema formation in the major generalized edematous states: congestive heart failure, the nephrotic syndrome, and hepatic cirrhosis with ascites (which refers to the accumulation of fluid within the peritoneal space).
- The mechanisms by which the three major classes of diuretics (loop diuretics, thiazide-type diuretics, and potassium-sparing diuretics) inhibit sodium reabsorption in the different nephron segments.
- The hemodynamic consequences of fluid removal during the treatment of edema.

Pathophysiology of Edema Formation

Edema is defined as a palpable swelling produced by expansion of the interstitial fluid volume. Two basic steps are involved in edema formation:

- An *alteration in capillary hemodynamics* that favors the movement of fluid from the vascular space into the interstitium.
- The *renal retention of dietary sodium and water*, thereby expanding the extracellular fluid volume.

The central role of the kidneys in the development of edema can be appreciated from the following observations. Edema does not become clinically apparent until the interstitial volume has increased by at least 2.5 to 3 L. Since the normal plasma volume is only about 3 L, patients would develop life-threatening hemoconcentration and shock if the edema fluid were derived only from the plasma.

These complications do not occur because compensatory sodium and water retention by the kidney maintain the plasma volume. Let us assume, for example, that there is increased movement of fluid from the vascular space into the interstitium because of a rise in capillary hydraulic pressure (the importance of which will be discussed later). The ensuing plasma volume depletion reduces tissue perfusion, leading to the activation of the renin–angiotensin–aldosterone and sympathetic nervous systems. These and other sodium-retaining forces (such as a reduction in renal perfusion pressure; see Chapter 2) limit further sodium and water excretion. Some of the retained fluid stays in the vascular space, returning the plasma volume and tissue perfusion toward normal. However, the primary rise in intracapillary pressure results in most of the retained fluid entering the interstitium and eventually becoming apparent as edema. The net effect is a marked expansion of the total extracellular volume (as edema) with maintenance of the plasma volume at near-normal levels.

This example illustrates an important point that applies to patients with congestive heart failure and hepatic cirrhosis: Renal sodium and water retention is an *appropriate* compensation in that it restores tissue perfusion, even though it also augments the degree of edema. On the other hand, removing the edema fluid with a diuretic will improve symptoms but may diminish tissue perfusion, occasionally to clinically significant levels.

The hemodynamic effects are somewhat different when the primary abnormality is *inappropriate* renal fluid retention. This problem most often occurs in patients with primary renal disease and is often associated with elevated blood pressure. In this setting, both the plasma and interstitial volumes are expanded and there are no deleterious hemodynamic effects from removal of the excess fluid. This is an example of *overfilling* of the vascular tree in contrast to the *underfilling* that occurs if there is primary movement of fluid out of the vascular space.

Capillary Hemodynamics

Starling's Law
The exchange of fluid between the plasma and the interstitium is determined by the hydraulic and oncotic pressures in each compartment. The relationship between these parameters can be expressed by Starling's law (Fig. 4.1),

$$Net\ filtration = LpS\ (\Delta\ hydraulic\ pressure - \Delta\ oncotic\ pressure)$$
$$= LpS\ [(P_{cap} - P_{if}) - \sigma(\Pi_{cap} - \Pi_{if})] \qquad \text{(Eq. 1)}$$

where Lp is the unit permeability or porosity of the capillary wall, S is the surface area available for filtration, P_{cap} and P_{if} are the capillary and interstitial fluid hydraulic pressures, Π_{cap} and Π_{if} are the capillary and interstitial fluid oncotic pressures (which are primarily determined by albumin), and σ represents the reflection coefficient of proteins across the capillary wall (with values ranging from 0 if completely permeable to 1 if completely impermeable). In addition to these forces, the degree of fluid accumulation in the interstitium is also determined by the rate of fluid removal by the lymphatic vessels.

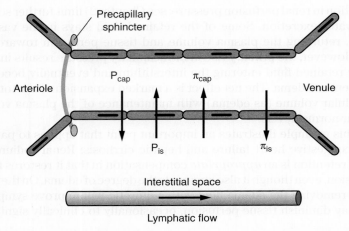

FIGURE 4.1. Schematic representation of the effect of the hydraulic pressure (P) and the oncotic pressure (π) in the capillary (cap) and the interstitium (is) on fluid movement between the vascular space and the interstitium. The *arrows* point in the direction in which that parameter will cause fluid to move. The resistance at the precapillary sphincter is an important regulator of the capillary hydraulic pressure, allowing it to remain relatively constant despite changes in the arterial perfusion pressure.

QUESTION 1   **Sodium salts have a much higher concentration than albumin in the capillary [280 mmol (which includes the anions accompanying sodium) vs. 1 mmol for albumin]. Why are sodium salts not considered in the calculation of the plasma oncotic pressure?**

Capillary Hydraulic Pressure. Although generated by cardiac contraction, the capillary hydraulic pressure is relatively insensitive to alterations in arterial pressure. The stability of capillary pressure is due to variations in resistance at the precapillary sphincter, which determine the extent to which the arterial pressure is transmitted to the capillary (Fig. 4.1). If the arterial pressure is increased, for example, the precapillary sphincter constricts, preventing any significant change in capillary hemodynamics. This response, which is called *autoregulation*, is under local control, being mediated both by stretch receptors in the vascular wall and by local metabolic factors. The efficiency of autoregulation explains why patients with systemic hypertension do not routinely develop edema.

In contrast, the resistance at the venous end of the capillary is not well regulated. Consequently, an increase in venous pressure produces a similar change in capillary hydraulic pressure, thereby predisposing to edema formation.

Interstitial Oncotic Pressure. The major effective interstitial solutes are mucopolysaccharides and, more importantly, filtered proteins, particularly albumin. The degree of accumulation of filtered proteins is determined by two factors: the permeability of the capillary wall and the rate of removal by the lymphatics. If, for example, there were no lymphatic removal, then the interstitial protein concentration would eventually equal that in the plasma even though the capillary wall might have a very low permeability to proteins.

The net effect is that the interstitial oncotic pressure is in part dependent upon the plasma protein concentration. This relationship has important implications for the possible role of hypoalbuminemia in the development of edema. A reduction in the plasma albumin concentration and therefore in the plasma oncotic pressure will favor fluid movement from the vascular space into the interstitium. Over time, however, less albumin will be filtered and the interstitial oncotic pressure (Π_{if}) will fall. As a result, the transcapillary oncotic pressure gradient ($\Pi_{cap} - \Pi_{if}$) may be unchanged and the oncotic pressure gradient favoring edema formation will not occur.

Normal Values in Different Organs. The normal values for Starling's forces in experimental animals and humans are uncertain, largely because of difficulties in measurement of these parameters (with the exception of the plasma oncotic pressure, which can be determined from a blood sample). Despite these difficulties, important differences in the magnitude of Starling's forces have been identified in different organs, such as skeletal muscle and subcutaneous tissue (the sites of peripheral edema) and the liver (the site of ascites formation in hepatic disease). In skeletal muscle capillaries, the most important forces are the mean capillary hydraulic pressure (17 mm Hg), which pushes fluid out of the capillary, and the plasma oncotic pressure (26 mm Hg), which pulls fluid into the vascular space. The effect of the plasma oncotic pressure is partially counteracted by the interstitial oncotic pressure, which is thought to average from 10 to 15 mm Hg. When the effects of the interstitial hydraulic pressure are accounted for, the net effect is a small mean gradient of about 0.3 to 0.5 mm Hg favoring filtration out of the vascular space; this fluid is returned to the systemic circulation by the lymph vessels.

In comparison, the hepatic sinusoids have very different characteristics. The sinusoids are highly permeable to proteins; as a result, the capillary and interstitial oncotic pressures are roughly equal and there is essentially no transcapillary oncotic pressure gradient. Thus, the hydraulic pressure gradient favoring filtration is virtually unopposed. To some degree, filtration is minimized by a lower capillary hydraulic pressure than in skeletal muscle, since approximately two-thirds of hepatic blood flow is derived from the portal vein, a low-pressure system. Nevertheless, there is still a larger gradient favoring filtration; however, edema does not normally occur, because the filtered fluid is again removed by the lymphatics.

Edema Formation

The development of edema requires a relatively large alteration in one or more of Starling's forces in a direction that favors an increase in net filtration. This is most often due to an elevation in capillary hydraulic pressure; less frequently, edema results from enhanced capillary permeability, reduced plasma oncotic pressure, or lymphatic obstruction (Table 4.1).

For the reasons described above, increased capillary hydraulic pressure is usually induced by a rise in venous pressure. A persistent elevation in venous pressure leading to edema can occur by one or both of two

TABLE 4.1

Major Causes of Edematous States

I. **Increased capillary hydraulic pressure**
  A. **Increased plasma volume due to renal sodium retention**
    1. Congestive heart failure
    2. Primary renal sodium retention:
       – Renal disease including nephrotic syndrome
       – Drugs including nonsteroidal anti-inflammatory drugs, estrogens
       – Early hepatic cirrhosis
       – Pregnancy and premenstrual edema
       – Idiopathic edema, when diuretic induced
  B. **Venous obstruction**
    1. Ascites in hepatic cirrhosis or hepatic venous obstruction
    2. Acute pulmonary edema
    3. Local venous obstruction, as with deep vein thrombosis

II. **Decreased plasma oncotic pressure (primarily when the plasma albumin concentration is below 1.5–2.0 g/dL)**
  A. **Protein loss from nephrotic syndrome or gastrointestinal**
  B. **Reduced albumin synthesis from hepatic disease or malnutrition**

III. **Increased capillary permeability**
  A. **Allergic reactions**
  B. **Sepsis or inflammation**
  C. **Burns or trauma**
  D. **Interleukin-2 therapy**
  E. **Adult respiratory distress syndrome**

IV. **Lymphatic obstruction or increased interstitial oncotic pressure**
  A. **Nodal enlargement due to malignancy**
  B. **Postmastectomy**
  C. **Malignant ascites**
  D. **Hypothyroidism (perhaps due to binding of filtered proteins by excess interstitial mucopolysaccharide accumulation)**

basic mechanisms: (1) when the blood volume is expanded, augmenting the volume in the venous system, and (2) when there is venous obstruction. Examples of edema due to volume expansion include congestive heart failure and renal disease. Examples of edema due at least in part to venous obstruction include ascites formation in hepatic cirrhosis and acute pulmonary edema following a sudden impairment in cardiac function (as with a myocardial infarction).

The following discussion will be limited to the three most common forms of generalized edema: congestive heart failure, hepatic cirrhosis, and renal disease—including the nephrotic syndrome. The latter refers to glomerular diseases associated with increased glomerular permeability leading to heavy proteinuria, hypoalbuminemia (due in part to albumin loss in the urine), and edema.

 Experimental and clinical studies have shown that edema occurs only when there is a relatively large increase of more than 10 mm Hg in the gradient favoring filtration. What safety factors prevent persistent interstitial fluid accumulation as edema when there is a lesser change in Starling's forces?

Renal Sodium Retention

The second step in edema formation is expansion of the extracellular fluid volume by renal sodium retention. This process results from one of two basic mechanisms: (1) primary renal sodium retention or (2) an appropriate response to a decrease in the effective circulating volume.

Primary Renal Sodium Retention

A primary defect in renal sodium excretion can occur with advanced renal failure or with glomerular diseases such as acute glomerulonephritis or the nephrotic syndrome. Figure 4.2 shows an example of the role of the kidney in an animal model of unilateral nephrotic syndrome induced by injection of a toxin to the glomerular epithelial cells in one renal artery. Only the diseased kidney retained sodium, indicating the intrarenal rather than systemic neurohumoral factors must be of primary importance. Micropuncture studies, in which the fluid at different nephron segments were analyzed, showed that delivery of filtered sodium to the end of the distal tubule was the same in both kidneys. Thus, the decrease in sodium excretion probably resulted from increased sodium reabsorption in the collecting ducts. How this might occur is not known.

Compensatory Response to Effective Circulating Volume Depletion

Sodium and water retention leading to edema more commonly represents an *appropriate compensatory response* to effective circulating volume depletion, with the urine sodium concentration often being less than

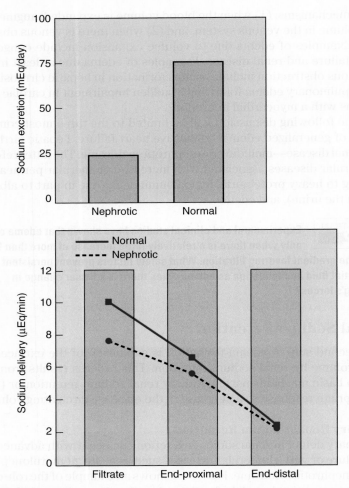

FIGURE 4.2. Sodium excretion is reduced in nephrotic kidneys by approximately two-thirds (*top*). Micropuncture studies (in which samples are taken via micropipettes from different nephron segments) of sodium handling in unilateral nephrotic syndrome in the rat. Although less sodium is filtered in the nephrotic kidney (due to reduced GFR), less is reabsorbed so that the quantity of sodium remaining in the tubular lumen at the end of the distal tubule is the same in the two kidneys (*bottom*). Thus, sodium reabsorption must be increased in the collecting ducts to account for the two-thirds reduction in total sodium excretion in the nephrotic kidney when compared to the normal kidney.

15 mEq/L. As reviewed in Chapter 2, the effective circulating volume is an unmeasurable entity that refers to the arterial volume (normally about 700 mL in a 70-kg man) that is effectively perfusing the tissues.

Congestive heart failure is a common clinical example of a reduction in the effective circulating volume depletion leading to edema.

Myocardial dysfunction initially lowers the cardiac output, resulting in increased release of the three *hypovolemic hormones*: renin (which leads to the production of angiotensin II and aldosterone), norepinephrine, and antidiuretic hormone. These hormones have the following effects that limit sodium and water excretion and promote edema formation:

- A reduction in GFR due to renal vasoconstriction.
- Enhanced proximal sodium reabsorption mediated by angiotensin II and norepinephrine.
- Increased collecting tubular sodium and water reabsorption due to aldosterone and ADH, respectively.

Compensated State. If the cardiac disease is not severe, then fluid retention can restore relatively normal systemic hemodynamics (at least at rest). The increase in plasma volume will enhance venous return to the heart, thereby raising the intracardiac filling pressures and (via the Frank–Starling relationship described below) increasing the cardiac output toward normal. In this new compensated state, the systemic blood pressure, plasma renin activity and aldosterone concentration, and urinary sodium excretion may return to baseline levels, at the price of persistent plasma volume expansion, hypertension, and edema (Fig. 4.3).

Renal Disease and Nephrotic Syndrome

Edema in most forms of renal disease is due to volume expansion induced by an inability to excrete dietary sodium. There are two settings in which this is most likely to occur: (1) with advanced renal failure where the marked reduction in GFR is limiting, and (2) with glomerular diseases such as acute glomerulonephritis or the nephrotic syndrome (see Chapter 9). As depicted in Figure 4.2, the GFR may be reduced in glomerular diseases (reduced filtered sodium in filtrate) but the sodium retention is primarily due to increased tubular reabsorption, primarily in the collecting ducts.

It is not clear why edema is relatively unusual in tubulointerstitial and vascular diseases. The most likely explanation is that the primary process (with tubulointerstitial disorders) and ischemic injury (with vascular disease) impair tubular sodium reabsorption.

It is important to appreciate that urinary sodium excretion is determined by the difference between the filtered load (GFR × plasma sodium concentration) and tubular reabsorption. Thus, a mild to moderate reduction in GFR alone is usually not sufficient to interfere with sodium homeostasis, since it can be counterbalanced by a reduction in tubular sodium reabsorption. The factor in glomerular disease that is responsible for the increase in collecting duct sodium reabsorption has not

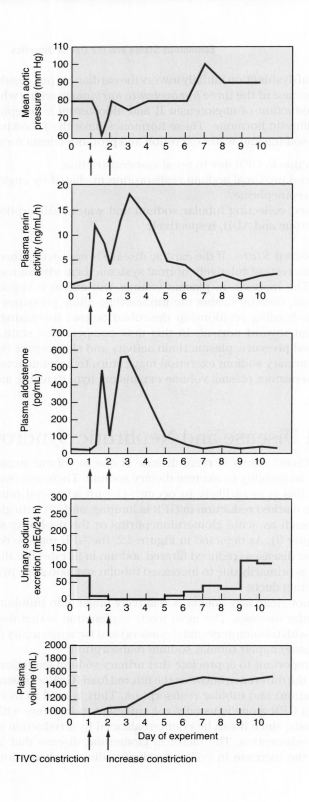

been identified. Both decreased responsiveness to atrial natriuretic peptide and increased activity of the Na^+–K^+-ATPase pump that drives active sodium transport have been observed.

 Compare the changes in plasma renin activity and plasma atrial natriuretic peptide levels that will be seen in edema due to a low cardiac output in congestive heart failure and to *primary* sodium retention in acute glomerulonephritis.

Nephrotic Syndrome

The nephrotic syndrome refers to those disorders in which there is increased glomerular permeability to macromolecules, leading to a constellation of findings, including heavy proteinuria (protein excretion generally above 3.5 g/day vs. a normal level of less than 150 mg), hypoalbuminemia, and edema. It had been thought that the mechanism of edema formation in this setting was different from that in other renal diseases, being due to hypoalbuminemia-induced underfilling of the vascular space rather than overfilling from primary renal sodium retention.

It is important to emphasize, however, that the distribution of fluid between the vascular space and the interstitium is dependent on the transcapillary oncotic pressure gradient ($\Pi_{cap} - \Pi_{if}$)], not on the plasma oncotic pressure alone. Figure 4.4 illustrates the relationship between the plasma and interstitial oncotic pressures in patients with minimal change disease, a common cause of the nephrotic syndrome that can usually be cured with corticosteroid therapy. Thus, patients could be studied both during active disease and after remission has been induced. As can be seen, the fall in the plasma albumin concentration with active disease was associated with a parallel decline in the interstitial albumin concentration due to less entry of albumin into the interstitium. As a result, the transcapillary oncotic gradient is near normal and therefore should not be responsible for the development of edema. Studies in animals suggest that the renal disease itself leads to sodium retention via increased collecting duct sodium reabsorption (Fig. 4.2).

Thus, edema in the nephrotic syndrome is more likely to result from overfilling of the vascular space unless the plasma albumin concentration

---

FIGURE 4.3. Sequential changes in mean aortic pressure, plasma renin activity, plasma aldosterone concentration, urinary sodium excretion, and plasma volume in dogs with chronic thoracic inferior vena cava constriction, a model of congestive heart failure. The initial reduction in venous return to the heart leads to a reduction in cardiac output, hypotension, activation of the renin–angiotensin–aldosterone system, and a fall in sodium excretion. The ensuing fluid retention raises venous return to the heart, thereby allowing systemic hemodynamics and hormone activation to be normalized.

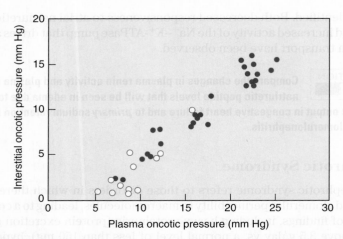

FIGURE 4.4. Relationship between plasma and interstitial oncotic pressures in patients with the nephrotic syndrome due to minimal change disease. The patients were studied during active disease (when they had a low plasma albumin concentration; *open circles*) and when they were in remission (*dark circles*). The oncotic pressure in the interstitium changed in parallel with that in the plasma, resulting in little or no change in the transcapillary oncotic pressure gradient. As a result, hypoalbuminemia alone should not have been responsible for edema in these patients.

falls below 1.5 to 2 g/dL (normal is from 4 to 5 g/dL). There are several clinical observations that are compatible with this hypothesis. Perhaps, the most compelling is the finding in minimal change disease that correction of the glomerular permeability defect with corticosteroids leads to a substantial rise in sodium excretion (with partial resolution of the edema) *before any significant elevation in the plasma albumin concentration.* It is therefore likely that the renal disease, rather than hypoalbuminemia, was responsible for the initial sodium retention.

Congestive Heart Failure

Congestive heart failure can be produced by a variety of disorders, including coronary artery disease, hypertension, valvular disease, and cardiomyopathies. The edema in this setting is due to an elevation in venous pressure that produces a parallel rise in capillary hydraulic pressure. However, two different mechanisms may be involved:

■ In acute pulmonary edema due to a myocardial infarction or ischemia, the sudden decrease in left ventricular function results in an elevation in the left ventricular end-diastolic pressure. This pressure is then transmitted *back* through the left atrium and pulmonary veins to the pulmonary capillaries. Thus, pulmonary edema in this setting is due to a form of venous obstruction.

■ In chronic heart failure, the sodium retention is, as described above and illustrated in Figure 4.3, due to activation of sodium-retaining neurohumoral systems by the reduction in cardiac output.

The sequential hemodynamic effects in chronic heart failure can be appreciated from the Frank–Starling relationship in Figure 4.5. The upper curve represents the normal relationship between stroke volume and the left ventricular end-diastolic pressure (LVEDP); note that increasing LVEDP increases the stroke volume (and, if heart rate is unchanged, the cardiac output). This effect is thought to be mediated by a stretch-induced enhancement of cardiac contractility.

The development of mild cardiac dysfunction (*middle curve*) will tend to lower both stroke volume and cardiac output (*line AB*). The ensuing renal sodium and water retention can reverse these abnormalities, since the increments in plasma volume and LVEDP will augment cardiac contractility (*line BC*). At this point, the patient is in a new steady state of *compensated heart failure* in which further sodium retention does not occur similar to that depicted in Figure 4.3. However, the restoration of tissue perfusion in this setting has occurred only after there has been an elevation in the LVEDP, perhaps to a level sufficient to produce pulmonary edema.

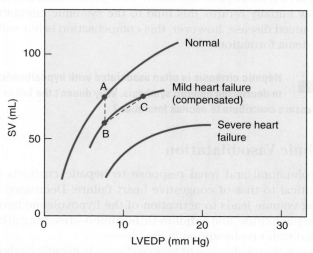

FIGURE 4.5. Frank–Starling curves relating stroke volume (SV) to left ventricular end-diastolic pressure (LVEDP) with normal cardiac function and with mild and severe heart failure. Decreased stroke volume leads to decreased cardiac output (at constant heart rate), activation of sodium-retaining hormones leading to increased plasma volume. These changes will restore stroke volume (and cardiac output) at the expense of elevated LVEDP.

The findings are different with severe heart failure (*lower curve*, Fig. 4.5). In this disorder, the myocardial dysfunction is so severe that increasing the LVEDP cannot normalize the stroke volume. As a result, the cardiac output will also be low and there will a continuing tendency to sodium retention.

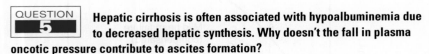 **Diuretics are usually given to remove some of the edema fluid in patients with congestive heart failure. The relief of pulmonary congestion is associated with fewer symptoms of shortness of breath and often with an improved sense of well-being. What do you think happens to the cardiac output in this setting? If it occurred, how would you detect a clinically significant reduction in the cardiac output?**

Hepatic Cirrhosis and Ascites

There are two major changes induced by hepatic cirrhosis that promote sodium retention and the subsequent deposition of most of this excess fluid in the peritoneum as ascites: vasodilatation that lowers systemic vascular resistance and postsinusoidal obstruction induced by hepatic fibrosis. As renal sodium and water retention expand the plasma volume, the postsinusoidal obstruction results in a preferential elevation in hepatic sinusoidal pressure, thereby causing fluid to move out of the sinusoids across the hepatic capsule into the peritoneum. Increased lymphatic flow initially returns this fluid to the systemic circulation; with more advanced disease, however, this compensation is not sufficient to prevent edema formation.

QUESTION 5 **Hepatic cirrhosis is often associated with hypoalbuminemia due to decreased hepatic synthesis. Why doesn't the fall in plasma oncotic pressure contribute to ascites formation?**

Splanchnic Vasodilatation

The neurohumoral and renal response to hepatic cirrhosis is essentially identical to that of congestive heart failure: Decreased effective circulating volume leads to activation of the hypovolemic hormones—renin, norepinephrine, and antidiuretic hormone—resulting in increased sodium and water reabsorption in the kidney.

However, the mechanism of hypoperfusion in hepatic cirrhosis is different from that in congestive heart failure. In the latter disorder, primary myocardial dysfunction lowers the cardiac output; the subsequent fall in systemic blood pressure (which is equal to the product of the cardiac output and systemic vascular resistance) then activates the appropriate neurohumoral systems. In comparison, the primary hemodynamic

changes in hepatic cirrhosis are splanchnic vasodilatation and the formation of multiple arteriovenous fistulas throughout the body (such as the
spider angiomas on the skin). The mechanism by which hepatic cirrhosis
produces these hemodynamic alterations is not known. Nevertheless,
the ensuing reduction in systemic vascular resistance lowers the systemic blood pressure, again leading to activation of the sodium-retaining
systems.

In contrast to the low cardiac output in congestive heart failure,
the cardiac output in hepatic cirrhosis is often elevated (discussed in
Chapter 2; Table 2.2). However, much of the cardiac output is circulating
ineffectively, bypassing the capillary circulation through the arteriovenous fistulas. Thus, the output reaching the capillary circulation (including the glomerular capillaries) is actually reduced despite the high total
output.

These changes—vasodilatation in the splanchnic circulation and
neurohumorally mediated vasoconstriction in the renal and musculoskeletal circulations—become progressively more severe with more
advanced hepatic disease. The renal manifestations of these hemodynamic changes include reductions in renal blood flow and GFR, and
sodium excretion that may eventually fall below 10 mEq/day. Patients
with advanced hepatic failure may also develop renal failure due primarily to intense renal vasoconstriction rather than structural renal disease.
This disorder is called the hepatorenal syndrome and is discussed further
in Chapter 11.

The importance of splanchnic vasodilatation-induced underfilling on
the impairment in renal function in hepatic cirrhosis can be illustrated
by the response to an infusion of ornipressin, an analog of antidiuretic
hormone. Ornipressin is a preferential vasoconstrictor in the splanchnic
circulation that, in patients with hepatic cirrhosis, leads sequentially to
elevations in systemic vascular resistance and mean arterial pressure; reductions in the plasma renin activity and norepinephrine concentration;
and elevations in renal blood flow, glomerular filtration rate, and urinary
sodium excretion (Fig. 4.6).

Physical Examination and Site of Edema Formation

The conditions described above can produce edema at three sites: peripheral edema in the subcutaneous tissue that, due to gravity, is generally
most prominent in the legs after the patient has been standing; pulmonary
edema; and ascites. Patients with peripheral edema complain of swollen
legs and difficulty in walking due to the increased fluid deposition in the
legs. Peripheral edema can be detected by the presence of pitting (a persistent indentation) after pressure is applied to the edematous area. The

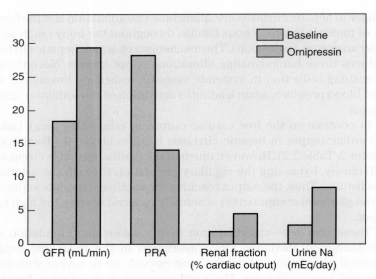

FIGURE 4.6. Effect of infusion of ornipressin, an analog of antidiuretic hormone that causes preferential splanchnic vasoconstriction, in patients with advanced hepatic cirrhosis and functional renal failure (the hepatorenal syndrome). Ornipressin raised the glomerular filtration rate (GFR) from 18 to 29 mL/min, lowered the plasma renin activity (PRA) from 28 to 14 (normal equals <3 on a regular salt intake), raised the fraction of the cardiac output from 2% to 5% (normal equals 20%), and raised urinary sodium excretion from 3 to 9 mEq/day. Thus, ornipressin only induced partial correction of these abnormalities; it is not known if a greater response would be seen with less severe disease or with a higher dose.

pitting results from movement of the excess interstitial water away from the area in which pressure is being applied.

Peripheral edema can produce symptoms and is cosmetically undesirable. It is not, however, life threatening as is pulmonary edema in severe cases. Patients with pulmonary edema complain of shortness of breath that is more prominent on exertion and when lying flat (called orthopnea). The physical examination typically reveals an ill patient who is breathing more rapidly than usual. The excess alveolar fluid can be detected by the finding of wet rales on auscultation of the chest. Patients with heart failure also may have gallop rhythms and murmurs on examination of the heart.

The third major type of edema—ascites—causes an increased abdominal girth as the major symptom. Patients may also complain of shortness of breath if the intra-abdominal pressure is sufficiently high to cause upward pressure on the diaphragm. Abdominal distension and a visible fluid wave on percussion of the abdomen are the primary physical findings in this setting.

Site of Edema Formation

Each of the major edematous states is associated with increased capillary hydraulic pressure. Where this occurs will determine the site of edema formation. In congestive heart failure and renal disease, there is generalized expansion of the vascular volume with a diffuse elevation in intracapillary pressures. As a result, peripheral edema, ascites, and pulmonary edema all may be seen.

In other conditions, however, there is a preferential rise in venous pressure in one circulation, causing localized edema formation. The major examples are congestive heart failure with isolated left ventricular dysfunction, in which pulmonary edema may be the predominant finding, and hepatic cirrhosis, in which postsinusoidal obstruction causes the excess fluid to be primarily deposited as ascites.

 A patient who has chronically abused alcohol presents with massive ascites. The differential diagnoses include alcohol-induced cardiomyopathy and alcohol-induced hepatic cirrhosis. How could you distinguish between these disorders on physical examination by estimation of the jugular venous pressure, which is roughly equal to that in the right atrium (normal value equals 1 to 7 cm H_2O)?

Diuretics and Treatment of Edema

Diuretics are used in a variety of conditions to lower the plasma volume by increasing the excretion of sodium and water. The three major classes of diuretics—loop diuretics, thiazide-type diuretics, and potassium-sparing diuretics—act by inhibiting sodium reabsorption in different sites in the nephron. Each diuretic reduces sodium movement from the urinary space into the tubular cell across the luminal membrane. They act in different nephron segments because each segment has a different sodium entry mechanism that is specifically inhibited (Table 4.2)—the transporters and channels involved in tubular sodium reabsorption are reviewed in Chapter 1:

- Loop diuretics (such as furosemide and bumetanide) inhibit sodium chloride reabsorption in the thick ascending limb of the loop of Henle by competing for the chloride site on the Na^+–K^+–$2Cl^-$ cotransporter in the luminal membrane.
- Thiazide-type diuretics (such as hydrochlorothiazide and chlorthalidone) inhibit sodium chloride reabsorption in the distal tubule by competing for the chloride site on the Na–Cl cotransporter in the luminal membrane.

TABLE 4.2

Characteristics of Major Classes of Diuretics

	Type	Site of Action and Transporter Inhibited	Percent Filtered Na Excreted
	Loop diuretics	Thick ascending limb of loop of Henle; compete for chloride site on luminal $Na^+–K^+–2Cl^-$ cotransporter	35–40%
	Thiazide-type diuretics	Distal tubule; compete for chloride site on luminal Na–Cl cotransporter	5–8%
	Potassium-sparing diuretics	Collecting tubules; close luminal sodium channels	2–3%

■ Potassium-sparing diuretics (such as amiloride, triamterene, and the aldosterone antagonist spironolactone) inhibit sodium reabsorption in the collecting ducts by affecting the open probability and/or numbers of the epithelial cell apical sodium channel. The normal movement of cationic sodium through these channels makes the lumen electronegative, thereby creating an electrical gradient that promotes the secretion of potassium from the cell into the lumen. Thus, closing the sodium channels with these diuretics indirectly inhibits potassium secretion (hence the name potassium-sparing). This is important clinically, since distal potassium secretion accounts for most of urinary potassium excretion (see Chapter 7).

Diuretic Potency

The ability of a diuretic to increase urinary sodium excretion is dependent upon the interplay of three factors: diuretic dose, the quantity of sodium normally reabsorbed at the diuretic-sensitive site, and the ability of the more distal segments to reabsorb the excess sodium.

Diuretic Dose

Virtually all diuretics act *within the tubular lumen* to impair the sodium entry mechanism. Therefore, these drugs are *dependent* upon glomerular

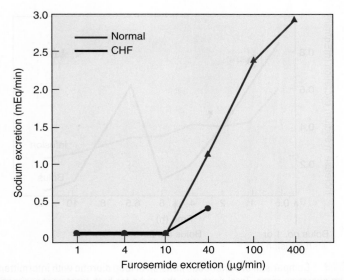

FIGURE 4.7. Relationship between the rate of excretion of furosemide (a loop diuretic) and the associated increase in the rate of urinary sodium excretion in normal subjects and in patients with congestive heart failure (CHF). There is no diuresis below a furosemide excretion rate of 10 μg/min. This is followed by a dose-dependent increase in sodium excretion with a maximum effect occurring when furosemide excretion exceeds 400 μg/min. At the same rate of furosemide excretion, patients with CHF tend to have a lesser diuresis due to increased sodium reabsorption in other nephron segments.

filtration for delivery to the appropriate nephron segment. Not surprisingly, there is a dose–response curve in which the increment in sodium excretion is related to the rate of diuretic excretion (i.e., the rate of diuretic presentation to its tubular site of action); this curve has three components (Fig. 4.7). At low doses, there is an insufficient rate of diuretic excretion to significantly impair sodium reabsorption. Once a threshold rate of diuretic excretion is reached, there is a direct relationship between increased availability of the diuretic and the degree to which sodium reabsorption is inhibited. Finally, there is also a maximum rate of diuretic excretion at which the diuretic-sensitive transporter is completely inhibited. Exceeding this dose will produce no further diuresis but may increase the incidence of drug-induced side effects. Diuretics can also be administered as a continuous infusion to provide more sustained inhibition of the diuretic-sensitive transporter (Fig. 4.8).

Quantity of Sodium Reabsorbed at Diuretic-Sensitive Site

Over 99% of the filtered sodium undergoes tubular reabsorption in normal subjects. Approximately 55% to 60% occurs in the proximal tubule, 30% to 35% in the loop of Henle, 5% in the distal tubule, and 4% in the

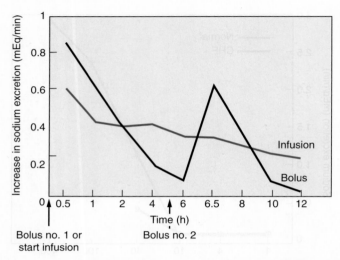

FIGURE 4.8.   Comparison of continuous infusion of loop diuretic with intermittent bolus on sodium excretion rates. Total dose was the same for both treatment regimens. Total sodium excretion was 30% higher with the continuous infusion, but the naturetic effect declined over time with both regimens.

collecting ducts. Thus, a loop diuretic is more potent than a thiazide or potassium-sparing diuretic because more sodium is normally reabsorbed at that site.

Increased Reabsorption in Other Nephron Segments

A variable proportion of the increased sodium delivered out of the diuretic-sensitive segment can be reabsorbed in the more distal segments. Let us consider what happens following the administration of a loop diuretic. The extra sodium leaving the loop first enters the distal tubule. Transport in this segment is flow dependent; thus, increasing sodium delivery to the distal tubule results in increased sodium reabsorption, thereby limiting the diuresis. There is also some flow dependence in the collecting ducts, further decreasing the net rise in sodium excretion.

These responses increase over time. In the patient with congestive heart failure, for example, fluid loss decreases cardiac-filling pressures and eventually lowers the cardiac output (as in going from point C to point B on the *middle curve* in Fig. 4.5). This decline in tissue perfusion leads to increased activation of the renin–angiotensin–aldosterone and sympathetic nervous systems, resulting in increased sodium reabsorption in the proximal tubule (due to angiotensin II and norepinephrine) and the collecting ducts (due to aldosterone). In addition, the chronic increase in sodium delivery to, and transport in, the distal

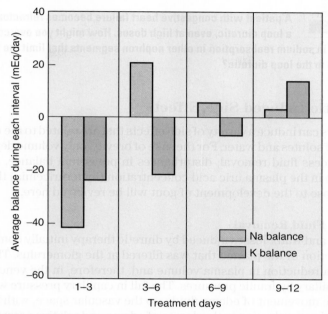

FIGURE 4.9. Reestablishment of the steady state after the administration of a high dose of a thiazide diuretic to normal subjects. There is a negative balance (*bars* going downward below the zero point) of sodium for 3 days and of potassium for 6 to 9 days before intake and output come back into balance due to activation of counterregulatory forces.

tubule induces a hypertrophic response that enhances distal reabsorptive capacity.

The net effect of all of these counterregulatory responses, assuming the diuretic dose is constant, is the reestablishment of a steady state in which sodium intake and output are equal. (This process is discussed in detail in Chapter 2.) Although the pronatriuretic action of the diuretic leads to initial sodium loss, this is gradually counteracted by the above antinatriuretic factors. In general, all of the sodium loss occurs within the first week of diuretic therapy unless the dose is then increased (Fig. 4.9).

These observations are very important clinically, since they mean that all of the clinical improvements and risk of fluid and electrolyte complications associated with a given dose of a diuretic will occur within the first 2 to 3 weeks. Once the patient is beyond this point, repeat measurement of blood tests at every visit to detect the possible presence of worsening renal function (due to excessive fluid loss) or potassium depletion is not necessary unless there has been some change in the patient's condition (such as worsening heart disease or superimposed gastrointestinal losses due to vomiting or diarrhea).

A patient with congestive heart failure becomes refractory to a loop diuretic, even at high doses. How might you overcome the increase in sodium reabsorption in other nephron segments that limit the net response to the loop diuretic?

Diuretic-Induced Side Effects

Diuretics can induce a variety of side effects that are related to the urinary losses of solutes and water. For the sake of brevity, only volume depletion from excess fluid removal, disturbances in potassium balance, and an increase in the plasma uric acid concentration (hyperuricemia) that can predispose to the development of gout will be reviewed here.

Excess Fluid Removal

The salt and water losses induced by diuretic therapy initially come from that fraction of the plasma that was filtered at the glomerulus. This will lead to a reduction in plasma volume and, therefore, in the venous and intracapillary hydraulic pressures. The fall in capillary pressure will promote the movement of edema fluid into the vascular space, with the net effect being a reduction in the degree of edema and relative preservation of the plasma volume. If, however, too much fluid is removed, the plasma volume and eventually the cardiac output and tissue perfusion will fall. Although cerebral, coronary, splanchnic, or musculoskeletal perfusion or the total cardiac output cannot be easily measured in ambulatory patients, renal perfusion can be estimated by following the BUN and plasma creatinine concentration. If these values are stable as an edematous patient is diuresed, a clinically significant reduction in tissue perfusion has not occurred. On the other hand, an otherwise unexplained elevation in these parameters is an indication to withhold further diuretic therapy.

Decreased tissue perfusion can occur even in patients who remain markedly edematous. How this occurs can be appreciated by returning to the Frank–Starling relationship in Figure 4.5. Fluid loss with diuretic therapy will move the patient from point C down toward point B. The reduction in stroke volume and cardiac output resulting from the fall in cardiac stretch may lower renal perfusion and raise the BUN and creatinine concentrations even though the filling pressures remain high enough for edema to persist.

Rate of Fluid Removal. A somewhat related issue is the rate at which edema fluid can be safely removed without inducing clinically significant plasma volume depletion. The answer to this question varies with the underlying disorder. With sodium retention in congestive heart failure or renal failure, the associated plasma volume expansion raises the filling pressures in *all* peripheral capillaries as evidenced on physical examination by an elevation in jugular venous pressure (which reflects the pressure in the right atrium). As a result, edema fluid can be mobilized from all of these capillaries as the venous and intracapillary pressure fall following fluid loss. The net effect is that there is little or no rate limitation to fluid removal in these settings. Patients with advanced congestive heart failure and marked edema can lose 5 kg overnight without developing signs of decreased tissue perfusion.

Hepatic cirrhosis with ascites represents an important exception to this rule. In this disorder, the primary defect is postsinusoidal obstruction leading to an isolated elevation in hepatic sinusoidal pressure. Thus, ascites formation occurs across the sinusoids and ascites mobilization following diuretic therapy can only occur via the peritoneal capillaries. (The hepatic capsule prevents mobilization back into the hepatic sinusoids.)

Fluid movement into the peritoneal capillaries is a rate-limited process with a maximum of 500 to 900 mL/day. Thus, the rate of fluid loss should not exceed 500 mL/day in patients with hepatic cirrhosis and ascites unless there is also peripheral edema that can be mobilized. As shown in Figure 4.10, more rapid fluid loss can lead to plasma volume depletion and a rise in the BUN in patients without peripheral edema.

 Ascites can also be removed by paracentesis in which a needle or catheter is inserted into the peritoneal space. What initial effect would this method of fluid removal have on the plasma volume? By what mechanism might paracentesis lower the plasma volume?

Potassium Balance

Urinary potassium excretion is primarily derived from the secretion of potassium from the cortical collecting duct cell into the lumen; in comparison, most of the filtered potassium is reabsorbed in the proximal tubule and loop of Henle (see Chapter 7). Distal potassium secretion is primarily dependent upon two factors: aldosterone, which increases the number of open sodium and potassium channels in the luminal membrane, and the distal delivery of sodium and water. The loop and thiazide-type diuretics affect both of these processes: Distal delivery is increased, since less sodium and water are reabsorbed in the loop of Henle and distal tubule, respectively, and fluid losses lead to activation of the renin–angiotensin–aldosterone system. Thus, potassium excretion tends to increase and hypokalemia (a fall in the plasma potassium concentration) is a not uncommon complication.

The findings are different with the potassium-sparing diuretics, which act *at the potassium secretory site* rather than proximal to it.

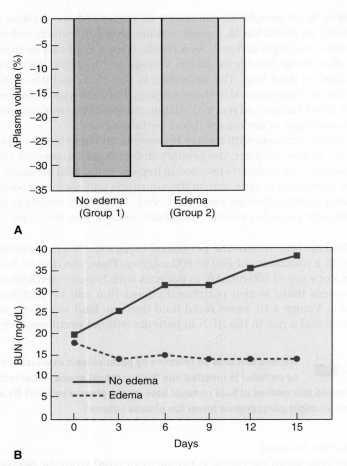

FIGURE 4.10. Effect of fluid removal by diuresis at a rate of 1 to 1.5 L/day in patients with hepatic cirrhosis and ascites (Group 1 with peripheral edema or Group 2 without peripheral edema). Substantial plasma volume reductions were achieved in both groups (**A**), but plasma volume depletion as determined by elevated BUN concentrations only occurred in the relatively rapidly diuresed patients with no edema (**B**).

The decrease in sodium reabsorption induced by these agents makes the lumen less electronegative (since less cationic sodium is removed), thereby diminishing the electrical gradient favoring the passive entry of cellular potassium into the lumen. The net effect is an initial fall in potassium excretion and an elevation in the plasma potassium concentration. In the clinical setting, the potassium-sparing diuretics are most often used to minimize potassium losses induced by the loop or thiazide-type diuretics.

Hyperuricemia

Uric acid handling in the kidney involves four steps: filtration across the glomerulus, reabsorption of almost all of the filtered uric acid in the early parts of the proximal tubule, secretion of uric acid back into the lumen in the later proximal tubule, and a variable degree of postsecretory reabsorption in the late proximal tubule. The mechanism by which these processes occur is incompletely understood, but uric acid reabsorption appears to be indirectly linked to that of sodium.

Diuretics affect this process by reducing tissue perfusion. The ensuing elevations in angiotensin II and norepinephrine production increase proximal sodium and water reabsorption, thereby increasing net uric acid reabsorption. As a result, there is an initial reduction in uric acid excretion and an elevation in the plasma uric acid concentration. This side effect can be induced by any of the diuretics.

CASE DISCUSSION The patient presented at the beginning of the chapter has generalized edema that could be due to one of the three major causes of edema: congestive heart failure, hepatic cirrhosis or renal disease. Heart failure and renal failure are excluded by the normal jugular venous pressure and the normal BUN and plasma creatinine concentration, respectively. The acute onset and lack of ascites as a major site of edema formation or other findings of chronic liver disease rule out hepatic cirrhosis. The presence of the nephrotic syndrome is evidenced by the heavy proteinuria and hypoalbuminemia.

ANSWERS TO QUESTIONS

1 To generate an osmotic pressure, solutes must be unable to cross the separating membrane. Sodium salts are freely permeable across the capillary wall and therefore are considered ineffective osmoles at this site (see Chapter 2; Fig. 2.2). Protein movement, on the other hand, is largely restricted by the size- and charge-selective properties of the capillary wall.

2 Three safety factors protect against the development of edema. Most important is increased lymphatic flow that can initially remove the excess filtrate. Fluid entry into the interstitium also will raise the interstitial hydraulic pressure and lower the interstitial oncotic pressure, both of which will retard further movement of fluid out of the vascular space. The fall in interstitial oncotic pressure occurs by dilution and by lymphatic-mediated removal of interstitial proteins.

3 Volume expansion in acute glomerulonephritis leads to suppression of the release of renin and increased secretion of atrial natriuretic peptide.

In comparison, the low cardiac output in congestive heart failure is associated with activation of the renin–angiotensin system. However, atrial natriuretic peptide levels will also be increased, since intracardiac filling pressures are increased due to the cardiac disease.

4 Decreasing the plasma volume with diuretic therapy will relieve pulmonary congestion by lowering the intracardiac filling pressures. This fall in LVEDP often lowers the stroke volume and therefore the cardiac output. In most cases, the fall in cardiac output is not clinically significant and the patient is substantially improved. Given the difficulty in routine measurement of the cardiac output or cerebral, coronary, splanchnic, or musculocutaneous blood flow, the simplest way to monitor the adequacy of tissue perfusion is by following the BUN and plasma creatinine concentration. An otherwise unexplained elevation in these parameters suggests a significant reduction in blood flow to the kidneys and presumably to other organs as well. On the other hand, a stable ratio suggests that tissue perfusion is being maintained as the edema fluid is being removed.

5 The hepatic sinusoid is freely permeable to albumin. As a result, the plasma and hepatic interstitial oncotic pressures are essentially equal and do not play an important role in the regulation of fluid movement across the sinusoid.

6 Edema in congestive heart failure is due to increased venous pressure resulting from sodium retention and plasma volume expansion. Because of the cardiac disease, intracardiac filling pressures are increased (as in Fig. 4.5) and the jugular venous pressure should be elevated. In comparison, the postsinusoidal obstruction in hepatic cirrhosis results in the deposition of much of the excess fluid in the peritoneum. As a result, the jugular venous pressure is usually normal or low normal.

7 One way to treat resistant edema is to block sodium transport at several sites within the nephron. Thus, the addition of a thiazide-type diuretic to a loop diuretic often produces a good diuretic response. Addition of a potassium-sparing diuretic also might be helpful in this setting by modestly enhancing the natriuresis while minimizing the amount of potassium lost.

8 In contrast to diuretic therapy, which removes fluid initially from the plasma, paracentesis has no direct effect on the plasma volume since the ascitic fluid is in an extravascular space. However, recurrent ascites formation, which is promoted by the associated reduction in intraperitoneal pressure, can lead to a late reduction in plasma volume. Many physicians are now using paracentesis rather than diuretics as a rapid and safe therapy in patients with marked ascites.

SUGGESTED READINGS

Brater DC. Diuretic therapy. N Engl J Med 1998;339:387.

Ellison DG. The physiologic basis of diuretic synergism: its role in treating diuretic resistance. Ann Intern Med 1991;114:886.

Fernandez-Seara J, Prieto J, Quiroga J, et al. Systemic and renal hemodynamics in patients with liver cirrhosis and ascites with and without functional renal failure. Gastroenterology 1989;97:1304.

Gines P, Guevara M, Arroyo V, et al. Hepatorenal syndrome. Lancet 2003;362:1819.

Ichikawa I, Rennke HG, Hoyer JR, et al. Role for intrarenal mechanisms in the impaired salt excretion of experimental nephrotic syndrome. J Clin Invest 1983;71:91.

Martin-Llahi M, Pepin MN, Guevara M, et al. Terlipressin and albumin vs. albumin in patients with cirrhosis and hepatorenal syndrome: a randomized study. Gastroenterology 2008;134(5):1352–1359.

Pockros PJ, Reynolds TB. Rapid diuresis in patients with ascites from chronic liver disease: the importance of peripheral edema. Gastroenterology 1986;90:1827.

Sherlock S. The kidneys in hepatic cirrhosis: victims of portal-systemic venous shunting (portal-systemic nephropathy). Gastroenterology 1993;104:931.

Valentin JP, Diu C, Muldowney WP, et al. Cellular basis for blunted volume expansion natriuresis in experimental nephrotic syndrome. J Clin Invest 1992;90:1302.

5

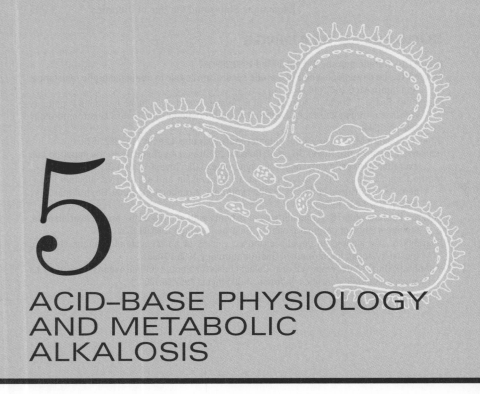

ACID–BASE PHYSIOLOGY AND METABOLIC ALKALOSIS

CASE PRESENTATION

A 32-year-old woman develops severe vomiting due to viral gastroenteritis. This problem persists for 2 days, with the patient able to eat only small amounts of hot soup. Physical examination in the doctor's office reveals a blood pressure of 110/70 supine and 95/60 erect, the estimated jugular venous pressure is below 5 cm H_2O, and skin turgor is moderately reduced. The patient's weight is 2.1 kg below her previous baseline.

Initial blood and urine tests reveal the following:

BUN	= 31 mg/dL (9–25)
Creatinine	= 1.2 mg/dL (0.8–1.4)
Na	= 141 mEq/L (136–142)
K	= 3.2 mEq/L (3.5–5)
Cl	= 90 mEq/L (98–108)
Total CO_2	= 36 mEq/L (21–30)
Arterial pH	= 7.50 (7.37–7.43)
PCO_2	= 48 mm Hg (36–44)
Urine Na	= 10 mEq/L (variable)
Urine pH	= 5.0 (variable)

OBJECTIVES

By the end of this section, you should have an understanding of each of the following issues:

- The basic principles of acid–base physiology, including the role of the bicarbonate–carbon dioxide buffer system.
- How the kidney maintains acid–base homeostasis by adjusting the rate of net acid excretion to equal the daily acid load.
- The characteristics of the different acid–base disorders and the compensatory responses they initiate.
- The factors responsible for the generation and continuation of metabolic alkalosis.
- The mechanisms by which metabolic alkalosis can be corrected by promoting the urinary excretion of the excess bicarbonate.

Introduction

As with other components of extracellular fluid, the hydrogen concentration is maintained within narrow limits. However, this process must be extremely sensitive, since the normal extracellular hydrogen concentration is 40 nEq/L, roughly one-millionth the milliequivalent per liter concentrations of sodium, potassium, and chloride.

The maintenance of this extremely low hydrogen concentration is essential for normal cell function. Hydrogen ions are highly reactive, particularly with negatively charged portions of protein molecules. Thus, proteins gain or lose hydrogen ions when there is a change in the hydrogen concentration, leading to alterations in protein function.

These effects of hydrogen are determined by the intracellular hydrogen concentration. Although this parameter cannot be measured clinically, it varies in parallel with (although it is not identical to) the concentration of hydrogen in the extracellular fluid. Thus, the state of acid–base balance can usually be estimated from the plasma (usually arterial) hydrogen concentration or pH (which is equal to $-\log [H^+]$).

Acids and Bases

An understanding of acid–base balance begins with the following definitions. An acid is a substance that can donate hydrogen ions and a base is a substance that can accept hydrogen ions. These properties are independent of charge. Thus, H_2CO_3 (carbonic acid), HCl (hydrochloric acid), NH_4^+ (ammonium), and $H_2PO_4^-$ (dibasic phosphate) all can act as acids:

$$
\begin{array}{lcl}
H_2CO_3 & \leftrightarrow & H^+ \quad + \quad HCO_3^- \\
HCl & \leftrightarrow & H^+ \quad + \quad Cl^- \\
NH_4^+ & \leftrightarrow & H^+ \quad + \quad NH_3 \\
H_2PO_4^- & \leftrightarrow & H^+ \quad + \quad HPO_4^{2-} \\
\textit{Acid} & & \textit{Base}
\end{array}
$$

There are two classes of acids that are physiologically important: carbonic acid and noncarbonic acids. Each day, the metabolism of carbohydrates and fats results in the generation of approximately 15,000 mmol of CO_2. Although CO_2 is not an acid, it combines with H_2O to form H_2CO_3. Thus, there would be a progressive accumulation of acid if the endogenously produced CO_2 were not excreted. This is prevented by the loss of CO_2 via alveolar ventilation.

On the other hand, noncarbonic acids are primarily generated from the metabolism of proteins. In particular, the oxidation of sulfur-containing amino acids results in the formation of H_2SO_4 (sulfuric acid). In comparison to the very high rate of CO_2 production, only about 50 to 100 mEq of noncarbonic acid is produced each day. Elimination of this acid is a two-step process:

■ Initial combination with extracellular bicarbonate and intracellular buffers to minimize the change in the free hydrogen concentration.
■ The subsequent excretion of this acid by the kidney.

Law of Mass Action

Although the concept of buffering should be familiar to the reader, it is useful to review the law of mass action and the derivation of the Henderson–Hasselbalch equation. The law of mass actions states that the velocity of a reaction is proportional to the concentration of the reactants. Thus, for the reaction,

$$HPO_4^{2-} + H^+ \leftrightarrow H_2PO_4^-$$

the velocity with which the reaction moves to the right is equal to

$$v_1 = k_1[HPO_4^{2-}][H^+]$$

where k_1 is the rate constant for the reaction. Similarly, the velocity with which the reaction moves to the left is equal to

$$v_2 = k_2[H_2PO_4^-]$$

At equilibrium, v_1 equals v_2. As a result,

$$k_1[HPO_4^{2-}][H^+] = k_2[H_2PO_4^-]$$

Solving for k_2:

$$k_2 = k_1[HPO_4^{2-}][H^+] \div [H_2PO_4^-]$$

If the two rate constants are combined into one, K_a, which is the apparent ionization of dissociation constant for this acid,

$$K_a = k_2 \div k_1$$

$$= ([HPO_4^{2-}][H^+]) \div [H_2PO_4^-]$$

or

$$[H^+] = K_a[H_2PO_4^-] \div [HPO_4^{2-}] \qquad \text{(Eq. 1)}$$

If the negative logarithm of each side is taken, then

$$-log[H^+] = -log\,K_a - log([H_2PO_4^-] \div [HPO_4^{2-}])$$

If $-log\,[H^+]$ is called the pH, $-log\,K_a$ is defined as the pK_a, and $-log\,[a/b]$ is converted to $+log\,[b/a]$, then Eq. 1 becomes the Henderson–Hasselbalch equation:

$$pH = pK_a + log([HPO_4^{2-}] \div [H_2PO_4^-]) \qquad \text{(Eq. 2)}$$

This equation can be written more generally for any weak acid as

$$pH = pK_a + log([base] \div [acid]) \qquad \text{(Eq. 3)}$$

Thus, knowing the base-to-acid ratio for any weak acid in a solution such as the extracellular fluid is sufficient to estimate the pH in that solution.

HPO_4^{2-} is able to act as a buffer in the physiologic pH range because it is able to take up extra hydrogen ions, thereby minimizing the elevation in the free hydrogen concentration or the reduction in pH.

Bicarbonate–Carbon Dioxide System

As will be described below, HPO_4^{2-} is one of the major urinary buffers and plays an important role in net acid excretion. In comparison, the state of systemic acid–base balance is estimated clinically by use of the bicarbonate–carbon dioxide buffering system. This buffer system can be described by the following reactions:

$$CO_2 \underset{\text{gas phase}}{\leftrightarrow} CO_2 + H_2O \xrightarrow[\text{aqueous phase}]{} H_2CO_3 \leftrightarrow H^+ + HCO_3^- \qquad \text{(Eq. 4)}$$

The pK_a for carbonic acid is 3.8, so at normal pH, the H_2CO_3 concentration is 340 times less than the concentration of dissolved CO_2 in the aqueous phase and 6800 times less than the HCO_3^- concentration. As a result, H_2CO_3 can be ignored and Eq. 4 simplifies to

$$CO_2 + H_2O \leftrightarrow H^+ + HCO_3^- \qquad \text{(Eq. 5)}$$

TABLE 5.1

Normal Acid–Base Values				
	pH	[H+] (nEq/L)	PCO$_2$(mm Hg)	[HCO$_3^-$] (mEq/L)
Arterial	7.37–7.43	37–43	36–44	22–26
Venous	7.32–7.38	42–48	42–50	23–27

The Henderson–Hasselbalch equation for this system can be expressed by the following equation:

$$pH = 6.10 + log\left([HCO_3^-] \div [0.03 \times PCO_2]\right) \qquad \text{(Eq. 6)}$$

where 6.10 is the pK_a for this equation and 0.03 times the partial pressure of carbon dioxide is equal to the concentration of dissolved carbon dioxide. The normal range of values for these parameters is listed in Table 5.1.

The lower pH (and higher hydrogen concentration) in venous blood is due to the addition of metabolically produced carbon dioxide in the capillary circulation. The range of pH that is compatible with survival is between 7.80 and 6.80 (equivalent to a range of hydrogen concentrations between 16 and 160 nEq/L).

Most hospital laboratories measure the total CO_2 concentration in the plasma rather than the bicarbonate concentration. This test is performed by adding a strong acid to a blood sample and measuring via a colorimetric reaction the quantity of CO_2 generated. Most of the CO_2 will be generated from the combination of the added acid with bicarbonate to form carbonic acid; however, the dissolved CO_2 ($0.03 \times PCO_2$) will also be measured. As a result, the total CO_2 concentration normally exceeds the bicarbonate concentration by 1 to 1.5 mEq/L.

Acidosis and Alkalosis

The extracellular pH is abnormal in a variety of clinical conditions. A reduction in pH (or elevation in the hydrogen concentration) is called *acidemia*; an elevation in pH (or reduction in hydrogen concentration) is called *alkalemia*. Processes that tend to lower or raise the pH are called *acidosis* and *alkalosis*, respectively.

In general, acidosis causes acidemia and alkalosis causes alkalemia. However, exceptions can occur when there is a mixed acid–base disturbance in which more than one abnormality is present. From Eq. 6, pH of the bicarbonate–carbon dioxide system is determined by the ratio of base (bicarbonate concentration) to acid (PCO_2). Therefore, acidosis can be induced either by a reduction in the plasma bicarbonate concentration or an elevation in the PCO_2. The former is called metabolic acidosis and, since the PCO_2 is regulation by ventilation, the latter is called respiratory acidosis. In contrast, alkalosis can be induced either by a rise in the plasma bicarbonate concentration (metabolic alkalosis) or a decline in the PCO_2 (respiratory alkalosis).

Response to the Daily Acid Load

Acid can be generated from a variety of sources, most of which come from the metabolism of sulfur-containing amino acids (such as methionine and cystine) or cationic amino acids (such as arginine or lysine).

$$Methionine \rightarrow glucose + urea + SO_4^{2-} + 2H^+$$

$$Arginine \rightarrow glucose\,(or\,CO_2) + urea + H^+$$

On the other hand, hydrogen ions are consumed by the metabolism of anionic amino acids (such as glutamate and aspartate) and by the oxidation or utilization of organic anions (such as citrate and lactate).

$$Lactate^- + H^+ \rightarrow glucose + CO_2$$

A normal Western diet results in the net production of 50 to 100 mEq of hydrogen per day in adults. The homeostatic response to this acid load involves two steps: buffering and renal excretion.

Buffering

Survival of the organism is dependent upon the body buffers. It is essential to remember that the normal hydrogen concentration is 40 nEq/L. If, for example, 80 mEq of acid were freely distributed through the total body water (approximately 40 L in an average adult man), then the body water hydrogen concentration would rise by 2 mEq/L, almost one million times normal. The pH in this setting would be below 3.0, a level that would not be compatible with life.

Fortunately, this marked acidemia does not occur because the rise in free hydrogen concentration is limited by the combination of hydrogen ions with bicarbonate in the extracellular fluid, HPO_4^{2-} and protein anions in the cells, and carbonate (CO_3^{2-}) in bone.

If, for example, 2 mEq/L of hydrogen were added to the extracellular fluid, the buffering reaction for the bicarbonate–carbon dioxide system would be driven to the left:

$$CO_2 + H_2O \leftarrow H^+ + HCO_3^-$$

Almost all of the excess hydrogen ions would be buffered by bicarbonate, lowering the plasma bicarbonate concentration from the normal value of 24 mEq/L down to 22 mEq/L. Each milliequivalent of bicarbonate that is buffered also generates 1 mmol of carbon dioxide. Thus, the dissolved CO_2 concentration would rise from 1.2 mmol/L (0.03×40) to 3.2 mmol/L, which is equivalent to a PCO_2 of 107 mm Hg. From the Henderson–Hasselbalch equation, the new pH would be 6.93, rather than the normal value of 7.40:

$$pH = 6.10 + log(22 \div [0.03 \times 107]) = 6.93$$

This is much better than a pH below 3.0 if there were no buffering, but it is still a marked change clinically. The relative inefficiency of this system occurs because the pK_a is 6.10, more than 1.0 pH units (the range in which a buffer is most effective) from the extracellular pH of 7.40.

However, bicarbonate does act as a very effective buffer in the body because the PCO_2 can be controlled independently via respiration. If, for example, ventilation were stimulated so that the PCO_2 remained constant at 40 mm Hg, then

$$pH = 6.10 + log(22 \div [0.03 \times 40]) = 7.36$$

However, the system is even more efficient because even mild degrees of acidemia stimulate ventilation to better protect the pH by reducing the PCO_2 below normal. A 2-mEq/L fall in the plasma bicarbonate concentration might result in a 2 mm Hg reduction in the PCO_2 to 38 mm Hg. In this setting, the pH would be essentially normal:

$$pH = 6.10 + log(22 \div [0.03 \times 38]) = 7.385$$

This example highlights a central theme in compensation for acid–base disturbances: The presence of a simple (single) acid–base disorder will result in compensation that corrects the pH toward 7.40 but not equal to 7.40. Therefore, measuring a pH of 7.40 in the setting of an acid–base abnormality implies that at least two processes are occurring.

Renal Acid Excretion

Despite the efficacy of extracellular and intracellular buffering, the body buffers (such as extracellular bicarbonate) would eventually become depleted if the dietary acid load were not eventually excreted in the urine. The following major steps are involved in this process in which 50 to 100 mEq of hydrogen ions must be excreted per day:

- Hydrogen excretion occurs by hydrogen secretion by the tubular cells in the proximal tubule, loop of Henle, and collecting ducts.
- The minimum urine pH that can be achieved is 4.5. Although this is 1000 times (three log units) more acidic than the plasma, the free hydrogen ion concentration in the urine is still only 40 μmol/L. Thus, 2500 L of urine would be required to excrete 100 mEq of hydrogen. This is not

possible physiologically, so hydrogen ions must be buffered in the tubular lumen, a process that primarily involves HPO_4^{2-} and ammonium (NH_4^+).

■ At a glomerular filtration rate of 180 L/day and a plasma bicarbonate concentration of 24 mEq/L, 4320 mEq of bicarbonate is filtered each day. From Eq. 5, each milliequivalent of bicarbonate lost leaves behind a free hydrogen ion. Thus, essentially *all of the filtered bicarbonate must be reabsorbed before the quantitatively much smaller daily acid load can be excreted.*

Cell Model for Proximal Bicarbonate Reabsorption and Hydrogen Secretion

A cell model for bicarbonate reabsorption and hydrogen secretion in the proximal tubule is depicted in Figure 5.1. Ions cannot freely move across the lipid bilayer of the cell membrane. As a result, transmembrane transport requires the presence of carriers or channels that span the membrane.

Hydrogen is secreted into the tubular fluid via the Na^+/H^+ exchanger at the apical membrane of the tubular cells. The energy for this process is indirectly provided by the $Na^+–K^+$-ATPase pump in the basolateral membrane; this pump maintains the cell sodium concentration at a low level and creates a cell-interior negative electrical potential (see Chapter 1). As a result, there is a highly favorable gradient for passive sodium entry into the cell at the apical membrane; this gradient is sufficient to drive hydrogen secretion. The combination of hydrogen with filtered bicarbonate generates carbonic acid (H_2CO_3). Under the influence of carbonic anhydrase located in the brush border of the apical membrane, carbonic acid rapidly dissociates into CO_2 and water. The water is rapidly reabsorbed through apical water channels (aquaporin-1) and the CO_2 diffuses across the plasma membrane. Intracellular carbonic anhydrase then catalyzes the reformation of carbonic acid that then dissociates into hydrogen and bicarbonate. This bicarbonate leaves the cell via a $Na^+–3HCO_3^-$ cotransporter in the basolateral membrane; the energy for this net movement of negative charge is provided by the cell-interior negative potential. This process removes bicarbonate from the lumen. However, the bicarbonate ion that is returned to the systemic circulation is the bicarbonate that was generated within the cell when hydrogen was secreted (Fig. 5.1). *The result is reabsorption of the filtered bicarbonate, but there is no net acid secretion occurring through this mechanism.* The net effect is that roughly 80% to 90% of the filtered bicarbonate is reabsorbed in the proximal tubule, with the tubular fluid pH falling from 7.40 in the filtrate to about 6.70 at the end of proximal tubule. Another 15% of bicarbonate is reabsorbed in the thick ascending limb of the loop of Henle using mechanisms similar to the proximal tubule (via carbonic anhydrase). The final site for bicarbonate reabsorption and hydrogen secretion is the distal

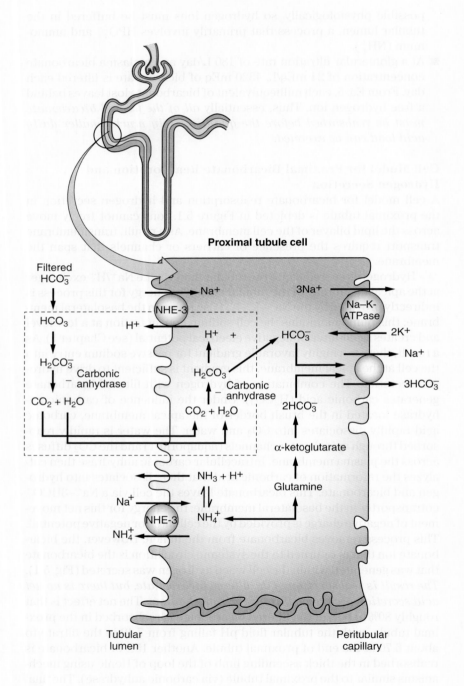

nephron through intercalated cells (Fig. 5.2). The excretion of hydrogen ion generates an equivalent amount of bicarbonate reabsorption through the basolateral anion exchanger AE1. These cells play no role in sodium reabsorption, which occurs in the adjacent principal cells in the cortical collecting duct (the model for which is depicted in Fig. 1.4) and in the inner medullary collecting duct.

Titratable Acidity. Bicarbonate reabsorption reclaims filtered bicarbonate but does not participate in the excretion of the dietary acid load. The latter process requires the combination of secreted hydrogen ions with buffers or the formation of ammonium (NH_4^+). Weak acids filtered at the glomerulus can act as buffers in the urine; their ability to do so is related both to the quantity of buffer present and to its pK_a. Monobasic phosphate (HPO_4^{2-}) is the most prevalent effective buffer in the tubular fluid. The pK_a is 6.80 for the phosphate buffering reaction:

$$HPO_4^{2-} + H^+ \leftrightarrow H_2PO_4^-$$

As a result, almost all of the filtered HPO_4^{2-} will be converted to $H_2PO_4^-$ as the tubular fluid pH falls below 5.8 (1.0 pH unit from the pK_a). Although there is some buffering via this mechanism in the proximal tubule, the majority of HPO_4^{2-} buffering occurs more distally as urine pH falls (Fig. 5.2).

Note that each secreted hydrogen ion that combines with a titratable acid leaves a bicarbonate ion within the cell (Fig. 5.2). This bicarbonate is returned to the systemic circulation (via the chloride–bicarbonate exchanger in the basolateral membrane) to replace a bicarbonate ion initially consumed by buffering of the dietary acid load. The energy for this process is derived from the favorable inward gradient for chloride, which has a high concentration in the extracellular fluid and a low concentration in the cells.

FIGURE 5.1. Major steps involved in acid secretion in the proximal tubule. Within *dotted line box* is the hydrogen and bicarbonate cycle between the cell and the tubular lumen. Hydrogen secretion from the cell into the tubular lumen primarily occurs via a Na^+–H^+ exchanger (which can also function as a Na^+–NH_4^+ exchanger) in the apical membrane. The hydrogen ions combine with filtered HCO_3^- to form carbonic acid. Luminal carbonic anhydrase (CA) catalyzes conversion of H_2CO_3 to CO_2 and H_2O that are reabsorbed through the apical membrane. Intracellular CA generates carbonic acid that dissociates into hydrogen and bicarbonate. Each hydrogen ion secreted generates a bicarbonate ion within the cell that is returned to the peritubular capillary by the Na^+–$3HCO_3^-$ cotransporter in the basolateral membrane. This transporter also serves as the mechanism by which changes in the plasma bicarbonate concentration are sensed by the cells. Ammonium is generated from metabolism of glutamine that can be secreted as NH_4^+, or NH_3 can diffuse into tubular lumen where it can be protonated in the distal nephron (Fig. 5.2).

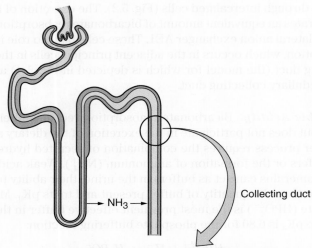

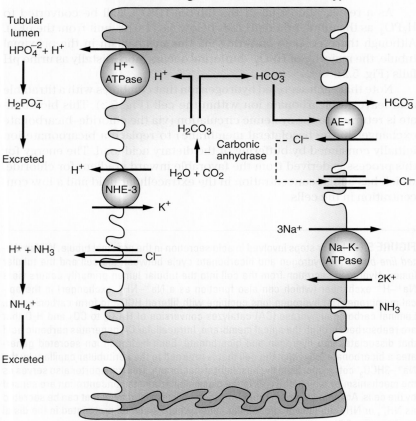

Cortical collecting duct—intercalated cell type A

Tubular lumen

$HPO_4^{-2} + H^+$

$\downarrow$

$H_2PO_4^-$

$\downarrow$

Excreted

H^+ - ATPase

H^+ HCO_3^-

H_2CO_3

HCO_3^-

AE-1

Carbonic anhydrase

Cl^-

H^+ $H_2O + CO_2$

NHE-3

Cl^-

K^+

Cl^-

$H^+ + NH_3$

Cl^-

$3Na^+$

Na–K-ATPase

$2K^+$

NH_3

NH_4^+

$\downarrow$

Excreted

Buffering by phosphate and, to a lesser degree, other buffers such as urate and creatinine is called titratable acidity because of the manner in which it is measured. Total buffering by these weak acids is equal to the quantity of a base, such as sodium hydroxide, that must be added to the urine to raise the pH back to 7.40, the value present in the filtrate.

Titratable acidity normally accounts for the excretion of 10 to 40 mEq of hydrogen per day. However, titratable acidity cannot be easily increased in the presence of an acid load, since this process is limited by the quantity of potential buffer (particularly phosphate) excreted in the urine. One important exception occurs in diabetic ketoacidosis where large quantities of β-hydroxybutyrate are excreted in the urine. In this setting, titratable acid excretion can be augmented by more than 50 mEq/day. Although the pK_a for β-hydroxybutyrate is approximately 4.80, it can act as an effective buffer in the distal nephron where the tubular fluid pH can fall to 5.0 in patients with ketoacidosis.

Ammonium Excretion. Ammonium excretion constitutes the major adaptive response to an acid load, because the rate of ammonium production can be varied according to physiologic needs. The normal rate of ammonium excretion is from 30 to 40 mEq/day, but can increase to over 300 mEq/day after a maximum acid load. This is in marked contrast to the limited ability to enhance titratable acid excretion.

Most of the urinary ammonium is formed in the proximal tubule by a process illustrated in Figure 5.1. Ammonium is generated within the cell, primarily from the metabolism of the amino acid glutamine to glutamate and then to α-ketoglutarate:

$$Glutamine \rightarrow NH_4^+ + glutamate \rightarrow NH_4^+ + \alpha\text{-}ketoglutarate^{2-}$$

Further metabolism of α-ketoglutarate generates two bicarbonate ions that are then returned to the systemic circulation, thereby regenerating the bicarbonate lost during the initial buffering of dietary acid.

Ammonium can accumulate in the urine via one of two mechanisms. In the proximal tubule, ammonium may leave the cell directly, by

---

FIGURE 5.2.   Model of hydrogen secretion in the distal nephron, which mostly occurs in the intercalated type A cells in the cortical collecting duct and in the cells in the outer medullary collecting duct. Hydrogen secretion primarily occurs via an active H^+-ATPase pump in the apical membrane and each milliequivalent of hydrogen secreted generates an equivalent amount of bicarbonate that is reabsorbed through the basolateral anion exchanger, AE1. A proton ATPase (H^+–K^+-ATPase, NHE3) is also present, but may play a greater role in potassium reabsorption during potassium depletion than in acid–base balance (see Chapter 7). Secreted hydrogen combines with ammonia (secreted from the peritubular interstitium into the lumen) to form ammonium that is trapped in the tubular lumen. Secreted hydrogen is also buffered by filtered HPO_4^{-2} to form $H_2PO_4^-$. Note that the intercalated type A cells are not involved in sodium reabsorption.

substituting for hydrogen on the Na^+/H^+ exchanger (Fig. 5.1). In the collecting ducts, on the other hand, lipid-soluble ammonia (NH_3) can passively diffuse into the lumen where it combines with a secreted hydrogen ion to form ammonium (Fig. 5.2). Cationic ammonium is lipid insoluble and is therefore "trapped" in the lumen, since back-diffusion across the luminal membrane cannot occur.

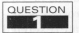 The pK_a for the reaction—$NH_3 + H^+ \leftrightarrow NH_4^+$—is approximately 9.0 in urine. If the urine pH is 5.0 in the collecting ducts, what is the ratio of urinary ammonia to ammonium? How does this promote further ammonium excretion?

Urine pH. Continued hydrogen secretion throughout the nephron results in a gradual reduction in the urine pH, which falls from 7.40 in the filtrate (in normal subjects) to 6.70 at the end of the proximal tubule to as low as 4.5 to 5.0 at the end of the collecting ducts after an acid load. The ability to maintain this 500 to 1000:1 hydrogen gradient between the collecting tubular lumen and the extracellular fluid requires that the apical membrane and tight junctions be highly impermeable to hydrogen ions or ammonium, thereby minimizing the degree of back-diffusion.

 Why must distal hydrogen secretion be mediated by an active H^+-ATPase pump rather than by Na^+–H^+ exchange?

Regulation of Renal Acid Excretion

The preceding section described the mechanisms by which hydrogen ions are secreted. From a clinical viewpoint, however, it is important to understand the factors that determine how much hydrogen is secreted. The extracellular pH normally plays the major role but, when present, effective circulating volume depletion and changes in the plasma potassium concentration can also affect acid secretion, possibly leading to alkalosis or acidosis.

Extracellular pH

Net acid excretion (primarily determined by the sum of titratable acidity and ammonium) varies inversely with the extracellular pH. With acidemia (low pH, high hydrogen concentration), for example, the pH can be returned toward normal by increasing net acid excretion. Each of the major factors involved in acid excretion participate in this response:

■ There is enhanced Na^+–H^+ exchange in the proximal tubule and loop of Henle, thereby raising hydrogen secretion in these segments. Both increased activity of the exchanger and, later, the synthesis of new exchangers are seen.

■ Ammonium production and secretion in the proximal tubule are enhanced due to elevations in both the uptake of glutamine by the tubular cells and the metabolism of glutamine within the cells.

■ H^+-ATPase activity in the collecting ducts increases due to the insertion of preformed cytoplasmic pumps into the apical membrane.

■ Increased activity of the Na:$3HCO_3$ exchanger in the basolateral membrane.

The net effect is more complete buffering by titratable acids, an elevation in ammonium secretion in the proximal tubule, and, due to a fall in urine pH, more efficient trapping of secreted ammonia as ammonium in the collecting ducts. The increase in net acid excretion will result in the return of an equivalent amount of new bicarbonate to the systemic circulation, thereby raising the extracellular pH toward normal.

 Suppose the minimum urine pH were 6.1, rather than 4.5 to 5.0. What effect would this have on titratable acid and ammonium excretion and on the extracellular pH?

A major signal for these physiologically appropriate changes is a parallel, although lesser, reduction in the renal tubular cell pH. It is important to consider how this might occur, since neither hydrogen ions nor bicarbonate ions can freely diffuse across the lipid bilayer of the cell membrane. Studies in experimental animals suggest that the bicarbonate exit step across the basolateral membrane—Na^+–$3HCO_3^-$ cotransport in the proximal tubule and Cl–HCO_3^- exchange in the collecting ducts—also serves as the mechanism by which changes in the plasma bicarbonate concentration are sensed by the cells. If, for example, an increased acid load lowers the plasma bicarbonate concentration, there will now be a greater concentration gradient for bicarbonate to diffuse out of the tubular cells. This loss of intracellular bicarbonate will lower the intracellular pH, providing the signal to increase hydrogen and ammonium secretion.

The mechanism is different if the change in extracellular pH is due to an alteration in the PCO_2 (that is, respiratory acidosis or alkalosis). In this setting, the alteration in intracellular pH is mediated by the diffusion of lipid-soluble CO_2 into or out of the cell.

We can now use this information to consider the renal response to the major acid–base disorders described above. Metabolic alkalosis (an elevation in pH due to a primary rise in the plasma bicarbonate concentration) will not be included here, because it is discussed in more detail later in this chapter.

Metabolic Acidosis. Metabolic acidosis is characterized by a fall in extracellular pH that is induced by a reduction in the plasma bicarbonate concentration, decreased renal acid excretion, bicarbonate loss in the gastrointestinal tract or the urine, or increased acid generation (see Chapter 6). The initial response to the net acid retention is buffering by extracellular bicarbonate and by the cell and bone buffers. Uptake of some of the excess hydrogen by the cells is accompanied in part by the loss of cell potassium and sodium into the extracellular fluid to maintain electroneutrality. Thus, metabolic acidosis is often associated with an elevation in the plasma potassium concentration above the level expected from the state of potassium balance. In some patients, the plasma potassium concentration is actually above normal (called hyperkalemia) even though body potassium stores are diminished (see Chapter 7 and Fig. 7.4). This cation shift is reversed with correction of the acidosis.

Although buffering is initially protective, the restoration of acid–base balance requires increased net acid excretion, a response that begins on the first day and reaches its maximum within 5 to 6 days as the changes in proximal and distal acidification described above increase in intensity. The elevation in acid excretion is mostly as ammonium, since titratable acidity is limited by the rate of phosphate excretion. Diabetic ketoacidosis represents one exception to this general rule, since urinary β-hydroxybutyrate can act as a titratable acid.

QUESTION 4 Suppose that metabolic acidosis is induced by an increased acid load due to bicarbonate loss in diarrhea. When the diarrhea resolves and the daily acid load returns to normal, what will be the signal to lower net acid excretion back to the baseline level?

In addition to the renal response, the extracellular pH in metabolic acidosis is also protected by a rise in alveolar ventilation, thereby lowering the PCO_2. From the Henderson–Hasselbalch equation, the pH is proportional to the *ratio* of the plasma bicarbonate concentration to the PCO_2. Thus, a fall in PCO_2 will protect the pH in the presence of a reduced plasma bicarbonate concentration. Empirical observations suggest that the PCO_2 falls by an average of 1.2 mm Hg for every 1-mEq/L decline in the plasma bicarbonate concentration. Thus, a plasma bicarbonate concentration of 14 mEq/L (10 mEq/L below normal) should be associated with a PCO_2 of approximately 28 mm Hg (12 mm Hg below normal) (Table 5.2).

QUESTION 5 Calculate what the pH will be with a plasma bicarbonate concentration of 14 mEq/L with and without the respiratory compensation. The PCO_2 will remain at the normal value of 40 mm Hg in the latter setting.

TABLE 5.2

Primary and Compensatory Changes in Different Acid–Base Disorders

Disorder	Primary Change	Compensatory Response
Metabolic acidosis	Fall in plasma bicarbonate concentration	Reduction in PCO_2 averaging 1.2 mm Hg per 1-mEq/L reduction in plasma bicarbonate concentration
Metabolic alkalosis	Rise in plasma bicarbonate concentration	Elevation in PCO_2 averaging 0.6–0.7 mm Hg per 1-mEq/L rise in plasma bicarbonate concentration
Respiratory acidosis	Elevation in PCO_2	**Acute**: Rise in plasma bicarbonate concentration averaging 1 mEq/L per 10 mm Hg elevation in PCO_2 **Chronic**: Increase in plasma bicarbonate concentration averaging 3.5 mEq/L per 10 mm Hg rise in PCO_2
Respiratory alkalosis	Reduction in PCO_2	**Acute**: Fall in plasma bicarbonate concentration averaging 2 mEq/L per 10 mm Hg decline in PCO_2 **Chronic**: Fall in plasma bicarbonate concentration averaging 4 mEq/L per 10 mm Hg decline in PCO_2

Respiratory Acidosis. Respiratory acidosis is induced by a rise in PCO_2 (hypercapnia) resulting from decreased alveolar ventilation and occurs in a variety of clinical setting associated with respiratory failure (a detailed discussion of the causes of respiratory acidosis is beyond the scope of this book). Although correction of this disorder requires the restoration of normal pulmonary function, the kidney can minimize the change in extracellular pH by increasing acid excretion (primarily as ammonium), thereby generating new bicarbonate ions in the plasma and raising the plasma bicarbonate concentration. This renal effect is presumably mediated by a fall in tubular cell pH as the excess CO_2 diffuses into the cells.

On average, the plasma bicarbonate concentration will initially rise in respiratory acidosis by approximately 1 mEq/L for every 10 mm Hg elevation in the PCO_2 by tissue buffering and then, over a period of 5 to 6 days, by 3.5 mEq/L for every 10 mm Hg rise in the PCO_2 due to the added effect of enhanced renal acid excretion. The net result is that the extracellular pH is generally well defended in chronic respiratory acidosis.

Tissue buffering results from the diffusion of CO_2 into cells, such as red blood cells. Combination of this CO_2 with H_2O within the cells generates H_2CO_3, which then dissociates into a hydrogen ion (that is buffered by cell proteins or hemoglobin) and a bicarbonate ion. The latter diffuses out of the cell into the extracellular fluid, thereby raising the plasma bicarbonate concentration.

Note that the responses to acute and chronic respiratory acidosis are different, due to the delayed increase in renal acid excretion. This is in contrast to the respiratory compensation in metabolic acidosis, which occurs rapidly over a period of hours.

Respiratory Alkalosis. Similar considerations, although the changes are in the opposite direction, apply to respiratory alkalosis. This disorder is characterized by a primary increase in alveolar ventilation that lowers the PCO_2 (hypocapnia) and is seen in many clincial settings including respiratory disorders such as pneumonia, anxiety, severe infection, and liver failure. The plasma bicarbonate concentration will initially fall by 2 mEq/L for every 10 mm Hg fall in PCO_2 due to tissue buffering. This will be followed over a period of several days by an intracellular alkalosis-induced decrease in net acid excretion due both to bicarbonate loss in the urine (as less is reabsorbed) and diminished ammonium excretion. The net effect is an average fall in the plasma bicarbonate concentration of 4 mEq/L for every 10 mm Hg decline in PCO_2, resulting in near-normalization of the extracellular pH in chronic respiratory alkalosis.

Effective Circulating Volume Depletion

Bicarbonate reabsorption also can be influenced by the effective circulating volume, with the most important effect being an elevation in bicarbonate reabsorptive capacity with volume depletion. This relationship is depicted in Figure 5.3. Raising the plasma bicarbonate concentration by an infusion of sodium bicarbonate leads to a plateau in bicarbonate reabsorption with a plasma level of about 26 mEq/L. This is an appropriate response, since excretion of bicarbonate above this level will help to maintain a normal plasma bicarbonate concentration.

In comparison, bicarbonate reabsorptive capacity can be increased by 4 mEq/L (to approximately 30 mEq/L) simply by the ingestion of a low-salt diet and can rise to above 35 mEq/L with more marked volume depletion. In this setting, the reabsorption of sodium bicarbonate is

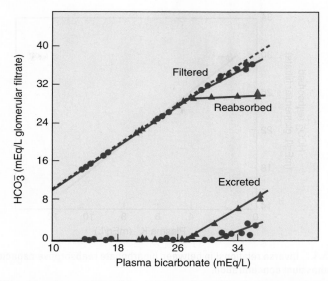

FIGURE 5.3. Filtration, reabsorption, and excretion of bicarbonate as a function of the plasma bicarbonate concentration and volume status in a patient receiving a sodium bicarbonate infusion to gradually raise the plasma bicarbonate concentration. When volume expansion was allowed to occur (*triangles*), bicarbonate reabsorptive capacity reached a plateau at a plasma bicarbonate concentration of 26 mEq/L, with the excess bicarbonate being excreted in the urine. In comparison, bicarbonate reabsorptive capacity exceeded 34 mEq/L and bicarbonaturia occurred at a higher plasma bicarbonate concentration if mild volume depletion were induced with a diuretic prior to the bicarbonate infusion (*circles*).

protective from the viewpoint of volume regulation, since it will tend to minimize the volume deficit.

The major setting in which this relationship assumes clinical importance is in metabolic alkalosis, since the elevation in bicarbonate reabsorptive capacity prevents correction of the alkalosis by excretion of the excess bicarbonate in the urine. Increased release of aldosterone (in response to volume depletion) and a reduction in the plasma—and therefore tubular fluid chloride concentration—play a contributory role in this response (see "Metabolic Alkalosis" below).

Plasma Potassium Concentration
Both bicarbonate reabsorption and ammonium excretion vary inversely with the plasma potassium concentration (Fig. 5.4). This relationship is mediated at least in part by transcellular cation shifts that lead to changes in intracellular pH. With potassium loss, for example, the fall in plasma potassium concentration is minimized by diffusion of potassium out of the cells (which contain approximately 98% of the body potassium). The major cell anions—proteins and organic phosphates such as ATP—are

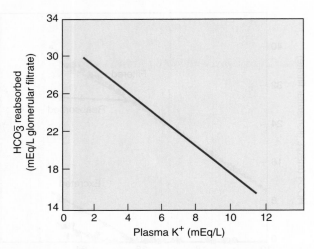

FIGURE 5.4.   Inverse relationship between bicarbonate reabsorptive capacity and the plasma potassium concentration.

too large to move out of the cells. Thus, electroneutrality is maintained by the movement of extracellular hydrogen and sodium into the cell (see Fig. 7.4). The net effect is an intracellular acidosis that will stimulate both bicarbonate reabsorption and ammonium excretion. The increased loss of acid will promote the development of metabolic alkalosis.

These changes are reversed with hyperkalemia, which is associated with an intracellular alkalosis and diminished acid excretion. The ensuing acid retention can lead to a mild metabolic acidosis.

Metabolic Alkalosis

Metabolic alkalosis illustrates the clinical importance of many of the principles described above. This disorder is characterized by a primary elevation in the plasma bicarbonate concentration and a rise in extracellular pH. Although the renal compensation to chronic respiratory acidosis also raises the plasma bicarbonate concentration, the extracellular pH is reduced in this setting.

Pathogenesis

Two questions must be addressed when approaching the patient with metabolic alkalosis:

■ What factors lead to the generation of the alkalosis by raising the plasma bicarbonate concentration?

■ What factors prevent excretion of the excess bicarbonate, thereby allowing the alkalosis to persist?

Generation of Metabolic Alkalosis

The most common mechanism responsible for the rise in the plasma bicarbonate concentration in metabolic alkalosis is the loss of hydrogen from the gastrointestinal tract (as with vomiting) or in the urine (as with diuretic therapy) (Table 5.3). From the buffering reaction for the bicarbonate–carbon dioxide system,

$$CO_2 + H_2O \leftrightarrow H^+ + HCO_3^-$$

the loss of hydrogen ions will result in the equimolar generation of bicarbonate.

Gastric secretions, for example, are highly acidic, containing high concentrations of hydrochloric acid. Under normal conditions, the effect of gastric acid is balanced by the secretion of an equal amount of pancreatic bicarbonate induced by entry of acid into the duodenum. However, there will be no stimulus for bicarbonate secretion if the gastric acid does not reach the duodenum due to vomiting or nasogastric suction. This results in loss of hydrogen ions *without* the appropriate bicarbonate

TABLE 5.3

Major Causes of Metabolic Alkalosis

 I. **Hydrogen loss**
   A. **Gastrointestinal loss**
      1. Removal of gastric secretions due to vomiting or nasogastric suction
      2. Antacids in advanced renal failure
   B. **Urinary loss**
      1. Loop or thiazide-type diuretics
      2. Primary mineralocorticoid excess (hyperaldosteronism)
      3. Posthypercapnic alkalosis
      4. Hypercalcemia and milk alkali syndrome
   C. **Movement of H^+ into the cells**
      1. Hypokalemia

 II. **Administration of bicarbonate or an organic ion that can be metabolized to bicarbonate, such as citrate in blood transfusions**

 III. **Contraction alkalosis**
   A. Loop or thiazide-type diuretics in edematous patients
   B. Vomiting or nasogastric suction in achlorhydria
   C. Sweat losses in cystic fibrosis

secretion resulting in equimolar retention of bicarbonate in the circulation for every mole of hydrogen ion lost.

Loop or thiazide-type diuretics, on the other hand, inhibit sodium reabsorption in the loop of Henle and the distal tubule, respectively (see Chapter 4). Some of the excess sodium is reclaimed in the principal cells in the cortical collecting duct under the influence of aldosterone (see Fig. 1.4), the secretion of which is increased by the diuretic-induced fluid loss. The reabsorption of cationic sodium creates a lumen-negative electrical potential, thereby favoring the urinary retention of hydrogen secreted by the adjacent intercalated cells (the mechanism of which is depicted in Fig. 5.2). Aldosterone also promotes hydrogen loss by directly stimulating the H^+-ATPase pump. Thus, in addition to secondary hyperaldosteronism resulting from volume depletion, metabolic alkalosis is also seen in conditions of primary aldosterone excess (such as an aldosterone-producing adrenal adenoma).

Other ways in which the plasma bicarbonate concentration can become elevated are the administration of bicarbonate (or an organic anion, such as citrate, that generates bicarbonate as it is metabolized), concurrent hypokalemia (since the transcellular potassium–hydrogen shift described above will cause an extracellular alkalosis and intracellular acidosis), and volume contraction.

A contraction alkalosis can be seen when a large quantity of relatively bicarbonate-free fluid is lost. This most commonly occurs with diuretic therapy in edematous states and can add to the effect of enhanced hydrogen loss induced by the diuretic. In this setting, the extracellular fluid volume contracts around a constant quantity of extracellular bicarbonate (since little or no bicarbonate is being lost); the net effect is a rise in the plasma bicarbonate concentration. Suppose, for example, that an edematous patient has an extracellular fluid volume of 20 L and a bicarbonate concentration of 24 mEq/L. The total quantity of extracellular bicarbonate is 480 mEq. If 5 L is lost by diuresis, then the extracellular fluid volume will fall to 15 L and, if no bicarbonate is lost, the plasma bicarbonate concentration will rise to 32 mEq/L. The steady state value will be somewhat lower due to buffering by the release of hydrogen ions from the cell buffers:

$$HCO_3^- + HBuf \rightarrow Buf^- + H_2CO_3 \rightarrow CO_2 + H_2O$$

An elevation in the plasma bicarbonate concentration also constitutes the compensatory renal response to a chronic elevation in the PCO_2 (hypercapnia). Although the extracellular pH is reduced in chronic respiratory acidosis, the restoration of normal ventilation (as with a mechanical respirator) can normalize the PCO_2 while the plasma bicarbonate concentration remains elevated. This phenomenon is called a posthypercapnic alkalosis and may persist if the excess bicarbonate cannot be excreted because of concurrent volume depletion.

Maintenance of Metabolic Alkalosis

Metabolic alkalosis cannot be induced by the administration of sodium bicarbonate to normal subjects since, as shown in Figure 5.3, the excess bicarbonate will be quantitatively excreted in the urine. One study showed that the administration of a massive quantity (1000 mEq) of sodium bicarbonate per day for 2 weeks produced only a minor elevation in the plasma bicarbonate concentration. Thus, persistence of metabolic alkalosis requires some concurrent abnormality that limits the renal excretion of bicarbonate.

The most common perpetuating factor is effective circulating volume depletion. As described above, bicarbonate reabsorptive capacity can exceed 35 mEq/L in hypovolemic subjects (Fig. 5.3) in an attempt to prevent further sodium losses. In addition to the effect of hypovolemia-induced hyperaldosteronism, there is evidence suggesting a major role of chloride depletion (with hydrogen in gastric secretions or after diuretic therapy) and reduced chloride delivery to the collecting ducts.

There are two major mechanisms by which chloride depletion can increase net distal bicarbonate reabsorption: increased hydrogen secretion and reduced bicarbonate secretion.

Increased Hydrogen Secretion. The collecting duct H^+-ATPase is associated with passive cosecretion of chloride to maintain electroneutrality (Fig. 5.2). A reduction in the tubular fluid chloride concentration will enhance the gradient for chloride secretion out of the cell, indirectly promoting hydrogen secretion.

Reduced Bicarbonate Secretion. Normally, elevated plasma bicarbonate concentration will result in decreased bicarbonate reabsorption. In addition, some of the urinary bicarbonate is derived from a subpopulation of intercalated cells (type B) in the cortical collecting duct that, in the presence of alkalemia, are able to secrete bicarbonate from the cell into the lumen (Fig. 5.5). In these cells, the site of the transporters for hydrogen and bicarbonate is the opposite of that seen in the hydrogen-secreting cells: The H^+-ATPase pump is located on the basolateral membrane, while the $Cl–HCO_3^-$ exchanger is located on the apical membrane. The energy for bicarbonate secretion is supplied by the favorable inward gradient for chloride. Thus, a reduction in the tubular fluid chloride concentration will diminish net bicarbonate secretion, thereby perpetuating the alkalosis.

Regardless of the mechanism, the role of chloride assumes clinical importance in both the diagnosis and the treatment of metabolic alkalosis.

 A 22-year-old man develops moderate gastrointestinal bleeding from a peptic ulcer. Will the associated volume depletion lead to the development of metabolic alkalosis?

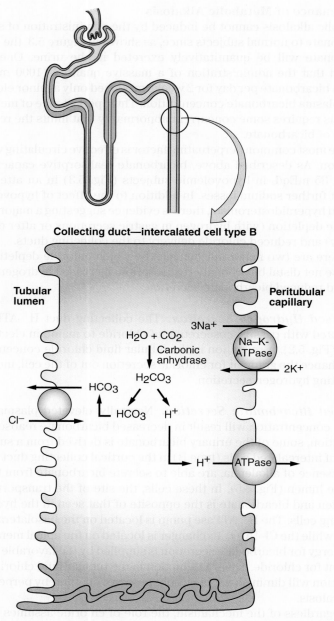

Collecting duct—intercalated cell type B

FIGURE 5.5.   Model of bicarbonate secretion in intercalated type B cells in the cortical collecting duct. The final step, bicarbonate secretion into the tubular lumen, is mediated by a chloride–bicarbonate exchanger located on the apical membrane; the H^+-ATPase pump in these cells is located on the basolateral membrane (CA = carbonic anhydrase).

Primary Hyperaldosteronism and Hypokalemia. Patients with primary hypersecretion of aldosterone develop both hypokalemia and metabolic alkalosis due to increased urinary excretion of potassium (see Chapter 7) and hydrogen. These patients tend to be mildly volume expanded due to aldosterone-induced sodium retention; thus, hypovolemia cannot be responsible for maintenance of the alkalosis. Studies in animals and humans suggest that it is hypokalemia that plays the major role since the plasma bicarbonate concentration will fall toward normal with the administration of potassium chloride.

It is presumed that the intracellular acidosis induced by potassium depletion leads to increased hydrogen secretion and enhanced bicarbonate reabsorptive capacity (Fig. 5.4). Potassium repletion will reverse these cation shifts, resulting in potassium movement into and hydrogen movement out of the cells. The net effect will be an elevation in intracellular pH (thereby decreasing bicarbonate reabsorption) and a direct reduction in the plasma bicarbonate concentration due to buffering by the hydrogen ions that leave the cell.

It is likely that hypokalemia also contributes to persistence of the alkalosis in other settings. As an example, potassium as well as hydrogen is lost with both vomiting and diuretic therapy. Thus, patients with these disorders tend to have hypokalemia as well as metabolic alkalosis. In this setting, correction of the potassium deficit will partially correct the alkalosis even though volume depletion persists.

Urine Chloride Concentration in Diagnosis of Metabolic Alkalosis

The cause of metabolic alkalosis is almost always evident from the history. If the diagnosis is in doubt, then the most likely diagnosis is surreptitious vomiting or diuretic ingestion, or one of the causes of primary overproduction of aldosterone (or some other mineralocorticoid).

Assessment of volume status is helpful in distinguishing between these possibilities. Vomiting or diuretic therapy should lead to volume depletion as opposed to volume expansion with excess mineralocorticoid. As described in Chapter 2, the urine sodium concentration can generally be used in this setting: A value below 25 mEq/L suggests hypovolemia (unless the diuretic is still-acting), whereas a value above 40 mEq/L suggests that the patient is normovolemic. The urine chloride concentration follows a similar pattern.

However, metabolic alkalosis represents one of the settings in which the *urine sodium and chloride concentrations may be dissociated.* Although volume depletion will cause sodium conservation, the obligation to excrete the excess bicarbonate may cause sodium wasting. As shown in Figure 5.3, for example, bicarbonate reabsorptive capacity may rise to 35 mEq/L with volume depletion. If, however, the plasma bicarbonate concentration is 42 mEq/L, then bicarbonate will be excreted in part with sodium.

Relation between Urinary Bicarbonate Sodium, Potassium, and Chloride

An understanding of the relationship between bicarbonate and other urinary electrolytes in metabolic alkalosis requires a brief review of transport in the different nephron segments. If bicarbonate is excreted because the filtered load exceeds reabsorptive capacity, then to maintain electroneutrality either sodium or potassium must accompany the bicarbonate. In the proximal tubule and loop of Henle, bicarbonate reabsorption occurs via Na^+–H^+ exchange (Fig. 5.1); inhibiting this transporter in metabolic alkalosis will deliver both sodium and bicarbonate to the distal nephron.

As described above, bicarbonate reabsorption or secretion in the cortical collecting duct occurs in the intercalated cells (Figs. 5.2 and 5.5); in comparison, the adjacent principal cells reabsorb sodium and chloride and secrete potassium in part under the influence of aldosterone (see Fig. 1.5). The process of sodium reabsorption through sodium channels in the apical membrane creates a lumen-negative potential that can be attenuated by the reabsorption of chloride or by the secretion of potassium.

In a hypovolemic patient with metabolic alkalosis, the associated secondary hyperaldosteronism will stimulate collecting duct sodium reabsorption. This process will continue until almost all of the chloride has been reabsorbed. At this point, nonreabsorbable bicarbonate is the major anion left in the tubular lumen. As a result, electroneutrality can be maintained with further sodium reabsorption only if it is accompanied by potassium secretion.

Thus, metabolic alkalosis with bicarbonaturia is a sodium- and potassium-wasting condition. In comparison, the urine chloride concentration will be appropriately reduced (less than 25 mEq/L) due both to hypovolemia and hypochloremia. The urine can be rendered virtually chloride-free in this setting, since there is *no impairment in the reabsorption of sodium chloride.*

A patient with unexplained metabolic alkalosis has a urine sodium concentration of 43 mEq/L. This could reflect lack of volume depletion, as in primary hyperaldosteronism, or volume depletion complicated by sodium wasting due to tubular dysfunction (most often induced by diuretic therapy) or due to bicarbonaturia as in Table 5.4. Other than having the laboratory measure the urine chloride concentration (which may not be readily available), what simple measurement can you make to confirm or exclude the presence of significant bicarbonaturia?

TABLE 5.4

Sequential Changes in Urinary Electrolyte Excretion in Metabolic Alkalosis Induced by Vomiting				
Time	Sodium	Potassium	Chloride	Bicarbonate
1–3 days	⇑	⇑	⇓	⇑
Late	⇓	⇓	⇓	⇓

Urinary Electrolytes in Metabolic Alkalosis

The range of urinary findings that can be seen in metabolic alkalosis can be illustrated by the sequential response to vomiting (Table 5.4). The initial loss of gastric secretions (hydrogen and potassium chloride) produces a high plasma bicarbonate concentration (since no stimulus for bicarbonate *secretion* in the duodenum) and therefore an elevation in the quantity of bicarbonate filtered. The associated volume depletion activates the renin–angiotensin–aldosterone system. However, the ability to maximally conserve bicarbonate takes several days to develop. As a result, some of the excess bicarbonate will be excreted with sodium and potassium, while only chloride will be appropriately conserved. The hypokalemia seen with vomiting is primarily due to increased urinary excretion during this period. The potassium concentration in gastric secretions is only from 5 to 10 mEq/L, thereby leading to only a modest amount of potassium loss.

The urinary findings change dramatically after several days if the degree of volume and chloride depletion is sufficient to increase net bicarbonate reabsorptive capacity to a level that allows essentially all of the filtered bicarbonate to be reabsorbed. In addition to enhanced reabsorption, the fall in tubular fluid chloride concentration will diminish the degree of bicarbonate secretion, since there is a less favorable gradient for luminal chloride to enter the cell and be exchanged for bicarbonate (Fig. 5.5).

The virtual elimination of bicarbonate from the urine at this time results in an acid urine pH that may be as low as 4.5 to 5.0 (as in the patient described at the beginning of this chapter). This phenomenon is called a *paradoxical aciduria*, since the urine pH should be high in metabolic alkalosis if the excess bicarbonate could be excreted. Sodium and potassium can also be appropriately conserved in this setting, in which there is no obligatory excretion with urinary bicarbonate (Table 5.4).

Treatment

In most cases, metabolic alkalosis can be corrected by administration of sodium chloride, potassium chloride (if the patient is hypokalemic), or hydrogen chloride (used only in patients with renal or cardiac failure). Therapy should also be directed against the underlying disease to diminish further hydrogen loss. As an example, the administration of an H_2-blocker to reduce the rate of gastric acid secretion may be beneficial in a patient with continued vomiting or nasogastric suction.

Sodium chloride and, if necessary, potassium chloride constitute the mainstays of therapy in patients with metabolic alkalosis due to vomiting, nasogastric suction, or diuretic use. This regimen will lower the plasma bicarbonate concentration in three ways: by reversing the contraction component; by removing the hypovolemic and hypokalemic stimuli to increased bicarbonate reabsorption; and by raising the tubular fluid chloride concentration, which will promote bicarbonate secretion in the cortical collecting duct (Fig. 5.5).

The therapeutic efficacy of volume repletion can be assessed at the bedside by monitoring the urine pH. The urine pH will exceed 7.0 and occasionally 8.0 when volume and chloride replacement are sufficient to allow excretion of the excess bicarbonate. Persistently acidic urine, on the other hand, indicates a continued elevation in bicarbonate reabsorption and the need for further fluid replacement.

The administration of sodium, potassium, or hydrogen must be given with chloride, the *only reabsorbable anion*. Consider the sequence of changes occurring with hydrochloric acid as compared to nitric acid (HNO_3). Both will initially buffer excess bicarbonate in the extracellular fluid and begin to correct the alkalosis:

$$HCl + NaHCO_3 \rightarrow NaCl + H_2CO_3 \rightarrow CO_2 + H_2O$$

$$HNO_3 + NaHCO_3 \rightarrow NaNO_3 + H_2CO_3 \rightarrow CO_2 + H_2O$$

However, the events within the kidney will be quite different. As sodium chloride is filtered, the sodium can be reabsorbed with the chloride, leading to volume expansion, and the increase in distal chloride delivery will promote bicarbonate secretion. In comparison, nitrate is a nonreabsorbable anion. Thus, sodium reabsorption in the collecting ducts must be accompanied by increases in hydrogen and potassium secretion to maintain electroneutrality. The net effects are persistence of the alkalosis due to excretion of much of the administered acid (as NH_4NO_3) and exacerbation of the potassium deficit.

Edematous States

The administration of sodium chloride is undesirable in edematous patients, since it will lead to more edema formation. Furthermore, congestive heart failure and hepatic cirrhosis are such sodium-avid states (see Chapter 4) that giving sodium chloride will not appreciably increase bicarbonate excretion.

Two options are available in this setting. First, hydrochloric acid can be given by intravenous infusion. However, this must be done with great care, since the highly acid solution is toxic to smaller veins. The simpler and preferable option is the administration of the carbonic anhydrase inhibitor acetazolamide, which decreases the activity of the Na^+–H^+ exchanger in the proximal tubule. (The role of carbonic anhydrase in this segment is discussed above.) The net effect is diminished sodium bicarbonate reabsorption in the proximal tubule, thereby promoting the excretion of both sodium and bicarbonate. The efficacy of this regimen can again be monitored by measuring the urine pH, which should exceed 7.0 if bicarbonate excretion is significantly increased.

CASE DISCUSSION The patient presented at the beginning of this chapter has alkalemia with a metabolic alkalosis and compensatory respiratory acidosis (vomiting-induced metabolic alkalosis with high arterial pH, elevated plasma bicarbonate concentration, compensatory rise in PCO_2 and hypokalemia). The differential causes are listed in Table 5.3 but the history clearly suggests vomiting-induced metabolic alkalosis in this case. The gastrointestinal loss of hydrogen is the initiating process and the decreased effective volume is necessary to maintain the alkalosis. By the time of presentation, the patient is sufficiently volume depleted so that all of the excess bicarbonate is reabsorbed in an attempt to prevent further urinary sodium losses. As a result, the urine sodium concentration is low (10 mEq/L) and the urine pH is paradoxically acidic (5.0). These findings correspond to the late phase in Table 5.4. In addition, the hypokalemia results in *intra*cellular acidosis from hydrogen shifts setting in motion mechanisms that increase bicarbonate reabsorption and hydrogen secretion. Fluid repletion with sodium chloride and potassium chloride will correct the alkalosis by allowing the bicarbonate to be lost in the urine as sodium bicarbonate. As this occurs, the urine pH will transiently rise above 7.0.

ANSWERS TO QUESTIONS

1 The four log unit difference between urine pH and the pK_a means that the ratio of ammonia to ammonium is 1:10,000.

$$5.0 = 9.0 + \log([NH_3]/[NH_4^+])$$

Thus, virtually all ammonia secreted into the lumen is converted to ammonium. The maintenance of a very low concentration of lipid-soluble ammonia promotes further ammonia diffusion into the lumen, where it can be trapped as ammonium. It is this continued supply of ammonia that allows this system to act as an effective "buffer" even though its pK_a is so far from the extracellular or urine pH.

The high urine pK_a also means that urinary ammonium is not measured as a titratable acid. Adding sodium hydroxide to raise the urine pH from 5.0 back up to the plasma level of 7.4 will not convert much ammonium back to ammonia. At a pH of 7.4, the ratio of ammonia to ammonium is 1:40 (1.6 log units). Thus, there is only 1 mEq of ammonia if there are 40 mEq of ammonium in the urine, and only 1 mEq out of 40 will be measured as a titratable acid. At a pH of 5.0, there is almost no ammonia.

2 The activity of the Na^+–H^+ exchanger is limited by the favorable inward concentration gradient for sodium, which is about 7:1 in the proximal tubule (140 mEq/L in the filtrate vs. about 20 mEq/L in the cells), but much less in the collecting ducts since the tubular fluid sodium concentration is so much lower. A urine pH of 5.0 (2.4 log units) represents a gradient of over 200:1, much greater than the inward gradient for sodium. Thus, an energy-requiring H^+-ATPase pump is necessary, not passive Na^+–H^+ exchange.

3 Buffering of titratable acids and the trapping of ammonium are pH dependent, and both processes become more efficient as the urine becomes more acidic. An inability to lower the urine pH normally, which is the primary defect in distal renal tubular acidosis (see Chapter 6), might prevent the daily acid load from being completely excreted, thereby resulting in hydrogen retention and metabolic acidosis. Note that at a urine pH of 6.1, which is the same as the pK_a of 6.1 for the bicarbonate–carbon dioxide system, the concentration of bicarbonate in the urine will be roughly equal to that of dissolved carbon dioxide: $0.03 \times 40 = 1.2$ mEq/L. This presents a negligible loss of bicarbonate. The urine pH has to be much higher, generally above 7.0, before there is a significant degree of bicarbonate wasting in the urine.

4 The stimulus to increased acid excretion is the fall in intracellular pH induced by the systemic acidemia. Once diarrhea stops and the daily hydrogen load declines to normal levels, the initially high rate of acid excretion will be greater than the rate of production, thereby raising the plasma bicarbonate concentration toward normal. This will lead to an elevation in the intracellular bicarbonate concentration (e.g., via the Na^+–$3HCO_3^-$ exchanger in the basolateral membrane in the proximal tubule). The ensuing increase in intracellular pH constitutes the signal to lower the rate of acid excretion.

5 The extracellular pH will be 7.32 with the compensatory hyperventilation, but much lower at 7.17 if there were no compensatory hyperventilation

and the PCO_2 remained constant:

$$7.32 = 6.10 + \log([14 \div (0.03 \times 28)])$$
$$7.17 = 6.10 + \log([14 \div (0.03 \times 40)])$$

6 Volume depletion will promote the *maintenance* of metabolic alkalosis by minimizing excretion of the excess bicarbonate in the urine. However, volume depletion will cause a metabolic alkalosis (i.e., cause the plasma bicarbonate concentration to rise) only if the fluid lost is relatively free of bicarbonate, as with vomiting or diuretic therapy. Bleeding, on the other hand, results in the loss of bicarbonate-containing plasma, which will not increase the plasma bicarbonate concentration.

7 The urine pH will tell if the high rate of sodium excretion is due to bicarbonaturia; as described in the answer to Question 3, the urine pH should be above 7.0 if there is a significant concentration of bicarbonate in the urine.

SUGGESTED READINGS

Galla JH. Metabolic alkalosis. J Am Soc Nephrol 2000;11:369.

Galla JH, Bonduris DN, Luke RG. Effects of chloride and extracellular fluid volume on bicarbonate reabsorption along the nephron in metabolic alkalosis in the rat. Reassessment of the classic hypothesis on the pathogenesis of metabolic alkalosis. J Clin Invest 1987;80:41.

Garg LC. Respective roles of H-ATPase and H–K-ATPase in ion transport in the kidney. J Am Soc Nephrol 1991;2:949.

Laski ME, Sabatini S. Metabolic alkalosis, bedside and bench. Semin Nephrol 2006;26(6):404–421.

Rose BD, Post TW. Clinical Physiology of Acid–Base and Electrolyte Disorders, 5th Ed. New York: McGraw-Hill, 2001.

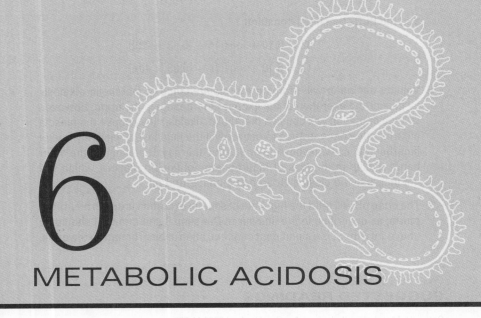

6

METABOLIC ACIDOSIS

CASE PRESENTATION A 58-year-old man has a massive acute myocardial infarction and presents to the hospital in shock. Physical examination reveals that the patient is confused, has cool clammy extremities, and is putting out no urine. The blood pressure is 80/50, well below his baseline level of 140/95. While being examined, the patient has a cardiopulmonary arrest. Mechanical ventilation is begun and a small amount of sodium bicarbonate is given to treat the acidemia noted after the following blood values are obtained:

Arterial pH = 7.30 (7.37–7.43)
PCO_2 = 32 mm Hg (36–44)
Na = 141 mEq/L (136–142)
K = 4.5 mEq/L (3.5–5)
Cl = 99 mEq/L (98–108)
Total CO_2 = 15 mEq/L (21–30)

It is assumed that the tissue pH is being relatively well maintained.

OBJECTIVES

By the end of this section, you should have an understanding of each of the following issues:

- The normal renal response to an acid load and how this becomes impaired in renal failure.
- Use of the anion gap in the differential of metabolic acidosis.
- The difference between measurement of arterial and mixed venous pH when tissue perfusion is markedly reduced in lactic acidosis.
- The general principles involved in the therapy of the different types of metabolic acidosis, including the mechanism by which bicarbonate administration might be deleterious in lactic acidosis.

Introduction

Metabolic acidosis is a relatively common clinical disorder characterized by a primary reduction in the plasma bicarbonate concentration, a low extracellular pH (or elevated hydrogen concentration), and compensatory hyperventilation, resulting in a fall in the PCO_2. A fall in the plasma bicarbonate concentration, however, is not diagnostic of metabolic acidosis, since it also results from the renal compensation to chronic respiratory alkalosis. In the latter disorder, however, the extracellular pH is elevated, not reduced as in metabolic acidosis.

Two basic mechanisms can lead to metabolic acidosis: increased acid production or an impairment in renal acid excretion (Table 6.1). This chapter will review the pathophysiologic characteristics of several of the most common causes of metabolic acidosis as well as the basic principles of therapy in each of these disorders. This will be followed by a review of the approach to differential diagnosis with emphasis on the anion gap.

As will be discussed, the plasma bicarbonate concentration can increase to normal in metabolic acidosis in one of three ways:

- Excretion of the excess acid in the urine.
- Administration of exogenous alkali, most often sodium bicarbonate.
- In organic acidoses (lactic acidosis and ketoacidosis), metabolism of the organic anion during correction of the underlying disorder results in the regeneration of bicarbonate. With lactate, for example,

$$Lactate^- + 3O_2 \rightarrow 2CO_2 + 2H_2O + HCO_3^-$$ (Eq. 1)

Decreased Acid Excretion

As described in Chapter 5, metabolism of dietary foodstuffs (particularly sulfur-containing amino acids) results in the generation of 50 to 100 mEq

TABLE 6.1

Major Causes of Metabolic Acidosis

Increased acid production
A. Lactic acidosis

B. Ketoacidosis, most often due to uncontrolled diabetes mellitus

C. Ingestions
   1. Aspirin
   2. Ethylene glycol, a component of antifreeze and solvents
   3. Methanol (wood alcohol), a component of shellac and de-icing solutions

D. Loss of bicarbonate
   1. Gastrointestinal—diarrhea, pancreatic, biliary or intestinal fistulas, ureterosigmoidostomy
   2. Renal—type 2 (proximal) renal tubular acidosis

Decreased acid excretion
A. Renal failure—decreased NH_4^+ excretion

B. Type 1 (distal) renal tubular acidosis

C. Type 4 renal tubular acidosis (hypoaldosteronism) (discussed in Chapter 7)

of acid each day on a regular diet. This acid is then excreted in the urine as ammonium and titratable acidity. If the acid load is increased, the renal response is to increase acid excretion, primarily as ammonium (Fig. 6.1).

Metabolic acidosis due to an inability to excrete the daily acid load most commonly occurs in patients with acute (recent onset) or chronic renal failure. Although type 1 (distal) and type 2 (proximal) renal tubular acidosis (RTA) are relatively rare conditions, a brief review of their pathophysiology helps to illustrate the different ways in which the acid secretory process can be impaired and the implications that these defects have for treatment of acidemia. See Table 6.2 for an overview of the clinical features of renal tubular acidosis. Type 4 RTA (hypoaldosteronism) will be discussed in Chapter 7, since hyperkalemia rather than metabolic acidosis is the most prominent finding.

Renal Failure

The loss of functioning nephrons in progressive kidney disease requires an adaptation in tubular function to maintain acid–base balance. Initially, net acid excretion is maintained by increased ammonium excretion per

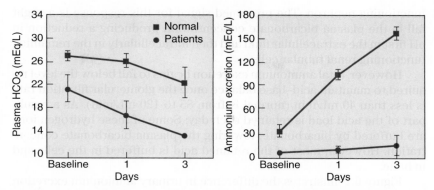

FIGURE 6.1. Effect of an acid load on the plasma bicarbonate concentration (*left panel*) and urinary ammonium excretion (*right panel*) in normal subjects (*squares*) and patients with renal failure (*circles*). Normal subjects show a fourfold increase in ammonium excretion with a fall in the plasma bicarbonate concentration from 27 down to 22 mEq/L. The patients with renal failure began with a low plasma bicarbonate concentration of 21 mEq/L but excreted less ammonium than did the normal subjects prior to the acid load. The administration of acid produced a much smaller rise in ammonium excretion in renal failure.

TABLE 6.2

Overview of Renal Tubular Acidosis			
	Type 1—Distal	**Type 2—Proximal**	**Type 4 (See Chapter 7)**
Basic abnormality	Impaired distal acidification	Diminished proximal bicarbonate reabsorption	Aldosterone resistance or deficiency
Urine pH	>5.3	Variable; >5.3 if above reabsorption threshold	<5.3
Plasma bicarbonate	Variable; can be <10 mEq/L	Usually 14–20 mEq/L	Usually >15
Plasma potassium	Usually reduced or normal, but can be elevated	Normal or reduced	Elevated
Complications	Nephrocalcinosis, renal stones	Rickets or osteomalacia	None

functioning nephron. The presumed signal for this response is a slight fall in the plasma bicarbonate concentration producing a reduction in pH first in the extracellular fluid and then intracellularly in the remaining functioning renal tubular cells.

However, total ammonium excretion begins to fall below the level required to maintain acid–base balance once the glomerular filtration rate is less than 40 mL/min (normal is from 85 to 120 mL/min). As a result, part of the acid load is retained each day: Some of these hydrogen ions are buffered by bicarbonate, lowering the plasma bicarbonate concentration. However, most of the retained acid is buffered in the cells and in bone.

Figure 6.1 illustrates the difference in urinary ammonium excretion between normal subjects and those with renal failure. The patients with renal failure began at baseline with a mild metabolic acidosis (plasma bicarbonate concentration equals 21 mEq/L) that is associated with a lower rate of ammonium excretion than that seen in normal subjects (Fig. 6.1, baseline values). After administration of an oral acid load, the differences in ammonium excretion are much more pronounced (25 vs. 160 mEq/day). If, however, total ammonium excretion is divided by the GFR (a rough index of the number of functioning nephrons), then ammonium excretion *per functioning nephron* is increased in the two groups. Thus, the impaired acid excretion in renal failure is due to *too few functioning nephrons*, rather than due to a defect in tubular function.

Other aspects of renal acid excretion are generally intact in renal failure. The urine pH is usually below 5.3, suggesting that the distal nephron can secrete hydrogen ions and maintain a high pH gradient; the limitation in net acid excretion results from the lack of availability of ammonia as a buffer.

 In the face of reduced net ammonium excretion, why doesn't the kidney adapt by increasing acid excretion as titratable acidity?

Treatment

The metabolic acidosis in chronic renal failure generally produces few overt symptoms, since the efficiency of bone and cell buffering maintains the plasma bicarbonate concentration between 12 and 20 mEq/L. However, these buffering processes may have adverse long-term effects, leading to loss of bone mineral (due to release of bone calcium as hydrogen ions are buffered by bone carbonate [CO_3^{2-}]) and to breakdown of muscle protein. Furthermore, the increase in ammonium production per nephron may enhance the rate of progressive renal injury (see Chapter 11). As a result, sodium bicarbonate is used to correct the metabolic acidosis of chronic renal failure.

What is the maximum amount of bicarbonate that would need to be given each day to prevent hydrogen retention in renal failure?

Type 1 Renal Tubular Acidosis

In type 1 (distal) RTA, the decrease in net acid excretion results from an inability to lower the urine pH below 5.5 to 6.0, rather than from diminished ammonium production (see Table 6.2). The higher urine pH (meaning that fewer free hydrogen ions are present) reduces the efficiency of both hydrogen buffering by titratable acids and ammonia trapping in the tubular lumen as ammonium.

Three different mechanisms can account for the decreased hydrogen secretion in the collecting ducts in this disorder (see Fig. 5.2 for a model of distal acidification):

- Direct impairment of the apical membrane H^+-ATPase pump through a number of acquired or genetic defects. Mutations in the basolateral chloride–bicarbonate exchanger that reduced the return of bicarbonate to the circulation (see Fig. 5.2) also results in type 1 RTA.
- Increased permeability of the apical membrane or tight junction, thereby allowing the back-diffusion of hydrogen ions out of the tubular lumen down a very favorable concentration gradient. As an example, the hydrogen concentration in the tubular lumen is 200 times higher than that in the extracellular fluid when the urine pH is 5.1 (2.3 pH units lower than the extracellular fluid).
- Decreased sodium reabsorption in the adjacent principal cells in the cortical collecting duct. The normal reabsorption of cationic sodium creates a lumen-negative electrical potential that promotes both the retention of secreted hydrogen ions in the lumen and the secretion of potassium. Thus, impaired sodium reabsorption results in metabolic acidosis and, due to decreased urinary potassium excretion, an elevation in the plasma potassium concentration (hyperkalemia).

The presence of type 1 RTA should be suspected in any patient with an otherwise unexplained normal anion gap metabolic acidosis (see below) and a urine pH that is persistently above 5.5. The principles of therapy are similar to those in chronic renal failure; that fraction of the daily acid load that is not excreted must be buffered by exogenous bicarbonate.

Type 2 Renal Tubular Acidosis

An entirely different defect is present in type 2 (proximal) RTA (Table 6.2). This disorder is characterized by an impairment in proximal bicarbonate reabsorption, leading initially to bicarbonate loss in the urine. This finding, however, is transient. Suppose that bicarbonate reabsorptive capacity is reduced from the normal level of approximately 26 mEq/L (see Fig. 5.3) down to 17 mEq/L. Filtered bicarbonate will be lost in the urine until the plasma bicarbonate concentration falls to 17 mEq/L. At this point, all of the filtered bicarbonate can now be reabsorbed and the patient is able to excrete the daily acid load. In other words, a new steady state is present in which the patient is similar to normal (acid in equals acid out) except that the plasma bicarbonate concentration is reduced by 9 mEq/L. Thus, type 2 RTA is a *self-limiting* disorder. Nevertheless, the resulting acidemia can contribute to bone mineral loss and the development of Rickets in children and osteomalacia in adults.

The defect in type 2 RTA does create a problem for therapy. As soon as exogenous alkali raises the plasma bicarbonate concentration, the filtered bicarbonate load will exceed reabsorptive capacity and most of the bicarbonate will be lost in the urine. Thus, very high doses have to be given (10 to 15 mEq/kg per day) to stay ahead of bicarbonate losses and to correct the acidemia.

Increased Acid Generation

The development of acidemia is gradual in renal failure or type 1 RTA, since it is induced by the retention of some fraction of the 50 to 100 mEq daily acid load that is not excreted. In contrast, acute and severe metabolic acidosis can occur when there is a marked increase in acid production (Table 6.1). As an example, exercising to exhaustion can, within a period of minutes, enhance lactic acid production, reducing the plasma bicarbonate concentration to as low as 5 mEq/L in some cases, with the arterial pH falling to as low as 6.80. There are two major mechanisms of increased acid generation leading to metabolic acidosis. These are divided into processes that reduce bicarbonate *and* chloride concentrations (anion gap acidosis) and processes in which the bicarbonate concentration is reduced, but chloride becomes elevated (hyperchloremic metabolic acidosis).

Anion Gap in Diagnosis of Metabolic Acidosis due to Increased Acid Generation

The etiology of metabolic acidosis is often evident from the history and routine laboratory data (such as a chronic elevation in the plasma creatinine concentration in renal failure; or hyperglycemia, ketonuria, and ketonemia in diabetic ketoacidosis). In addition, calculation of the anion gap is a routine part of the evaluation of such a patient because it divides the different causes in Table 6.1 into two categories: a high and normal anion gap metabolic acidosis (Table 6.3).

The anion gap is equal to the difference between the plasma concentrations of the major cation (sodium) and the major measured anions

TABLE 6.3

Major Causes of Metabolic Acidosis According to the Anion Gap

Increased anion gap[a]
  A. Advanced renal failure—phosphate, sulfate, urate, hippurate

  B. Lactic acidosis—lactate

  C. Ketoacidosis—β-hydroxybutyrate

  D. Ingestions
    1. Aspirin—ketones, lactate, salicylate
    2. Ethylene glycol—glycolate, oxalate
    3. Methanol—formate
    4. Paraldehyde—organic anions
    5. Toluene; hippurate (usually presents with normal anion gap)
    6. Sulfur; SO_4^{2-}
    7. Pyroglytamic (5'-oxoproline) acidemia associated with acetaminophen use

  E. Massive rhabdomyolysis (severe muscle injury)

Normal anion gap or hyperchloremic metabolic acidosis
  A. Renal bicarbonate loss—type 2 (proximal RTA)—hereditary, drug associated (ifosfamide, tenofivir) or malignancy associated (multiple myeloma)

  B. Gastrointestinal loss of bicarbonate—diarrhea

  C. Renal dysfunction
    1. Some cases of chronic renal failure
    2. Type 1 (distal RTA) drugs, amphotericin, lithium, Sjogren syndrome, hypercalciuria
    3. Type 4 RTA (Hypoaldosteronism; see Chapter 7)

  D. Ingestions
    1. Ammonium chloride
    2. Some hyperalimentation fluids

[a]The substances after the dash represent the major retained anions in the increased anion gap acidoses.

(chloride and bicarbonate):

$$Anion\ gap = [Na^+] - ([Cl^-] + [HCO_3^-]) \qquad \text{(Eq. 2)}$$

The approximate normal values for these ions are 140, 108, and 24 mEq/L, respectively, leading to a normal anion gap of 6 to 10 mEq/L. The negative charges on the plasma proteins (particularly albumin) comprise most of this anion gap, as the charges on the other cations (potassium, calcium, and magnesium) and anions (phosphate, sulfate, and organic anions such as lactate and urate) tend to balance out.

The normal value for the anion gap must be adjusted downward in the presence of hypoalbuminemia. The approximate correction factor is a reduction in the anion gap of 2.5 mEq/L for every 1.0-g/dL reduction in the plasma albumin concentration (normal equals 4 to 4.5 g/dL). The factors that can affect the anion gap can be more easily appreciated if Eq. 2 is rewritten. In addition to being equal to the difference between measured cations and anions, the anion gap is also equal to the difference between the *unmeasured* anions and cations:

$$Anion\ gap = Unmeasured\ anions - unmeasured\ cations$$

A clinically significant increase in anion gap is almost always due to a rise in the concentration of unmeasured anions. This can be induced by a high plasma albumin concentration (resulting from hemoconcentration in hypovolemic subjects) or, more commonly in metabolic acidosis, to the accumulation of a variety of different anions (such as lactate). In theory, an elevated anion gap can also be produced by a fall in unmeasured cations (as in hypocalcemia, hypokalemia, or hypomagnesemia); however, these cations are normally present in relatively low concentrations and a reduction in concentration only raises the anion gap by 1 to 3 mEq/L.

In addition to hypoalbuminemia resulting in a lower anion gap, the accumulation of unmeasured cations will have a similar effect. With hypercalcemia, hyperkalemia, and hypermagnesemia, the gap will be reduced, and this can also be seen with lithium intoxication and in some cases of multiple myeloma that produce cationic paraproteins.

These relationships can be applied to the different causes of metabolic acidosis, in which the excess acid is rapidly buffered by extracellular bicarbonate. If the acid is HCl, then

$$HCl + NaHCO_3 \rightarrow NaCl + H_2CO_3 \rightarrow CO_2 + H_2O \qquad \text{(Eq. 3)}$$

(Refer to Eq. 5.3 for description of $H_2CO_3 \rightarrow CO_2 + H_2O$.)

With the addition of HCl, there is a mEq-for-mEq replacement of extracellular bicarbonate by chloride. As a result, there is no change in the anion gap, since the sum of the chloride and bicarbonate concentrations is unchanged and there is no change in the concentration of unmeasured anions. This disorder is called a normal anion gap or, due to the elevation in the plasma chloride concentration, a *hyperchloremic acidosis*.

Gastrointestinal or renal loss of sodium bicarbonate (as with diarrhea or type 2 RTA) indirectly produces the same result (see Table 6.3). Volume depletion induced by the sodium loss activates sodium-retaining mechanisms such as the renin–angiotensin–aldosterone system. The ensuing sodium chloride retention results in the net exchange of chloride for bicarbonate and no increase in the anion gap.

On the other hand, if hydrogen ions accumulate with any anion other than chloride, extracellular bicarbonate will be replaced by an unmeasured anion (A^-) (Table 6.3):

$$HA + NaHCO_3 \rightarrow NaA + H_2CO_3 \rightarrow CO_2 + H_2O \qquad \text{(Eq. 4)}$$

In this setting, the accumulation of A^- leads to an elevation in the anion gap. In the absence of an ingestion or chronic renal failure, an anion gap above 25 mEq/L (15 mEq/L above normal) in a patient with metabolic acidosis is almost always due to lactic acidosis or ketoacidosis. Lesser elevations also point to these disorders, but the diagnostic accuracy is not as high since other unmeasured anions may accumulate.

Furthermore, the distinction between a normal and a high anion gap acidosis is not always absolute. Patients with diarrhea, for example, typically develop a normal anion gap acidosis. However, the anion gap may begin to rise if the diarrhea is severe due to hemoconcentration (which raises the plasma albumin concentration) and concurrent lactic acidosis (due to hypoperfusion).

Lactic Acidosis

Lactic acid is derived from the metabolism of pyruvic acid in a reaction catalyzed by the enzyme lactate dehydrogenase and involving the conversion of NADH into NAD^+. Normal subjects produce from 15 to 20 mmol/kg of lactic acid per day. However, the normal plasma lactate concentration is only from 0.5 to 1.5 mEq/L, since almost all lactate produced is converted in the liver and, to a lesser degree, in the kidney to glucose (via the gluconeogenetic pathways) or back to pyruvate and then to carbon dioxide and water. Excess lactate can accumulate when there is increased lactate production and/or reduced lactate utilization. Lactic acidosis (defined as a plasma lactate concentration above 4 to 5 mEq/L) occurs when tissue oxygen delivery is reduced well below tissue needs. This can occur in settings such as maximal exercise or during a grand mal seizure, but is most often due to hypovolemic, septic, or cardiogenic shock. In these settings, pyruvate is preferentially converted to lactate and the reduction in hepatic and renal perfusion then minimizes the rate of lactate utilization, since as noted in Eq. 1, lactate metabolism requires the presence of oxygen.

Arterial Versus Mixed Venous pH

In most clinical conditions, the extracellular pH is measured from an arterial blood specimen, although carefully drawn venous blood can also be used. (The normal values are listed in Table 5.1.) It is assumed that the values obtained reflect those present in the tissues. Cardiovascular collapse represents the one clinical setting in which this assumption may be inaccurate, because of an often marked reduction in pulmonary blood

TABLE 6.4

Simultaneously Obtained Arterial and Mixed Venous Blood Values During Cardiopulmonary Resuscitation

	pH	PCO₂ (mm Hg)	[HCO₃⁻] (mEq/L)
Arterial	7.41	32	20
Mixed venous	7.15	74	24

flow. This problem can be illustrated in Table 6.4, which depicts simultaneously drawn arterial and mixed venous values in patients undergoing cardiopulmonary resuscitation. As can be seen, the results from arterial blood suggest that the pH is being well maintained; in comparison, there is a dramatic mixed venous acidemia due mostly to a much higher PCO_2 in venous blood.

This difference can be explained in the following way. The below normal PCO_2 (32 mm Hg) in arterial blood indicates only that blood entering the pulmonary circulation is cleared of much of the carbon dioxide that it contains. However, total CO_2 removal is diminished in this setting because of the marked reduction in total blood flow. Thus, some of the metabolically produced CO_2 accumulates in the tissues, raising the mixed venous PCO_2. The net effect is that arterial blood may give a misleading estimate of the state of acid–base balance and this defect becomes more prominent over time. Furthermore, this problem may be exacerbated by the administration of sodium bicarbonate.

Role of Bicarbonate in Treatment of Lactic Acidosis

The primary goal of therapy in lactic acidosis is the restoration of normal tissue perfusion by, for example, fluid administration in hypovolemic shock. The attainment of adequate oxygenation will allow lactate to be metabolized, thereby regenerating bicarbonate and correcting the acidemia (see Eq. 1).

Some patients, however, have severe acidemia with an arterial pH below 7.15. In this setting, it has been proposed that the acidemia itself might cause both myocardial depression and systemic vasodilatation, further reducing oxygen delivery. As a result, raising the extracellular pH by the administration of bicarbonate might directly improve cardiovascular function and tissue perfusion.

However, both experimental and human studies have suggested that bicarbonate therapy is often relatively ineffective in lactic acidosis, producing only *a transient elevation in the plasma bicarbonate concentration and possibly worsening the intracellular acidosis.* The inability to raise the pH in this setting appears to be due in part to an associated increase in net lactic acid production that counterbalances the effect of the added bicarbonate.

How this might occur is related to the above discussion on the importance of tissue CO_2 accumulation induced by the reduction in pulmonary blood flow. Buffering of excess acid by exogenous bicarbonate generates more CO_2, potentially worsening the mixed venous acidemia:

$$HCO_3^- + H^+ \rightarrow CO_2 + H_2O$$

This rise in PCO_2 also intensifies the intracellular acidosis, since CO_2 is lipid soluble and rapidly diffuses into the cells. The fall in intracellular pH in cardiac cells can decrease cardiac contractility, further reducing tissue perfusion and increasing lactic acid production. In addition, lactate utilization will be diminished as the intracellular acidosis diminishes hepatic lactate utilization.

These findings make the optimal therapy of lactic acidosis uncertain. Many physicians feel that there is little indication for sodium bicarbonate therapy, particularly during cardiopulmonary arrest. Other physicians, however, give small amounts of sodium bicarbonate to maintain the arterial pH above 7.15; the mixed venous pH should be monitored in this setting, if possible.

 The administration of a solution containing sodium carbonate (Na_2CO_3) may be more effective than sodium bicarbonate in lactic acidosis. Consider the buffering reaction for carbonate to explain why this might occur.

Diabetic Ketoacidosis

From an acid–base viewpoint, diabetic ketoacidosis (DKA) shares a number of similarities to lactic acidosis. Both disorders are due to increased endogenous acid production. In DKA, the combination of insulin deficiency and glucagon excess leads to increased hepatic synthesis of ketoacids, particularly β-hydroxybutyric acid and to a lesser degree acetoacetic acid. Two factors are required for increased ketoacid production:

■ The delivery of the precursor-free fatty acids to the liver must be increased. This effect is due to enhanced lipolysis, which is primarily mediated by low insulin levels, thereby removing the normal antilipolytic action of insulin.

■ Hepatic metabolism must be altered so that fatty acyl CoA is metabolized to ketoacids (a mitochondrial process) rather than to triglycerides (a cytosolic process). The rate-limiting step in ketoacid synthesis is the entry of fatty acyl CoA into the mitochondria, which is regulated by the cytosolic enzyme carnitine palmitoyl transferase. The activity of this enzyme is indirectly enhanced by the high glucagon levels in DKA, thereby allowing ketogenesis to proceed.

The acidemia may be severe but, as in lactic acidosis, is largely reversible by treatment of the underlying disorder. The administration of insulin stops further ketoacid synthesis and allows the excess ketoacids to be metabolized. The metabolism of ketoacid anions, as with lactate and other organic anions, results in the regeneration of bicarbonate and spontaneous correction of the acidemia.

 Some of the excess ketoacid anions in DKA are excreted in the urine. Documentation of ketonuria (with a dipstick) is part of the way in which the diagnosis is confirmed. What effect will these urinary losses have on the correctibility of the acidemia following insulin administration?

Salicylate Intoxication

Aspirin (acetylsalicylic acid) is rapidly converted into salicylic acid in the body. Most patients begin to show signs of intoxication [such as tinnitus (ringing in the ears), vertigo, and nausea] when the plasma salicylate level exceeds from 40 to 50 mg/dL, well above the therapeutic range of 20 to 35 mg/dL. Increasing doses of aspirin produce a progressively greater risk of toxicity because of saturation of protein binding sites on albumin. As a result, more drug remains in the physiologically active unbound form.

There are two major acid–base disturbances that can occur in this setting: respiratory alkalosis due to direct stimulation of the respiratory center and metabolic acidosis due to interference with oxidative metabolism, leading to the accumulation of organic acids such as lactate and ketoacids.

The more serious neurologic toxicity of salicylates, including seizures and death, is related to the cerebral tissue salicylate concentration. Thus, a reduction in the brain level is the first goal of therapy.

 The distribution of both the lipid-soluble salicylic acid (HS) and the lipid-insoluble salicylate anion (S⁻) between the brain and the extracellular fluid is depicted in Figure 6.2. How can you manipulate the reaction—$H^+ + S^- \leftrightarrow HS$—so that the total cerebral accumulation of salicylate is diminished? The pK_a for this reaction is 3.0:

$$pH = 3.0 + \log\left([S^-] \div [HS]\right)$$

How would you use the same principle to maximize the rate of salicylate excretion in the urine?

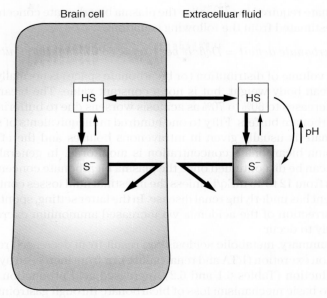

FIGURE 6.2. Schematic representation of the equilibrium distribution of salicylic acid (HS) and salicylate (S⁻) between the extracellular fluid and the brain cell. HS is lipid soluble and has an equal concentration in both compartments. In comparison, S⁻ is charged and does not achieve equal concentrations across the cell membrane. Since the pK_a is 3.0, almost all of the total salicylate in both compartments exists as the salicylate anion. By increasing extracellular fluid pH, there is a shift in equilibrium toward salicylate. The resulting lower HS levels in the extracellular fluid favors diffusion out of the brain cell. Similar effects occur with urinary alkalinization permitting increased excretion.

Diarrhea

The intestinal fluids below the stomach, including pancreatic and biliary secretions, are relatively alkaline with a net base concentration of 50 to 70 mEq/L. As a result, diarrhea or the loss of pancreatic or biliary secretions can lead to metabolic acidosis. For each mole of bicarbonate lost, there is retention of equivalent amount of hydrogen ions. This is analogous to retention of HCl (see Eq. 3) and demonstrates that the buffering of the retained hydrogen ion with bicarbonate leads to increased chloride concentrations. This can also occur with surreptitious laxative abuse, which should be considered in any patient with an otherwise unexplained normal anion gap metabolic acidosis.

Treatment

Alkali therapy is indicated only in patients with moderate to severe metabolic acidosis and continuing fluid loss. In theory, the quantity of bicarbonate required to normalize the plasma bicarbonate concentration can be estimated from the following equation:

$$Bicarbonate\ deficit = Deficit\ per\ liter \times volume\ of\ distribution$$

The volume of distribution (or bicarbonate space) is normally about 50% of lean body weight, but is not a constant value. The bicarbonate space increases to 60% to 70% as acidosis worsens due to buffering from nonbicarbonate buffers. Fifty to one hundred milliequivalents of sodium bicarbonate is usually given in intravenous boluses and the effect on the plasma bicarbonate concentration is monitored. In general, alkali therapy can be discontinued once the plasma bicarbonate concentration exceeds from 12 to 15 mEq/L unless the intestinal fluid losses continue or the patient has underlying renal disease. In the latter setting, spontaneous renal correction of the acidemia via increased ammonium excretion is less likely to occur.

In summary, metabolic acidosis can result from decreased renal hydrogen ion excretion (RTA and renal failure), or from increased hydrogen ion production (Tables 6.1 and 6.2). Increased acid production occurs from two basic mechanism: loss of bicarbonate through gastrointestinal or renal losses (diarrhea, and type 2 RTA) that results in hyperchloremic metabolic acidosis, and acid generation associated with an unmeasured anion (ketoacids, lactic acids, and ingestions) that result in increased anion gap acidosis (Table 6.3).

Urine Anion Gap

The urine anion gap follows the same principles of the serum anion gap described above, and may be helpful diagnostically in some cases of normal anion gap acidosis. The major measured cations and anions in the urine are sodium, potassium, and chloride. Urinary bicarbonate and ammonium concentrations are not readily measurable. Analogous to Eq. 2,

$$Urine\ anion\ gap = \left([Na^+] + [K^+]\right) - [Cl^-] \qquad \text{(Eq. 5)}$$

$$Urine\ anion\ gap = Unmeasured\ anions - unmeasured\ cations$$

In normal subjects excreting between 20 and 40 mEq of ammonium per liter, ammonium (NH_4^+) is the major unmeasured urinary cation, and the urine anion gap typically has a positive value or is near zero. With metabolic acidosis, however, the excretion of NH_4^+ (and of chloride to maintain electroneutrality) should increase markedly resulting in a strongly negative value of -20 to -50 mEq/L. The negative value occurs from the high levels of chloride that now exceed the sum of sodium and potassium. In comparison, the acidemia of renal failure and for distal RTA is primarily due to impaired NH_4^+ excretion, and the urine anion gap typically retains its positive value (Fig. 6.3).

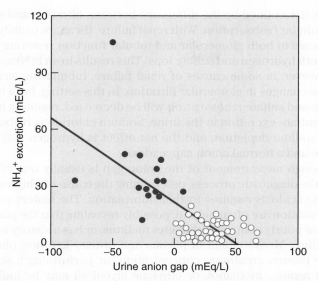

FIGURE 6.3. The relationship between the urine anion gap and the rate of NH_4^+ excretion in patients with metabolic acidosis due to diarrhea (*closed circles*) and in patients with impaired urinary acidification due to type 1 or 4 renal tubular acidosis (*open circles*).

Although helpful for distinguishing gastrointestinal from renal causes of normal anion gap acidosis, there are two circumstances in which the urine anion gap cannot be used. The first is in the presence of a high anion gap acidosis, where the excreted unmeasured anion (such as ketoacidosis) will counteract the effect of the NH_4^+. The second circumstance is volume depletion with avid sodium retention that will impair distal acidification (as discussed earlier).

Anion Gap in Renal Failure

It is important to emphasize that the increase in unmeasured anions with a high anion gap is only a clinical tool; it is the excess hydrogen ion, not the anion, that is responsible for the fall in the plasma bicarbonate concentration. This principle can be appreciated by considering the sequence of events initiated by the generation of sulfuric acid (from the metabolism of dietary proteins) in a patient with renal failure. The acid is rapidly buffered by bicarbonate and other buffers leading to the formation of sodium sulfate:

$$H_2SO_4 + 2NaHCO_3 \rightarrow Na_2SO_4 + 2H_2CO_3 \rightarrow 2CO_2 + 2H_2O$$

To maintain the steady state, both the hydrogen ions and sulfate must be excreted in the urine. Hydrogen excretion occurs primarily through ammonium production (Chapter 5), a tubular function. The excretion of sulfate is determined by the difference between filtration and some degree of tubular reabsorption. With renal failure, there are usually parallel impairments in both glomerular and tubular function resulting in retention of both hydrogen and sulfate ions. This results in an increased anion gap. However, in some causes of renal failure, tubular impairment exceeds the changes in glomerular filtration. In this setting, both hydrogen *secretion* and sulfate *reabsorption* will be decreased, resulting in normal sodium sulfate excretion in the urine. Sodium chloride is reabsorbed to prevent sodium depletion, and the net effect is hydrogen and chloride retention and a normal anion gap acidosis.

Although measurement of the anion gap is usually one of the first steps in the diagnostic process, determining the cause of a high anion gap metabolic acidosis requires further information. The history and physical examination are often helpful, possibly revealing that the patient is in shock, has poorly controlled diabetes mellitus, or has a history of chronic renal failure. Measurement of plasma and urinary ketones, plasma lactate, the plasma creatinine concentration, or performing a screen for ingested aspirin, methanol, or ethylene glycol all may be indicated in patients in whom the diagnosis is not apparent.

 A chronically ill patient develops a high fever, shaking chills, hypotension, and severe acidemia with the following arterial values:

Na^+	$= 140$ mEq/L
K^+	$= 4.6$ mEq/L
Cl^-	$= 115$ mEq/L
HCO_3^-	$= 12$ mEq/L
pH	$= 7.10$
PCO_2	$= 40$ mm Hg
Albumin	$= 1.5$ g/dL

What is the acid–base disturbance? The clinical picture suggests lactic acidosis but the physicians are confused by the anion gap of 13 mEq/L that is only a few mEq/L above normal despite a 12-mEq/L reduction in the plasma bicarbonate concentration. How can you explain this seeming discrepancy?

CASE DISCUSSION The patient presented at the beginning of the chapter has metabolic acidosis with an elevated anion gap of 27 mEq/L. In the setting of a cardiopulmonary arrest, lactic acidosis is almost certainly the underlying cause. There are, however, two problems with the patient's management. First, the assumption is that the tissue pH is being well maintained because the arterial pH is 7.30. There is a good chance that the mixed venous pH is much lower due to the reduction in pulmonary blood flow in this setting (see Table 6.4). Second, bicarbonate therapy is not indicated in almost any form of metabolic acidosis when the arterial pH is so minimally reduced. It may actually be deleterious during a cardiopulmonary arrest, since the carbon dioxide generated as excess hydrogen ions buffered by the administered bicarbonate may exacerbate the tissue and presumed intracellular acidosis.

ANSWERS TO QUESTIONS

1 Titratable acidity is limited by the rate of excretion of available buffers, particularly monobasic phosphate (HPO_4^{2-}). Phosphate excretion is primarily regulated by the state of phosphate balance, although there is a mild increase in metabolic acidosis. Thus, enhanced titratable acidity can make only a limited contribution to acid excretion if ammonium formation is reduced.

2 Patients with renal failure are unable to excrete some fraction of the daily acid load. The maximum alkali requirement would occur if none of this acid could be excreted; this is equal to the average acid load of 50 to 100 mEq/day.

3 Na_2CO_3 dissociates into $2Na + CO_3^{-2}$. The *initial* buffering reaction for carbonate CO_3^{-2} (1) generates bicarbonate rather than CO_2 (compare with the bicarbonate equation in Chapter 5, Eq. 5.3):

$$H^+ + CO_3^{2-} \rightarrow HCO_3^- + H^+ \rightarrow CO_2 + H_2O$$

Thus, there will be less CO_2 generation than with bicarbonate administration, thereby minimizing tissue CO_2 accumulation and possible worsening of the intracellular acidosis. However, animal studies of myocardial defibrillation have not found improvements in myocardial cell pH with administration, probably due to continued CO_2 production in the defibrillating cells.

4 Ketoacid anions, such as β-hydroxybutyrate, are primarily excreted with one of four cations: hydrogen, ammonium, sodium, and potassium. Excretion of the hydrogen or ammonium salt results in the loss of the acid as well as the anion, thereby correcting the acidosis. In contrast, excretion of the sodium or potassium salt results in the loss of "potential bicarbonate," since metabolism of the anion after insulin administration would have regenerated bicarbonate lost in the initial buffering of β-hydroxybutyric acid. As a result, the degree of normalization of the plasma bicarbonate concentration by insulin is limited by the quantity of ketoacid anion excreted.

5 In patients with an arterial pH below 7.40, the administration of bicarbonate to raise the pH to above 7.45 (thereby lowering the hydrogen concentration) will drive the reaction

$$H^+ + S^- \leftrightarrow HS$$

to the left. The reduction in the concentration of lipid-soluble HS in the extracellular fluid will promote the passive diffusion of HS out of the brain. Similar considerations apply to the urine. Water reabsorption will raise the HS concentration in the tubular lumen, promoting passive movement back into the extracellular fluid. Alkalinization of the urine will minimize back-diffusion by converting HS to the lipid-insoluble salicylate anion.

6 The acid–base disturbance is a mixed metabolic and respiratory acidosis. Although the PCO_2 is at the "normal" level of 40 mm Hg, this value is normal only at a plasma bicarbonate concentration of 24 mEq/L. Recall that compensation for primary processes will not correct to normal, so identifying a normal PCO_2 indicates a primary respiratory acidosis. At the plasma bicarbonate concentration of 12 mEq/L in this patient, there should be compensatory hyperventilation resulting in a PCO_2 of approximately 26 mm Hg (see Table 5.2 which lists the expected compensations in the different acid–base disorders). The pH would be much better protected at 7.27 if this had occurred.

The anion gap of 13 mEq/L seems to be only slightly elevated because it is assumed that the baseline anion gap in this patient is 9 mEq/L as in normal subjects. However, this patient has marked hypoalbuminemia, thereby decreasing the concentration of unmeasured anions. At a correction factor of 1.5 mEq/L for each 1-g/dL fall in the plasma albumin concentration, this almost 3-g/dL reduction should lower the anion gap by about 5 mEq/L. Thus, the baseline anion gap may have been approximately 6 mEq/L. Thus, an anion gap of 15 mEq/L represents an elevation of 9 mEq/L, indicating the presence of a high anion gap metabolic acidosis.

SUGGESTED READINGS

Adrogué HJ, Madias NE. Management of life-threatening acid–base disorders. N Engl J Med 1998;338:26.

Adrogué HJ, Rashad MN, Gorin AD, et al. Assessing acid–base status in circulatory failure: differences between arterial and central venous blood. N Engl J Med 1989;320:1312.

Batlle DC, Hizon M, Cohen E, et al. The use of the urine anion gap in the diagnosis of hyperchloremic metabolic acidosis. N Engl J Med 1988;318:594.

Emmett M. Anion-gap interpretation: the old and the new. Nat Clin Prac 2006;2:4.

Gabow PA. Disorders associated with an altered anion gap. Kidney Int 1985;27:472.

Rodriguez Soriano J. Renal tubular acidosis: the clinical entity. J Am Soc Nephrol 2002;13:2160.

Rose BD, Post TW. Clinical Physiology of Acid–Base and Electrolyte Disorders, 5th Ed. New York: McGraw-Hill, 2001.

Sabatini S, Kurtzman NA. Bicarbonate therapy in severe metabolic acidosis. J Am Soc Nephrol, 2009;20:692–695.

Weisfeld ML, Guerci AD. Sodium bicarbonate in CPR. JAMA 1991;266:2121.

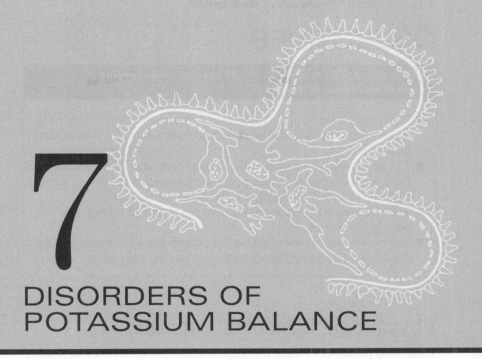

7

DISORDERS OF POTASSIUM BALANCE

A 49-year-old woman is found to have moderate hypertension that is known to be of recent onset. She is on no medication and complains only of mild muscle weakness. Physical examination reveals a blood pressure of 150/110 and proximal muscle weakness is noted.

Initial plasma and urine studies reveal the following:

Na	= 140 mEq/L (136–142)
K	= 3.1 mEq/L (3.5–5)
Cl	= 98 mEq/L (98–108)
Total CO_2	= 32 mEq/L (21–30)
Urine Na	= 80 mEq/L (variable)
K	= 60 mEq/L (variable)
Cl	= 100 mEq/L (variable)

OBJECTIVES

By the end of this section, you should have an understanding of each of the following issues:

■ The factors involved in the regulation of potassium balance, both in the transcellular distribution of potassium and in the excretion of potassium in the urine.
■ The major causes of hyperkalemia, with particular emphasis on the importance of impaired urinary potassium excretion in patients with a persistent elevation in the plasma potassium concentration.
■ The physiologic principles that govern the choice of therapies for reversing hyperkalemia.
■ The factors that can lower the plasma potassium concentration and the mechanisms by which urinary potassium wasting can occur.

Physiologic Effects of Potassium

Total body potassium stores are approximately from 3000 to 4000 mEq. Roughly 98% of the potassium is located in the cells; this distribution is in contrast to that of sodium, which is primarily limited to the extracellular fluid. The Na^+–K^+-ATPase pump in the cell membrane is responsible for the localization of potassium and sodium to separate compartments by transporting sodium out of and potassium into the cells in a 3:2 ratio (see Fig. 1.2). The net effect is that the potassium concentration in the extracellular fluid is only from 4 to 5 mEq/L, but it is as high as 140 mEq/L in the cells.

Potassium has two major physiologic functions. First, it plays an important role in regulating a variety of cell functions such as protein and glycogen synthesis. Second, the *ratio* (rather than the absolute values) of the potassium concentration in the cells ($[K^+]_{cell}$) to that in the extracellular fluid ($[K^+_{ecf}]$) is the major determinant of the resting membrane potential (E_m) across the cell membrane according to the following formula:

$$E_m = -61 \ log \frac{r[K^+]_{cell} + 0.01[Na^+]_{cell}}{r[K^+]_{ecf} + 0.01[Na^+]_{ecf}} \quad \text{(Eq. 1)}$$

where r is the 3:2 active transport ratio for the Na^+–K^+-ATPase pump and 0.01 is the relative membrane permeability of sodium to potassium. At the normal concentration of sodium and potassium in the cells and the extracellular fluid,

$$E_m = -61 \ log \frac{1.5(140) + 0.01(12)}{1.5(4.4) + 0.01(145)}$$

$$= -86 \ mV(cell\text{-}interior \ negative)$$

The resting membrane potential is important because it sets the stage for the generation of the *action potential* that is essential for normal neural and muscular function. Membrane excitability (or irritability) is equal to the difference between the resting and threshold potentials; the latter is the potential during depolarization at which an action potential is generated. Generation of the action potential is associated with a marked elevation in sodium permeability, resulting in sodium entry into the cells and complete depolarization of the cell membrane.

Changes in the plasma potassium concentration can have important effects on membrane excitability. From Eq. 1, a fall in the extracellular potassium concentration (*hypokalemia*) increases the magnitude of the resting potential (makes it more electronegative), a change that reduces membrane excitability by hyperpolarizing the membrane (i.e., increasing the difference between the resting and threshold potentials). However, changes in extracellular potassium have major effects on the state of activation of sodium channels. Hypokalemia removes the state of inactivation and inactivates sodium channels. The net effect is increased sodium entry into cells, making E_m less negative (closer to zero) and enhanced excitability that can lead to cardiac arrhythmias (see below).

Opposite changes are induced by a rise in the extracellular potassium concentration (*hyperkalemia*). The initial effect is to depolarize the membrane (make the potential less electronegative) and increase membrane excitability. This change, however, is transient, since depolarization also tends to inactivate the sodium channels in the cell membrane. Thus, persistent hyperkalemia is associated with decreased membrane excitability.

These effects on neuromuscular transmission are clinically important, because they are largely responsible for the most serious symptoms associated with disturbances in potassium balance: *muscle weakness* and potentially fatal *cardiac arrhythmias and disturbances in cardiac conduction*.

As with alterations in the plasma sodium concentration (see Chapter 3), the likelihood of inducing symptoms with alterations in potassium balance is related both to the degree and to the rapidity of change. As an example, the loss of potassium (as with severe diarrhea) will initially lower the plasma potassium concentration, have no effect on the cell potassium concentration, and therefore increase the ratio of cellular to extracellular potassium and make the resting potential more electronegative. However, the fall in the plasma potassium concentration creates a gradient that promotes potassium movement out of the cells; as this occurs, the concurrent reduction in the cell potassium concentration results in a smaller change in the ratio of cellular to extracellular potassium and therefore a lower likelihood of interfering with neuromuscular function and of inducing symptoms.

Regulation of Potassium Balance

In a normal adult with an extracellular fluid volume of 15 to 17 L and serum potassium concentration of 4 to 5 mEq/L, the total quantity of extracellular potassium is approximately from 60 to 80 mEq. This finding has important implications for the regulation of potassium balance. The ingestion of 40 mEq of potassium (as with a few large glasses of orange juice) could, if the ingested potassium initially remained in the extracellular space, double the extracellular fluid potassium concentration (measured clinically as the plasma potassium concentration) and lead to potentially serious symptoms. This does not occur because potassium regulation occurs in two steps (Table 7.1):

- Initial uptake of some of the ingested potassium into the cells, thereby limiting the rise in the plasma potassium concentration.
- Subsequent excretion of the excess potassium in the urine. On average, most of the potassium load will be excreted within 6 to 8 hours.

An understanding of the factors that regulate these two steps is clinically important, because an abnormality in one or both is present in many patients with an elevated plasma potassium concentration (*hyperkalemia*) and in some patients with a low plasma potassium concentration (*hypokalemia*).

TABLE 7.1

Major Factors Involved in Regulation of Potassium Balance

I. Potassium uptake by the cells
  A. Insulin
  B. Epinephrine (via the β_2-adrenergic receptors)
  C. Plasma potassium concentration

II. Urinary potassium excretion, which is primarily determined by secretion in the principal cells in the cortical collecting tubule
  A. Aldosterone
  B. Distal flow of sodium and water
  C. Plasma potassium concentration

Potassium Uptake by Cells

In normal subjects, three factors are of primary importance in promoting the transient movement of ingested potassium into the cells: a small elevation in plasma potassium concentration, insulin, and epinephrine (acting via the β2-adrenergic receptors). Basal levels of insulin and epinephrine appear to maintain the activity of the Na^+–K^+-ATPase pump and increases in levels of either hormone stimulate pump activity leading to increased cellular uptake. The physiologic importance of these hormones has been demonstrated by the responses to a β-adrenergic blocker. In these settings, the increment in the plasma potassium concentration after a dietary potassium load is greater and more prolonged than in normal subjects (Fig. 7.1). On the other hand, epinephrine released during a stress response drives potassium into the cells and can transiently lower the plasma potassium concentration by as much as 1 mEq/L. Other factors can also influence potassium entry into the cells as evidenced by the demonstration that the combination of β-blockade and insulin deficiency impairs but does not prevent this process.

Urinary Potassium Excretion

At a glomerular filtration rate (GFR) of 180 L/day (125 mL/min) and a plasma water potassium concentration of 4.5 mEq/L, the normal filtered

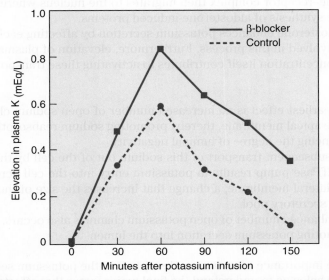

FIGURE 7.1. Sequential changes in the plasma potassium concentration after a potassium chloride infusion in controls (*solid circles*) and in subjects pretreated with propranolol, a β-adrenergic blocker (*solid squares*). The transient elevation in the plasma potassium concentration is significantly greater and more prolonged with propranolol.

load of potassium is 810 mEq. Although this is much greater than dietary intake [range equals 40 to 100 mEq on a typical diet (~1.5–4 g)], urinary potassium is *not* derived from glomerular filtration. Almost all of the filtered potassium is reabsorbed passively in the proximal tubule and thick ascending limb of the loop of Henle, with the rate of potassium excretion being primarily determined by potassium secretion from the cell into the lumen in the principal cells in the cortical collecting duct and outer medullary collecting duct.

A cell model for distal potassium secretion at these sites is depicted in Figure 7.2. Potassium secretion occurs through selective potassium channels in the apical membrane. Although the high cell potassium concentration favors diffusion into the lumen, this secretory process is markedly enhanced by the reabsorption of sodium through selective sodium channels in the apical membrane. The removal of cationic sodium from the lumen creates a lumen-negative electrical potential that promotes both potassium secretion through the apical potassium channels and chloride reabsorption between the cells across the tight junction.

Aldosterone plays a central role in the regulation of potassium excretion. A small rise in the plasma potassium concentration after a potassium load (of as little as 0.1 to 0.2 mEq/L) is sufficient to increase adrenal release of aldosterone. Aldosterone then enters the potassium-secreting cells in the distal nephron and combines with its cytosolic receptor; this hormone–receptor complex then migrates to the nucleus where it initiates the synthesis of aldosterone-induced proteins.

Aldosterone enhances potassium secretion by affecting each of the steps involved in this process. Furthermore, elevation of plasma potassium concentration itself contributes to activating these transport pathways:

- The earliest effect is an increased number of open sodium channels in the apical membrane, thereby promoting sodium reabsorption and enhancing the degree of luminal negativity.
- The subsequent transport of this sodium out of the cell by the Na^+–K^+-ATPase pump results in potassium entry into the cell across the basolateral membrane, a change that increases the size of the potassium secretory pool.
- An enhanced number of open potassium channels also occurs, further promoting potassium secretion into the lumen.

The importance of sodium reabsorption in the potassium secretory process helps us to understand the final major factor that affects potassium secretion: the distal delivery of sodium and water. At a constant aldosterone and plasma potassium concentration, increasing sodium delivery (as with a loop diuretic) will tend to enhance distal sodium

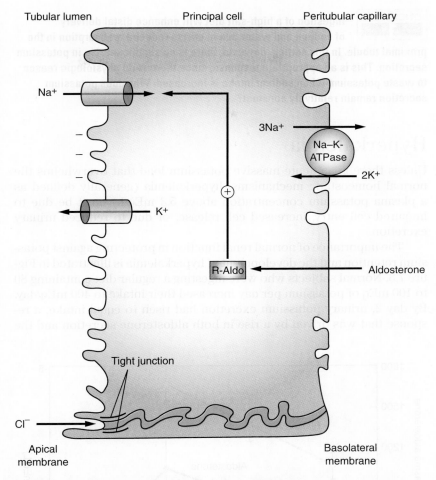

FIGURE 7.2. Schematic model of the transport pathways involved in potassium secretion in the principal cells in the cortical collecting duct and outer medullary collecting duct. Aldosterone enters the cell across the basolateral membrane and combines with its cytosolic receptor (R-Aldo), initiating a sequence of events that enhances sodium reabsorption and potassium secretion through apical membrane channels and chloride reabsorption between the cells across the tight junction.

reabsorption and thereby potassium secretion. Conversely, decreasing distal delivery will tend to diminish potassium secretion and predispose toward potassium retention and the development of hyperkalemia. A similar effect can be achieved by blocking the sodium channels with a potassium-sparing diuretic such as amiloride (see Chapter 4). The reduction in sodium entry into the cells will diminish potassium secretion as well.

QUESTION
1
Ingestion of a high-salt diet will enhance distal delivery of sodium and water due in part to reduced reabsorption in the proximal tubule. In this setting, however, there is no significant rise in potassium secretion. This is an appropriate response, since there is no physiologic reason to waste potassium when sodium intake is increased. Why does potassium secretion remain relatively constant?

Hyperkalemia

Unless there is an acute massive potassium load that overwhelms the normal homeostatic mechanisms, hyperkalemia (generally defined as a plasma potassium concentration above 5.3 mEq/L) must be due to impaired cell entry, increased cell release, or due to reduced urinary excretion.

The importance of normal renal function in protecting against potassium retention and the development of hyperkalemia is illustrated in Figure 7.3. Normal subjects who were ingesting a regular diet containing 80 to 100 mEq of potassium per day increased their intake to 400 mEq/day. By day 2, urinary potassium excretion had risen to equal intake, a response that was driven by a rise in both aldosterone secretion and the

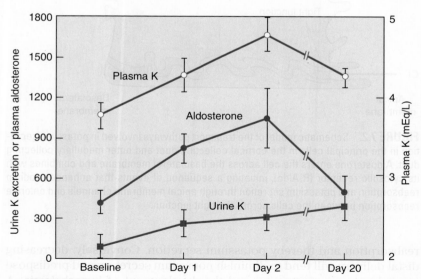

FIGURE 7.3.   Effect of increasing potassium intake from 100 to 400 mEq/day on urinary potassium excretion and the plasma aldosterone and potassium concentrations in normal subjects. Urinary excretion rises to equal intake by day 2 and persists through the study until day 20. A mild elevation in the plasma potassium concentration and an initial elevation in aldosterone release contribute to the reattainment of the steady state.

plasma potassium concentration (from 3.8 to 4.8 mEq/L). By day 20, potassium excretion had become much more efficient (a phenomenon called *potassium adaptation*) as 400 mEq is still being excreted, but the plasma aldosterone level had fallen almost to normal and the plasma potassium concentration had fallen to 4.3 mEq/L, only 0.5 mEq/L above baseline. This adaptation is mediated by increased $Na^+–K^+$-ATPase activity of the principal cells in the cortical and outer medullary collecting ducts. Enhanced pumping of potassium into these cells will increase the size of the intracellular potassium secretory pool.

This study illustrates an important physiologic principle: *hyperkalemia is always associated with an impairment in urinary potassium excretion.* We can therefore derive most of the differential diagnosis of persistent hyperkalemia simply by knowing the major factors (other than the plasma potassium concentration itself) that regulate potassium secretion: one of the causes of hypoaldosteronism, decreased distal urinary flow due to marked volume depletion (as in advanced heart failure) or advanced renal failure (too few functioning nephrons to excrete the potassium load). Impaired cell entry generally induces acute but not chronic hyperkalemia, since the extra potassium will ultimately be excreted in the urine if renal function is intact.

Etiology

The most common causes of hyperkalemia are listed in Table 7.2, according to the mechanism responsible. Several of these disorders will be reviewed briefly because of the pathophysiologic principles involved.

Metabolic Acidosis
Many of the excess hydrogen ions that accumulate in metabolic acidosis are buffered in the cells (see Chapter 5 and Fig. 7.4). The major extracellular anion chloride enters the cells to only a limited degree; as a result, electroneutrality is preserved in this setting by the movement of cellular potassium and sodium into the extracellular fluid. The net effect is a variable elevation in the plasma potassium concentration that averages 0.6 mEq/L (with a very wide range of 0.2 to 1.7 mEq/L) for every 0.1 pH unit fall in extracellular pH.

The actual plasma potassium concentration that is seen varies with the underlying disorder, although it will generally be elevated in relation to body potassium stores. Thus, the degree of hyperkalemia may be exacerbated in advanced chronic renal failure by the concurrent metabolic acidosis. On the other hand, a disorder such as diarrhea is commonly associated with potassium depletion due to gastrointestinal losses. As a result, hypokalemia is often present, but the metabolic acidosis will cause the plasma potassium concentration to be higher than it would be if the extracellular pH were normal. Correction of the acidemia in this

TABLE 7.2

Major Causes of Hyperkalemia

I. Increased potassium intake—may play a contributory role but not an independent cause of hyperkalemia unless a large amount is acutely ingested or infused

II. Decreased potassium entry into cells or increased potassium release from cells
    A. Metabolic acidosis
    B. Insulin deficiency and hyperglycemia in uncontrolled diabetes mellitus
    C. β-adrenergic blockade—may cause an enhanced rise in the plasma potassium concentration after a potassium load, but will not cause persistent hyperkalemia since the extra potassium will be excreted in the urine
    D. Increased tissue breakdown releasing potassium from cells, as with muscle breakdown (rhabdomyolysis) following trauma or a crush injury
    E. Exercise

III. Reduced potassium excretion in the urine
    A. Diminished distal delivery of sodium and water, typically associated with a significant decline in glomerular filtration rate
        1. Advanced renal failure, especially when the urine output is decreased
        2. Marked effective circulating volume depletion as in severe congestive heart failure
    B. Hypoaldosteronism
        1. Hyporeninemic hypoaldosteronism
        2. Angiotensin-converting enzyme inhibitors, which lower aldosterone release by inhibiting the formation of angiotensin II
        3. Nonsteroidal anti-inflammatory drugs, which act in part by removing the stimulatory effect of renal prostaglandins on the release of renin
        4. Potassium-sparing diuretics, which directly block sodium reabsorption and potassium secretion in the collecting tubules (see Chapter 4)
        5. Primary adrenal insufficiency

setting will unmask this phenomenon, leading to a further reduction in the plasma potassium concentration unless potassium supplements are also administered.

For reasons that are not well understood, the shift of potassium out of the cells is minimized in organic acidoses such as lactic acidosis or ketoacidosis. One possible contributory factor is that the organic anion may be able to follow hydrogen into the cells (perhaps as the undissociated, lipid-soluble intact acid), thereby removing the necessity for the redistribution of potassium. A transcellular shift of potassium does occur in diabetic ketoacidosis, frequently resulting in hyperkalemia at presentation

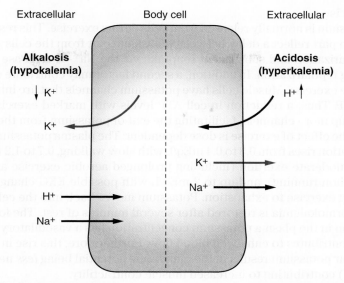

FIGURE 7.4. Reciprocal cation shifts of H$^+$, K$^+$, and Na$^+$ between the cells and the extracellular fluid. In the presence of a mineral acid load, H$^+$ moves into the cells where it is buffered. To maintain electroneutrality, K$^+$ and Na$^+$ leave the cell, resulting in an increased K serum concentration. The reverse occurs in the setting of a metabolic alkalosis.

even though body potassium stores are often markedly reduced due to the glucosuria-induced osmotic diuresis. However, factors other than metabolic acidosis appear to be primarily responsible in this setting.

Insulin Deficiency and Hyperglycemia

The redistribution of potassium out of the cells in uncontrolled diabetes mellitus is due in part to insulin deficiency. However, the associated hyperglycemia and hyperosmolality probably play a more important role. The elevation in plasma osmolality promotes the osmotic movement of water out of the cells, leading to the parallel movement of potassium into the extracellular fluid. Two factors contribute to this response. First, the loss of water raises the intracellular potassium concentration, thereby creating a favorable concentration gradient for passive potassium exit through selective *potassium channels* in the cell membrane. Second, the frictional forces between solvent (water) and solute results in potassium being carried out of the cell along with water through the aquaporins (*water channels*) in the cell membrane.

The administration of insulin reverses the insulin deficiency and hyperglycemia, leading to rapid movement of potassium into the cells. The plasma potassium concentration frequently falls to below normal as the underlying potassium depletion is unmasked.

Exercise

Potassium is normally released from cells during exercise. This response may in part reflect a delay between potassium exit from the cells during depolarization and subsequent reuptake via the Na^+–K^+-ATPase pump during repolarization. In addition, a second factor may contribute during severe exercise. Muscle cells have potassium channels that are inhibited by ATP. Thus, a reduction in cell ATP levels with marked exercise can open up more channels, facilitating the exit of potassium from the cells.

The effect of exercise is dose dependent: The plasma potassium concentration rises from 0.3 to 0.4 mEq/L with slow walking, 0.7 to 1.2 mEq/L with moderate exertion (including prolonged aerobic exercise as with marathon running), and up to 2 mEq/L with possible EKG changes following exercise to exhaustion. Potassium moves back into the cells and the normokalemia is restored after several minutes of rest. The local elevation in the plasma potassium concentration has a vasodilatory effect and contributes to enhanced blood flow. Furthermore, this rise in extracellular potassium results in the membrane potential being *less* negative (Eq. 1) contributing to increased muscle contractility.

Renal Failure

Potassium balance is generally well maintained even in moderate to advanced renal failure because increased potassium excretion per functioning nephron can balance the decline in the number of functioning nephrons. This represents another example of potassium adaptation that is mediated in part by enhanced Na^+–K^+-ATPase activity in the potassium-secreting cells.

The ability to maintain a normal plasma potassium concentration ultimately becomes impaired by two factors: There are now too few nephrons to excrete the dietary potassium load, and the urine output may fall, thereby decreasing distal sodium and water delivery. When hyperkalemia develops in a nonoliguric (urine output >400 mL/day) patient with mild to moderate renal failure, some other factor is generally superimposed such as an increased potassium load (due to enhanced intake or tissue breakdown) or one of the forms of hypoaldosteronism.

 A patient with advanced renal failure has an impairment in potassium excretion, leading to potassium retention. The plasma potassium concentration rises to 5.6 mEq/L and then stabilizes. What protective mechanisms allowed the steady state to be reattained? Why don't these adaptations return the plasma potassium concentration to normal?

Hypoaldosteronism

The major physiologic stimuli to the release of aldosterone are angiotensin II (generated in part by the release of renin from the kidney)

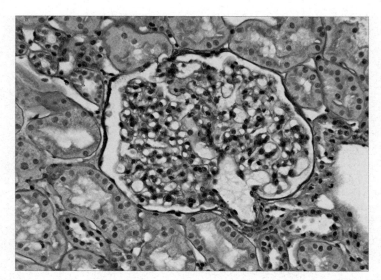

Color Fig. 1. Minimal change disease. The glomerulus shows a normal architecture, with open capillaries and no signs of active inflammation or sclerosis. (Periodic acid Schiff stain [PAS])

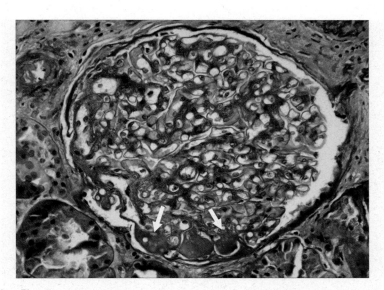

Color Fig. 2. Focal and segmental glomerulosclerosis (FSGS). This glomerulus is slightly enlarged and reveals a segmental area of the tuft with obsolescent capillaries that appear occluded by hyaline masses and occasional foam cells (arrows). There is also adhesion of the tuft to Bowman's capsule in the area of sclerosis. It is impossible by light microscopy alone to determine if this is an idiopathic form of FSGS with diffuse effacement of foot processes of the visceral epithelial cells or if it is adaptive and due hemodynamic changes. (PAS)

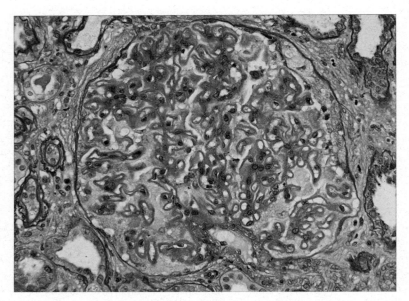

Color Fig. 3. Membranous nephropathy. This glomerulus reveals diffusely thickened basement membranes, open capillaries, and no signs of inflammation. (PAS)

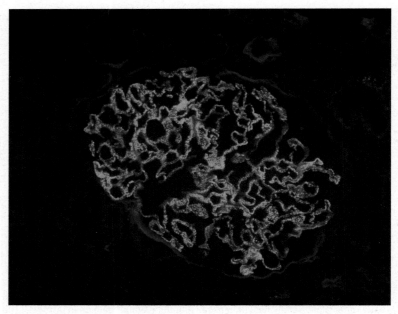

Color Fig. 4. Membranous nephropathy. This immunofluorescence microscopy image reveals diffuse granular deposits of IgG along the peripheral glomerular capillary walls. (fluorescein isothiocyanate-labeled antibody against gamma heavy chains of human IgG [FITC-anti-IgG])

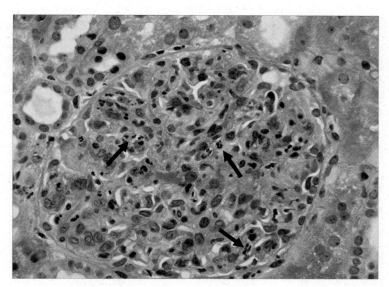

Color Fig. 5. Diffuse proliferative glomerulonephritis in a patient with acute post-streptococcal glomerulonephritis. This process is usually diffuse (it affects all glomeruli) and global, since the entire tuft is hypercellular. Most of the glomerular capillaries are occluded by inflammatory cells, many of them are neutrophils (arrows). (Hematoxylin and eosin stain [H&E])

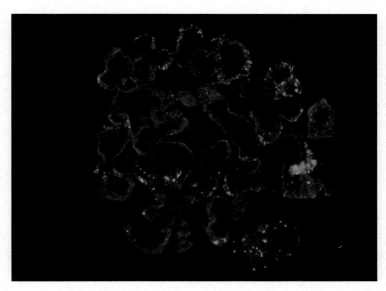

Color Fig. 6. Diffuse proliferative glomerulonephritis. There is sparse granular deposition of IgG along the peripheral capillary loops. The deposition of complement components, in particular C3 (not shown here), is usually more prominent and follows the same pattern of distribution. (FITC-anti-IgG)

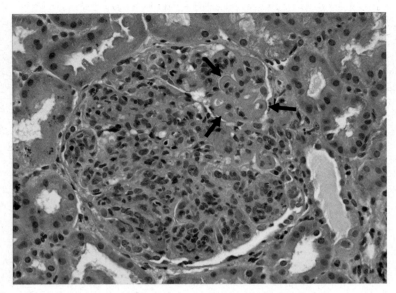

Color Fig. 7. Diffuse proliferative glomerulonephritis in a patient with diffuse lupus nephritis. In addition to the global hypercellularity depicted in this image, several loops reveal broad, eosinophilic deposits. These large and confluent subendothelial immune complexes are denominated "wire loops" (arrows) and are characteristic of diseases with a "serum sickness" pathophysiology. (H&E)

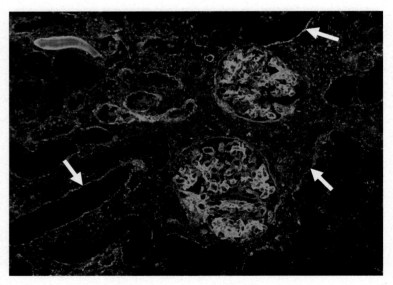

Color Fig. 8. Diffuse lupus nephritis. Fine granular deposits of IgG and complement components are present not only along the glomerular capillary walls, but also in the mesangium and along the tubular basement membranes (arrows). This image shows the location of the IgG deposits. (FITC-anti-IgG)

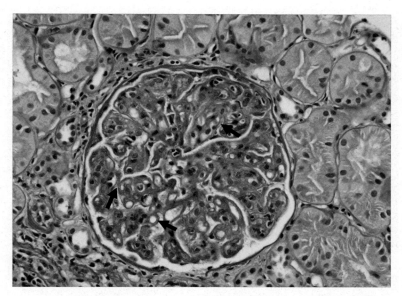

Color Fig. 9. Membranoproliferative glomerulonephritis in a patient with hepatitis C infection and circulating cryoglobulins. The glomerulus reveals diffuse hypercellularity of the tuft, mostly due to infiltration of the mesangial areas, and thickened capillary walls and basement membranes with "double contours" (arrows). (PAS)

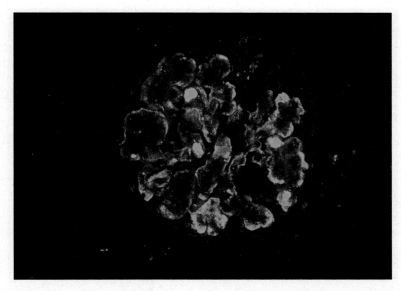

Color Fig. 10. Membranoproliferative glomerulonephritis in hepatitis C infection. There is coarse, irregular, and confluent deposition of IgM, IgG and complement components along the peripheral capillary loops; shown here is the distribution of IgM deposition. (FITC-anti-IgM)

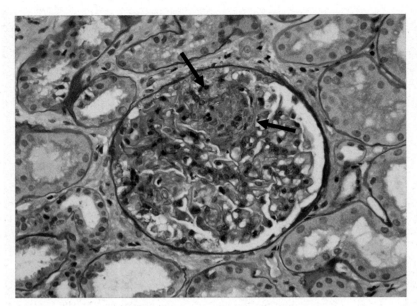

Color Fig. 11. Focal proliferative glomerulonephritis in a patient with gross hematuria and IgA nephropathy. There is segmental hypercellularity of the tuft (arrows) and mild diffuse expansion of the mesangial areas. (PAS)

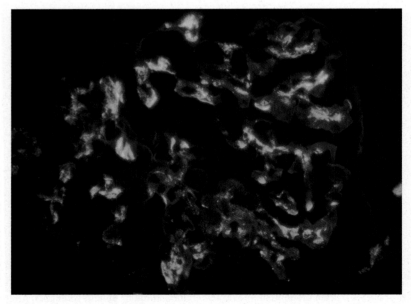

Color Fig. 12. IgA nephropathy. The mesangial areas reveal confluent and granular deposits of IgA; there is often also less intense IgG deposition and complement components in a similar distribution. (FITC-anti-IgA)

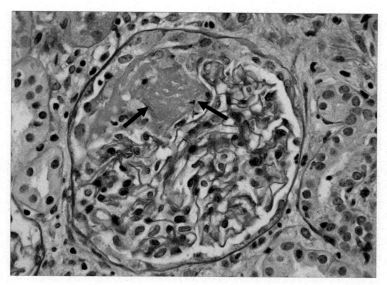

Color Fig. 13. Focal necrotizing glomerulonephritis in a patient with rapidly-progressive glomerulonephritis due to ANCA-associated polyangiitis. The glomerular tuft shows a segmental area of fibrinoid necrosis (arrows) and a small cellular crescent in the adjacent Bowman space. (PAS)

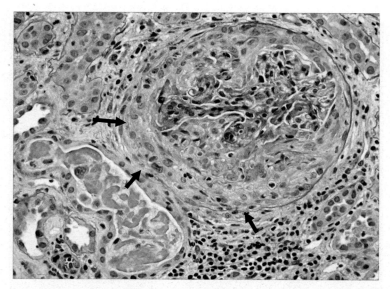

Color Fig. 14. Crescentic glomerulonephritis in a patient with anti-GBM disease and Goodpasture syndrome. The cellular crescent is large and surrounds the entire glomerular tuft. The glomerular capillaries appear compressed by the crescent. Notice also the focal discontinuities of the basement membrane of Bowman's capsule (arrows) and the associated inflammation that extends into the periglomerular interstitium. (PAS)

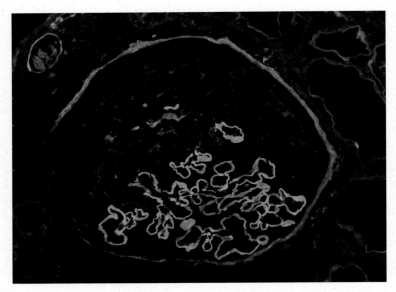

Color Fig. 15. Anti-GBM disease. There is diffuse and continuous linear or ribbon-like deposition of IgG along the glomerular basement membranes and less intense along Bowman's capsule. The distended Bowman's space is occupied by a cellular crescent (not stained with IgG). (FITC-anti-IgG)

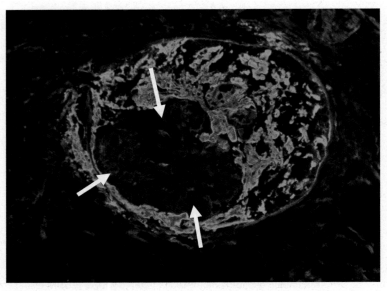

Color Fig. 16. Crescentic glomerulonephritis. This glomerulus shows prominent fibrin deposits between the inflammatory cells within the active cellular crescent. The central area not stained for fibrin (arrows) is occupied by the compressed glomerular tuft. (FITC-anti-fibrin)

and a rise in the plasma potassium concentration (see Chapter 2). Thus, hyperkalemia due to decreased aldosterone effect is usually due to renal disease (impairing renin secretion), adrenal dysfunction (impairing aldosterone release), or tubular resistance to aldosterone (Table 7.2).

The effect of hypoaldosteronism on the plasma potassium concentration can be appreciated from the experiments in Figure 7.5. Adrenalectomized dogs were given different levels of aldosterone replacement and the steady state plasma potassium concentration was noted at different levels of potassium intake. The horizontal dotted line shows the observed plasma potassium concentrations on 50 mEq/day potassium intake in animals treated with high (250 μg/day), normal (50 μg/day), or low (20 μg/day) aldosterone supplementation. As expected, in animals with lower than normal aldosterone supplementation, there were higher serum potassium levels. Another way to view the data is that for any given plasma potassium concentration, potassium excretion increases with higher aldosterone doses.

The diminished efficiency of potassium excretion with hypoaldosteronism does not prevent the reattainment of the steady state in which

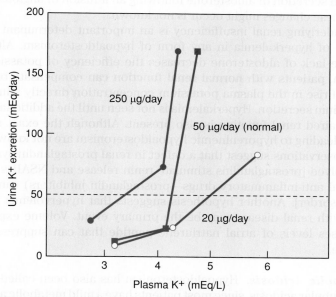

FIGURE 7.5. Mean values for plasma potassium concentration and steady state urinary potassium excretion (which is roughly equal to intake) in adrenalectomized dogs given high (250 μg/day), normal (50 μg/day), or low (20 μg/day) levels of aldosterone replacement. At any given level of potassium intake (such as the *dashed line* at 50 mEq/day), the plasma potassium concentration was lower with hyperaldosteronism and higher with hypoaldosteronism.

intake and excretion are roughly equal; however, a higher than normal plasma potassium concentration is required to counteract the decreased availability of aldosterone. This is similar to the studies in normal humans in Figure 7.3; a small rise in the plasma potassium concentration provides a sufficient signal to maintain potassium excretion at high levels without requiring a persistent increase in aldosterone secretion (Fig. 7.3; day 20).

Etiology. The most common causes of hypoaldosteronism in adults are the administration of a potassium-sparing diuretic and hyporeninemic hypoaldosteronism (Table 7.2). The latter disorder is, in the absence of an obvious etiology such as advanced renal failure or potassium-sparing diuretics, responsible for approximately 50% to 75% of cases of persistent hyperkalemia in adults. Most affected patients have diabetic nephropathy and a mild to moderate reduction in the GFR (creatinine clearance ranging between 20 and 75 mL/min).

The pathogenesis of hyporeninemic hypoaldosteronism is incompletely understood. In addition to a primary reduction in renin release, there is also evidence for an *intra-adrenal* defect characterized by decreased secretion of aldosterone following an infusion of angiotensin II. How these changes might occur is not known.

Underlying renal insufficiency is an important determinant of the degree of hyperkalemia in any form of hypoaldosteronism. Although relative lack of aldosterone decreases the efficiency of potassium secretion, patients with normal renal function can compensate because a small rise in the plasma potassium concentration directly stimulates potassium secretion. Hyperkalemia is not seen until the additional insult of impaired renal function is also present. Although the exact mechanisms leading to hyporeninemic hypoaldosteronism are not known, several observations suggest that a defect in renal prostaglandin synthesis is involved [prostaglandins stimulate renin release and NSAIDs (nonsteroidal anti-inflammatory drugs—prostaglandin inhibitors) can cause this disorder]. Another hypothesis suggests that hypervolemia associated with renal disease may be the primary event. Volume expansion increases levels of atrial natriuretic peptide that can suppress renin release.

Metabolic Acidosis. Hypoaldosteronism has also been called type 4 renal tubular acidosis, since most patients have a mild metabolic acidosis with the plasma bicarbonate concentration usually being between 17 and 21 mEq/L. Aldosterone can directly stimulate distal hydrogen secretion and reducing aldosterone will promote the development of metabolic acidosis. However, hyperkalemia appears to be of greater importance, since lowering the plasma potassium concentration induces partial or even complete normalization of the plasma bicarbonate concentration.

Can you derive a mechanism by which hyperkalemia could reduce acid and ammonium excretion? Consider where the excess potassium will be distributed and how electroneutrality will be maintained.

Symptoms

The symptoms associated with hyperkalemia are limited to muscle weakness (due to interference with neuromuscular transmission) and abnormal cardiac conduction. Disturbances in cardiac conduction induced by hyperkalemia can lead to cardiac arrest and death. As a result, monitoring of the EKG is an essential part of the management of this disorder. The approximate relationship between the plasma potassium concentration and the EKG is depicted in Figure 7.6, although there is marked variability among patients in the level at which particular changes will be seen. The earliest alteration is peaked and narrowed T waves due to more rapid repolarization; this change in T-wave configuration generally becomes apparent when the plasma potassium concentration exceeds from 6 to 7 mEq/L. Above 7 to 8 mEq/L, depolarization may become delayed (due to decreased excitability as described at the beginning of this chapter), leading to widening of the QRS complex and eventual loss of the P wave. The final changes are a sine wave pattern as the widened QRS complex merges with the T wave, followed by ventricular fibrillation or standstill.

Treatment

Treatment of hyperkalemia generally involves removal of the excess potassium from the body (Table 7.3). The major exception occurs in a disorder such as uncontrolled diabetes mellitus where the patient is actually potassium depleted and the elevation in plasma potassium concentration is due to a transcellular shift that can be reversed by therapy of the underlying disease.

Optimal treatment varies with the severity of the hyperkalemia. General principles include avoidance of potassium supplements and

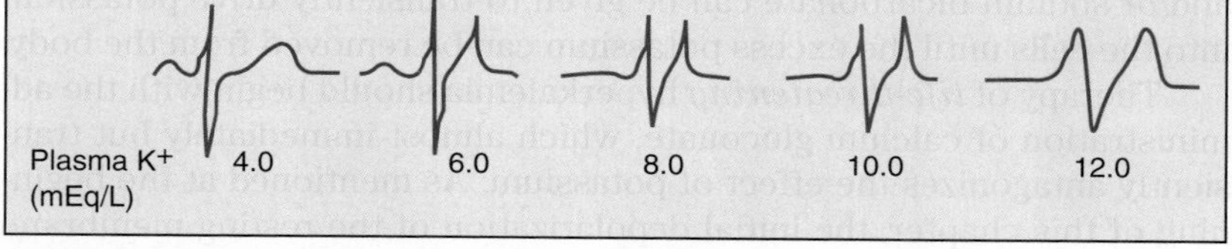

FIGURE 7.6. Electrocardiogram in relation to the plasma potassium concentration in hyperkalemia. The initial change is peaking and narrowing of the T wave, followed by widening of the QRS complex, loss of the P wave, and a sine wave pattern as the QRS complex merges with the T wave.

TABLE 7.3

Treatment of Hyperkalemia	
Mechanism	**Onset of Action**
I. Antagonism of membrane actions A. Calcium	Several minutes and then rapidly wanes
II. Increased potassium entry into cells A. Insulin and glucose B. β2-adrenergic agonists C. Sodium bicarbonate	Each of these modalities works within 30–60 minutes, lowers the plasma potassium concentration by 0.5–1.5 mEq/L, and lasts for several hours
III. Potassium removal from the body A. Diuretics B. Cation exchange resin C. Dialysis	Diuretics take several hours but patients with advanced renal failure may show little response Exchange resins take 2–3 hours Several hours

discontinuation of drugs that can lower aldosterone release (Table 7.2). Patients with a plasma potassium concentration below 6.0 mEq/L usually respond to the combination of a loop diuretic and a low-potassium diet. Asymptomatic patients with a plasma potassium concentration above 6.0 to 6.5 mEq/L can be treated with a cation exchange resin, given orally or by colonic enema. The most commonly used resin, sodium polystyrene sulfonate (Kayexalate), takes up potassium in the gut and releases sodium.

Indications for the other treatment modalities for hyperkalemia listed in Table 7.3 are for more marked or symptomatic hyperkalemia, where you cannot safely wait several hours for the resin to work. In this setting, insulin and glucose (10 units of insulin with at least 40 g of glucose to prevent hypoglycemia), a β2-adrenergic agonist (such as albuterol), and/or sodium bicarbonate can be given to transiently drive potassium into the cells until the excess potassium can be removed from the body.

Therapy of *life-threatening* hyperkalemia should begin with the administration of calcium gluconate, which almost immediately but transiently antagonizes the effect of potassium. As mentioned at the beginning of this chapter, the initial depolarization of the resting membrane potential induced by hyperkalemia inactivates the sodium channels in the cell membrane leading to a decrease in membrane excitability. Calcium reverses this effect and restores membrane excitability toward normal by a mechanism that is not well understood. In patients with severe renal failure or on dialysis, acute dialysis may be indicated for potassium removal.

Hypokalemia

Hypokalemia is most often induced by increased gastrointestinal or urinary losses, although increased entry into the cell can also occur (Table 7.4). A low-potassium diet alone generally has a relatively minor effect on the plasma potassium concentration, since urinary potassium excretion can be reduced to less than 15 to 25 mEq/day with potassium depletion. This response is mediated in part by a direct inhibitory effect of hypokalemia both on potassium secretion in the principal cells in the collecting ducts (Fig. 7.2) and on aldosterone release.

In addition, potassium can be reabsorbed by the acid-secreting intercalated cells in the cortical collecting duct. As shown in Figure 5.2, some of the hydrogen ions are secreted by a $H^+–K^+$-ATPase, which reabsorbs potassium as it secretes hydrogen. The activity of this transporter

TABLE 7.4

Major Causes of Hypokalemia

I. Decreased dietary intake—may play a contributory role but is rarely solely responsible for hypokalemia

II. Increased entry into the cells—generally produces only a transient reduction in the plasma potassium concentration
  A. Metabolic alkalosis
  B. Increased β-adrenergic activity, as with epinephrine release during a stress response

III. Enhanced gastrointestinal losses
  A. Vomiting
  B. Diarrhea
  C. Nasogastric Tube drainage

IV. Increased urinary losses—typically requires hyperaldosteronism and normal to enhanced distal flow
  A. Loop and thiazide-type diuretics
  B. Vomiting
  C. Primary mineralocorticoid excess, most often due to aldosterone-producing adrenal adenoma
  D. Secondary hyperaldosteronism due to renal artery stenosis
  E. Renal tubular acidosis

is increased with potassium depletion (the signal for which might be a reduction in the cell potassium concentration); the net effect is increased potassium reabsorption and an appropriately lower rate of potassium excretion.

Etiology

The major causes of hypokalemia are listed in Table 7.4. The transcellular shifts and increase in urinary potassium excretion generally involve mechanisms similar to but in the opposite direction from those described for hyperkalemia. As an example, a β-blocker may transiently raise the plasma potassium concentration after a potassium load (Fig. 7.1), while epinephrine released during a stress response can induce transient hypokalemia due to potassium movement into the cells.

Urinary Potassium Wasting
Two factors are generally required to cause hypokalemia by inappropriately increasing distal potassium secretion: enhanced secretion of aldosterone (as in left curve in Fig. 7.5), and normal or elevated delivery of sodium and water to the potassium secretory site. Loop and thiazide-type diuretics, for example, increase distal delivery by impairing sodium reabsorption in the loop of Henle or distal tubule, respectively, and they enhance the secretion of aldosterone by inducing volume depletion.

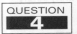 **Administration of a diuretic leads to potassium depletion because urinary excretion exceeds intake. What counterregulatory factors will tend to diminish potassium excretion and allow the steady state for potassium balance to be reestablished?**

Vomiting. Hypokalemia with vomiting is primarily due to urinary rather than gastrointestinal losses. Potassium wasting primarily occurs in the first few days, when the associated elevation in plasma bicarbonate concentration causes the filtered bicarbonate load to exceed reabsorptive capacity; as a result, more sodium bicarbonate is delivered out of the proximal tubule, which, in combination with volume depletion–induced hyperaldosteronism, will enhance potassium secretion (see Table 5.4).

Hypokalemia and Metabolic Alkalosis with and without Hypertension

Primary Hyperaldosteronism. Some patients have primary overproduction of aldosterone, most often due to an adrenal adenoma. Patients with this disorder initially retain sodium and remain slightly volume expanded and are usually hypertensive. Once again, increased aldosterone levels and adequate distal delivery lead to potassium wasting. The aldosterone stimulation of H^+-ATPase frequently results in metabolic alkalosis in addition to hypokalemia.

One rare cause of this disorder, excess ingestion of real licorice, has helped to shed important light on the mechanism by which mineralocorticoid activity is regulated in target cells, such as those in the collecting ducts. Licorice contains a steroid, glycyrrhetinic acid, that has slight aldosterone-like activity. More importantly, glycyrrhetinic acid inhibits the enzyme 11β-hydroxysteroid dehydrogenase. This enzyme, which is largely restricted in the kidney to the aldosterone-sensitive sites in the collecting ducts, promotes the conversion of cortisol to cortisone. This effect is physiologically important, because cortisol but not cortisone binds as avidly as aldosterone to the mineralocorticoid receptor. Although cortisol has a much higher plasma concentration than aldosterone, it does not normally have much mineralocorticoid activity since it is locally converted to inactive cortisone. Inhibiting this conversion with glycyrrhetinic acid allows normal levels of cortisol to induce an often marked elevation in net mineralocorticoid activity and hypokalemia.

Liddle syndrome is another disorder characterized by hypokalemia, metabolic alkalosis similar to hyperaldosteronism, but is independent of mineralocorticoids. This is an autosomal dominant condition characterized by a *gain of function* mutation in the collecting duct sodium channel (Fig. 7.2). It can be distinguished from hyperaldosteronism by the combination of *low* renin and aldosterone levels, and can be treated with sodium channel antagonists amiloride or triamterene (Chapter 4).

Bartter and Gitelman syndromes are rare hereditary disorders that present with hypokalemia, metabolic alkalosis but no hypertension. The pathogenesis is similar to that seen with loop and thiazide diuretics. Bartter syndrome has been described with mutations in any of the transporters of the thick ascending limb of Henle (Chapter 1). The genetic defects in Gitelman syndrome are in the thiazide sensitive Na–Cl cotransporter in the distal tubule. The sodium depletion in both disorders result in hyperreninemia and hyperaldosteronism. Consistent with functions of these nephron segments (Chapter 1), there are variable degrees of hypomagnesemia, and opposite effects on calcium excretion. Gitelman syndrome is associated with *hypocalciuria*; Bartter syndrome with *hyper*calciuria.

Renal Tubular Acidosis. The characteristics of the two major forms of renal tubular acidosis (RTA)—type 1 or distal RTA and type 2 or proximal RTA—are described in Chapter 6. Each can induce urinary potassium wasting and hypokalemia, although the mechanism is different. Patients with type 2 RTA have a reduced capacity for proximal bicarbonate re-absorption. They generally remain in normal or near-normal potassium balance if untreated, since the plasma bicarbonate concentration will have fallen to a low level at which all of the filtered bicarbonate can be reabsorbed. If, however, alkali therapy is given to raise the plasma bicarbonate concentration, the filtered load will exceed reabsorptive capacity and the ensuing increase in delivery of sodium bicarbonate to the potassium secretory site will stimulate potassium secretion.

A different mechanism is involved in type 1 RTA in which distal acidi-fication is impaired and the urine pH is persistently above 5.5, due in some cases to decreased activity of the H^+-ATPase pump. The lumen-negative potential generated by the reabsorption of sodium through sodium chan-nels in the apical membrane (Fig. 7.2) can be dissipated only by chloride reabsorption or by potassium or hydrogen secretion. The availability of chloride is limited and the impairment in hydrogen secretion means that potassium secretion must be increased to maintain electroneutrality as sodium is reabsorbed.

Symptoms

Most patients with chronic hypokalemia are asymptomatic and the low plasma potassium concentration is incidentally discovered on a blood test. If, however, the plasma potassium concentration is below 3 mEq/L, patients may complain of muscle weakness (induced in part by the change in resting membrane potential) and polyuria and polydipsia (in-creased thirst) due to resistance to antidiuretic hormone (nephrogenic di-abetes insipidus; see Chapter 3). The mechanism by which hypokalemia interferes with the action of ADH is not well understood, but there are decreased levels of aquaporin-2, the ADH-sensitive water channel. Hy-pokalemia can also predispose to EKG changes (such as depression of the ST segment, flattening of the T waves, and increased promi-nence of U waves) and to a variety of cardiac arrhythmias, particularly in patients taking digitalis or having acute coronary ischemia. In the latter setting, stress-induced epinephrine release can contribute by fur-ther reducing the plasma potassium concentration. Hypokalemia both increases automaticity and delays repolarization. As a result, a wide va-riety of arrhythmias can be seen, including premature atrial or ventric-ular beats, atrioventricular block, and even ventricular tachycardia or fibrillation.

Diagnosis

The cause of hypokalemia is usually evident from the history, with gas-trointestinal losses and diuretic therapy being most common. When the cause is not apparent, measurement of other laboratory tests is often helpful. For example, the most likely causes of unexplained hypokalemia in a normotensive patient are surreptitious vomiting, diarrhea, or diuretic therapy with a loop or thiazide-type diuretic.

 How might the plasma bicarbonate concentration, extracellular pH, and urinary potassium excretion help to distinguish between these disorders? Would the plasma renin activity be of any value?

In comparison, the major differential diagnosis in a hypertensive patient (as in the case at the beginning of this chapter) is surreptitious diuretic use, primary hyperaldosteronism, or renal artery stenosis (see Case Discussion below).

Treatment

Except for transient entry into the cells, the treatment of hypokalemia consists of the administration of potassium, usually as potassium chloride. An alternative in patients with chronic urinary potassium wasting due to continued diuretic therapy or nonoperable primary hyperaldosteronism is the administration of a potassium-sparing diuretic that closes the apical membrane sodium channels in Figure 7.2.

The total potassium deficit can only be approximated from the extracellular concentration, since almost all of the body potassium is located in the cells. In general, from 200 to 400 mEq of potassium must be lost to lower the plasma potassium concentration from 4.0 to 3.0 mEq/L and a similar quantity must be lost to reduce the plasma potassium concentration to 2.0 mEq/L. More severe hypokalemia is relatively rare, because potassium release from the cells can usually prevent a further fall in the plasma potassium concentration.

As with metabolic alkalosis (see Chapter 5), the administered potassium must be given with chloride or, if the patient also has metabolic acidosis, with bicarbonate. Consider, on the other hand, what would happen if potassium sulfate were given. The sulfate will be filtered and then partially reabsorbed in the proximal tubule. At the distal potassium secretory site depicted in Figure 7.2, sodium reabsorption makes the lumen electronegative; electroneutrality is maintained by potassium secretion, by chloride reabsorption—a process that largely occurs between the cells across the tight junction—or by hydrogen secretion in the adjacent intercalated cells. If nonreabsorbable sulfate rather than chloride is in the lumen, then sodium reabsorption will be matched in part by increased potassium and hydrogen secretion, thereby minimizing correction of the hypokalemia and concomitant metabolic alkalosis. If, however, potassium chloride were given, then distal sodium reabsorption can be matched by chloride reabsorption, thereby allowing the administered potassium to be retained.

CASE DISCUSSION

The patient presented at the beginning of the chapter has the recent onset of hypertension accompanied by hypokalemia, urinary potassium wasting (urinary potassium excretion should be below 25 mEq/day in the presence of hypokalemia), and metabolic alkalosis. The muscle weakness is probably due to the hypokalemia.

This constellation of findings is suggestive of hyperaldosteronism, which, in this setting, is most often due to one of three disorders:

- Primary hyperaldosteronism.
- Secondary hyperaldosteronism due to renal artery stenosis, a setting in which renal ischemia leads to enhanced renin secretion.
- Diuretic ingestion (which may be surreptitious) in a patient with underlying essential hypertension.

The diagnosis of surreptitious diuretic ingestion, which is not a rare disorder, can be established only by analyzing the urine for the presence of a diuretic. In this case, however, the recent onset of hypertension suggests one of the other two disorders since the onset of essential hypertension is not so abrupt.

Measurement of the plasma renin activity may be very helpful. Renin secretion is increased in renal artery stenosis but is markedly and appropriately suppressed by the volume expansion (induced by initial sodium retention) in primary hyperaldosteronism. The presence of renal artery stenosis, which is much more common, can be confirmed by performing a renal arteriogram in which radiocontrast media is injected directly into the renal arteries.

ANSWERS TO QUESTIONS

1 Volume expansion induced by the high-salt diet will decrease the activity of the renin–angiotensin–aldosterone system. The reduction in aldosterone secretion will tend to diminish potassium secretion, thereby counteracting the effect of increased distal flow. The decline in aldosterone levels will also diminish collecting duct sodium reabsorption, an appropriate response that will facilitate excretion of the excess sodium. The net effect is that aldosterone can contribute to the maintenance of sodium balance without interfering with potassium homeostasis.

2 Potassium is retained because the renal disease has impaired the efficiency of potassium excretion. The elevation in the plasma potassium concentration will tend to increase potassium excretion both by direct effects on the cortical collecting duct and by stimulating the release of aldosterone. The plasma potassium concentration will stabilize at a higher than normal concentration that is sufficient to increase the rate of excretion to match daily intake. These compensatory responses cannot

normalize the plasma potassium concentration, since a variable degree of chronic hyperkalemia is required to provide the signal for these adaptations to persist.

3 Since 98% of the body potassium is in the cells, most of the retained potassium will enter the cells. Electroneutrality will be maintained in part by the movement of cellular hydrogen and sodium out of the cells; the ensuing intracellular alkalosis in the renal tubular cells will diminish both acid secretion and ammonium generation (see Chapter 5).

4 The fall in the plasma potassium concentration itself will tend to diminish potassium secretion and increase potassium reabsorption by activating H^+–K^+-ATPase pumps in the luminal membrane of the cortical collecting duct. Within 1 to 2 weeks, these potassium-retaining forces will exactly balance the potassium-losing effect of the diuretic and a new steady state will be achieved. At this time, intake and output will again be equal but the plasma potassium concentration will be reduced due to the potassium lost before equilibrium was reestablished. In addition to the natriuretic response to the diuretic, increased urine flow and distal sodium delivery also return to match intake once steady state is obtained (Chapter 4).

5 Diarrhea tends to induce a metabolic acidosis (due to bicarbonate loss in the diarrheal fluid), leading to a low bicarbonate concentration and extra-cellular pH. In comparison, both diuretics and vomiting are associated with a high plasma bicarbonate concentration and metabolic alkalosis. Urinary potassium excretion should be persistently reduced (<25 mEq/day) with extrarenal losses due to diarrhea, but may be elevated with diuretics if the urine sample is obtained while the diuretic is still acting or with vomiting if the patient has bicarbonaturia (which should be associated with a urine pH above 7.0).

The plasma renin activity is of no diagnostic value in this setting. All three conditions lead to volume depletion and an appropriate increase in renin release.

SUGGESTED READINGS

Esposito C, Bellotti N, Fasoli G, et al. Hyperkalemia-induced ECG abnormalities in patients with reduced renal function. Clin Nephrol 2004;62:465.

Kaplan NM. The current epidemic of primary aldosteronism: causes and consequences. J Hypertens 2004;22:863.

Kassirer JP, Schwartz WB. The response of normal man to selective depletion of hydrochloric acid: factors in the genesis of persistent alkalosis. Am J Med 1966;40:10.

Rabelink TJ, Koomans HA, Hené RJ, et al. Early and late adjustment to potassium loading in humans. Kidney Int 1990;38:942.

Rose BD, Post TW. Clinical Physiology of Acid-Base and Electrolyte Disorders, 5th Ed. New York: McGraw-Hill, 2001.

Sterns RH, Cox M, Feig PU, et al. Internal potassium balance and the control of the plasma potassium concentration. Medicine 1981;60:339.

Young DB. Quantitative analysis of aldosterone's role in potassium regulation. Am J Physiol 1988;255:F811.

Young DB, Paulsen AW. Interrelated effects of aldosterone and plasma potassium on potassium excretion. Am J Physiol 1983;244:F28.

8

URINALYSIS AND APPROACH TO THE PATIENT WITH RENAL DISEASE

CASE PRESENTATION

A 67-year-old man has previously been well and has no past history of kidney disease. A plasma creatinine concentration drawn 3 months ago was relatively normal at 1.2 mg/dL and the urinalysis was unremarkable. Over the past month, the patient has noted easy fatigability and mild but persistent back pain. During the past week, his appetite began to diminish and he experienced a 3-lb weight loss.

Physical examination shows an ill-appearing man but no specific abnormalities are found. Laboratory data reveal the following:

BUN   = 110 mg/dL (9–25)
Creatinine   = 8.4 mg/dL (0.8–1.4)
Hematocrit   = 25% (previous value normal at 41%)
Urinalysis   = trace protein by dipstick, no cells or casts in
               the sediment

OBJECTIVES

> **By the end of this section, you should have an understanding of each of the following issues:**
>
> ■ The different types of proteinuria and how they are detected.
> ■ The distinction between glomerular and extraglomerular bleeding.
> ■ The difference between acute and chronic renal disease.
> ■ The general correlation between the different patterns of urinary findings and certain disease states.
> ■ The meaning of the urine sodium concentration and the fractional excretion of sodium, and how they are used to distinguish between prerenal disease and acute tubular necrosis as the cause of acute renal failure.

Patients with renal disease can present to the physician in a number of different ways. Some have symptoms that are directly related either to the urinary tract (such as flank pain or gross bleeding that turns the urine red) or to associated extrarenal findings induced by the renal disease (such as edema or hypertension). However, many patients are asymptomatic and the presence of underlying renal disease is incidentally discovered when routine laboratory tests reveal an elevated plasma creatinine concentration or an abnormal urinalysis.

The major types of renal disease are grouped according to the following commonly used functional classification:

■ Prerenal disease, in which reduced renal perfusion is the primary abnormality.
■ Postrenal disease, in which obstruction at some site in the urinary tract partially or completely blocks the flow of urine.
■ Intrinsic renal disease, which can be caused by glomerular, vascular, or tubulointerstitial disorders.

The major causes of renal disease, most of which will be discussed in the following chapters, are listed in Table 8.1.

Once the presence of renal disease has been documented, the primary goals are to establish the correct diagnosis and to assess the severity of the renal dysfunction. The initial approach to diagnosis begins with the history, physical examination, and careful evaluation of the urine. As will be seen, some urinary findings are virtually pathognomonic for a particular type of disease. Even a relatively normal urinalysis is a positive finding, since it can help to narrow the differential diagnosis. The severity of renal dysfunction is primarily assessed by estimating the glomerular filtration rate via measurement and serial monitoring of the plasma

TABLE 8.1

Most Common Causes of Renal Disease

I. **Postrenal—urinary tract obstruction; need to exclude early in the evaluation**
   A. **Prostatic disease**
   B. **Pelvic or retroperitoneal adenopathy or malignancy**
   C. **Renal or ureteric calculi (bilateral)**
   D. **Congential abnormalities**

II. **Prerenal**
   A. **True volume depletion caused by gastrointestinal, renal, skin, or third-space losses**
   B. **Congestive heart failure in which there is a primary reduction in cardiac output**
   C. **Hepatic cirrhosis in which splanchnic vasodilation leads to pooling in the splanchnic system and underperfusion of other organs**
   D. **Nonsteroidal anti-inflammatory drugs, which can induce renal vasoconstriction in susceptible subjects by blocking the synthesis of renal vasodilator prostaglandins**
   E. **Bilateral renal artery stenosis, often made worse by use of an angiotensin-converting enzyme inhibitor that interferes with autoregulation of the glomerular filtration rate**
   F. **Shock due to sepsis, fluid loss, or cardiac disease**

III. **Intrinsic Disease**
   A. **Glomerular disease**
      1. Glomerulonephritis
      2. Nephrotic syndrome
   B. **Vascular disease**
      1. Benign or malignant hypertensive nephrosclerosis
      2. Systemic vasculitis
      3. Thrombotic microangiopathy in the hemolytic–uremic syndrome, thrombotic thrombocytopenic purpura, and scleroderma
   C. **Tubular disease**
      1. Acute tubular necrosis
      2. Myeloma kidney
      3. Hypercalcemia (also causes afferent vasoconstriction)
      4. Polycystic kidney disease
   D. **Interstitial disease**
      1. Acute, usually drug-induced interstitial nephritis
      2. Acute pyelonephritis (infection of the renal parenchyma)
      3. Chronic pyelonephritis, usually due to vesicoureteral reflux
      4. Analgesic nephropathy

creatinine concentration and calculation of the estimated GFR (eGFR) or the measured creatinine clearance (see Chapter 1). The urinalysis is of variable importance in evaluating the severity and activity of the renal injury. In glomerular diseases, for example, the presence of heavy proteinuria and an active urine sediment with many red cells and casts generally reflects more severe disease than mild proteinuria or a few cells and casts.

However, this relationship between the urinary findings and disease severity does not always apply. When acute inflammation in the glomeruli (called glomerulonephritis) resolves, there may be a transition to chronic disease with marked scarring. At this time, the urinalysis typically becomes less abnormal (due to diminished inflammation) despite progressive nephron loss and eventually a decline in GFR.

Urinalysis

Analysis of the urine should be performed on a fresh specimen within 30 to 60 minutes after voiding. A midstream specimen is adequate after first cleansing the external genitalia to avoid contamination with local secretions. The stage in the menstrual cycle should also be noted, since active menses can lead to blood contamination of the urine sample.

The fresh urine should be centrifuged at 3000 r/min for 3 to 5 minutes. Most of the supernatant should then be poured into a separate tube and the sediment at the bottom of the tube resuspended by gently flicking the side of the tube. The sediment should be poured or transferred with a pipette onto a slide and covered with a cover slip. Both the supernatant and the sediment are now ready for detailed analysis.

Evaluation of the supernatant usually begins with a dipstick that can test for the following, as well as for protein excretion:

■ **pH**—The pH of the urine normally ranges between 5 and 6.5, depending primarily upon dietary intake. Measurement of the urine pH is generally of little clinical importance except in two settings. First, a urine pH above 7.5 to 8 suggests a urinary tract infection with a urea-splitting organism and the nitrite test should also be positive. The metabolism of urea can raise the urine pH by driving the reaction—$NH_3 + H^+ \leftrightarrow NH_4^+$—to the right, thereby lowering the free hydrogen concentration and raising the urine pH. Second, the urine pH should be below 5.3 (maximally acid) in a patient with metabolic acidosis, since excreting more acid will tend to normalize the extracellular pH. A urine pH above 5.5 in this setting suggests an impairment in the acidification process, due most often to one of the forms of renal tubular acidosis (see Chapter 6).
■ **Glucose**—Glucose is detectable in the urine primarily in patients with hyperglycemia due to inadequately controlled diabetes mellitus. In this setting, the filtered glucose load is increased to a level that

exceeds proximal glucose reabsorptive capacity, resulting in glucosuria. Rarely, glucosuria is noted with a normal plasma glucose concentration; this finding, called renal glucosuria, is indicative of a proximal tubular defect in glucose reabsorption and may be seen in combination with other proximal tubular defects (bicarbonaturia; see Chapter 6).

■ **Ketones**—Patients with uncontrolled diabetes mellitus also may have ketoacidosis. β-hydroxybutyric acid is the primary ketone formed, but acetoacetic acid and acetone are also present. Only the latter two compounds are detected by the dipstick, which will therefore tend to underestimate total ketone excretion.

■ **Nitrite**—Dietary nitrate is normally excreted in the urine. If, however, bacteria are present and there is adequate contact time (as in a specimen obtained when the patient first voids in the morning), then urinary nitrate can be partially converted to nitrite. Thus, a positive dipstick for nitrite is a reasonably good screening test for a urinary tract infection.

■ **Heme**—A positive test for heme is usually indicative of red cells being present in the urine, a finding that must be confirmed by examination of the urine sediment. In addition to hemoglobin in red cells, the dipstick can also detect free heme proteins as with hemoglobinuria due to intravascular hemolysis and myoglobinuria due to skeletal muscle breakdown (rhabdomyolysis). In the latter two conditions, however, the supernatant will be heme positive but there will few or no red cells in the urine sediment.

Proteinuria

The glomerular capillary wall allows the relatively free filtration of smaller, low molecular weight proteins (such as immunoglobulin light chains and amino acids), but restricts the filtration of larger macromolecules (such as albumin and IgG). The factors responsible for these permselective properties of the glomerular capillary wall are reviewed in Chapter 9. What is important for the purposes of this discussion is to be familiar with the three different types of proteinuria that may be seen:

■ **Glomerular proteinuria**—Glomerular proteinuria refers to an increase in the permeability of the glomerular capillary wall that leads to the abnormal filtration and subsequent excretion of larger, normally nonfiltered proteins such as albumin. This problem can be seen with any form of glomerular disease.

■ **Tubular proteinuria**—Low molecular weight proteins are normally filtered and then largely reabsorbed in the proximal tubule. (The small amounts of albumin that are filtered are also mostly reabsorbed at this site.) Tubulointerstitial diseases that impair tubular function can interfere with this reabsorptive process, resulting in increased excretion of these smaller proteins. Tubular proteinuria is not a clinically important disorder unless accompanied by other defects in proximal function, potentially leading to problems such as metabolic acidosis (from bicarbonate wasting) and hypophosphatemia and rickets (from phosphate wasting).

■ **Overflow proteinuria**—In some conditions, increased production of smaller proteins leads to a rate of filtration that exceeds normal proximal reabsorptive capacity. This most commonly occurs with overproduction of monoclonal immunoglobulin light chains in multiple myeloma and other plasma cell dyscrasias.

Limitations of the Dipstick

The dipstick commonly used in the initial evaluation of the urine is impregnated with a dye that changes color according to the quantity of proteins present, particularly albumin. Although the dipstick is reasonably accurate for the detection of glomerular proteinuria (see below), it will miss nonalbumin proteins such as immunoglobulin light chains. Likewise, periodic measurements of urinary microalbumin on random urine is the standard for monitoring patients for the development of diabetic nephropathy. However, this assay will also miss nonalbumin proteins in the urine that would be detected with a total protein determination or a urinary immunoelectrophoresis. An older beside test using sulfosalicylic acid added to the urine supernatant will detect all proteins, with the degree of turbidity noted being proportional to the protein concentration.

 What factor other than the rate of albumin excretion will affect the urine albumin concentration and therefore the intensity of the reaction on the urine dipstick? What else may be measured in the urine to correct for these variables?

Normal Values and Quantitation

Normal subjects usually excrete between 40 and 80 mg of protein per day, with the upper range of normal being 150 mg/day. A number of different proteins are excreted. Albumin, for example, accounts for less than 20 mg/day, while Tamm–Horsfall mucoprotein (uromodulin) accounts for 30 to 50 mg/day. The latter is a protein of uncertain function that may have an immunomodulatory role in preventing development of urinary tract infections and kidney stones. The protein is secreted by the cells in the thick ascending limb of the loop of Henle, and it constitutes the matrix for almost all urinary casts. Mutations in Tamm–Horsfall mucoprotein result in two autosomal dominant disorders: typical familial juvenile hyperuricemic nephropathy and type 2 medullary cystic kidney disease. Both disorders are characterized by hyperuricemia, medullary cysts, interstitial nephritis, and progressive renal failure.

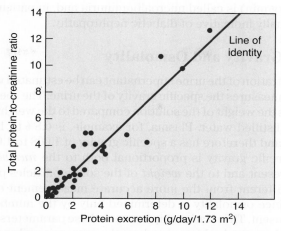

FIGURE 8.1.   Protein-to-creatinine ratio to estimate protein excretion. The relationship between estimates of protein excretion on random urine determinations of protein and creatinine with 24-hour measurements of total protein excretion.

Daily protein excretion has traditionally been measured by a 24-hour urine collection (the gold standard). There is, however, a much more convenient alternative to estimate the degree of proteinuria: calculation of the ratio of total protein to creatinine (in mg/mg) on a random urine specimen. By normalizing the protein concentration to the amount of creatinine in a random sample, variations in urine protein concentration (due to variable oral intake) are avoided. The fortuitous observation that the average daily creatinine excretion is approximately 1000 mg/day permits the ratio to approximate the 24-hour protein excretion rate. If, for example, a random urine specimen contains 210 mg/dL of protein and the creatinine concentration is 42 mg/dL, then the patient is excreting approximately 5 g/day per 1.73 m^2 ($210 \div 42 = 5$). Figure 8.1 shows that there is good correlation between random urine protein/creatinine ratios and 24-hour determinations.

Microalbuminuria. The dipstick is relatively insensitive to initial increases in glomerular permeability, since it will not begin to be positive until protein excretion exceeds from 300 to 500 mg/day. This is a particular problem in diabetics, since advanced glomerular injury will already be present by this time. An alternative that allows much earlier detection of glomerular injury is the direct measurement of albumin excretion (microalbuminuria). Like the urine protein/creatinine ratio, the microalbumin/creatinine ratio is a valid estimate of microalbumin excretion rates. The normal rate of albumin excretion is less than 20 mg/day (15 μg/min); persistent albumin excretion between 30 and 300 mg/day

(20 to 200 μg/min) is called microalbuminuria and, in patients with diabetes, is usually indicative of diabetic nephropathy.

Specific Gravity and Osmolality

The concentration of the urine supernatant can be estimated with a urometer, which measures the specific gravity of the urine. The specific gravity is defined as the weight of the solution compared to the weight of an equal volume of distilled water. Plasma, for example, is 0.8% to 1.0% heavier than water and therefore has a specific gravity of 1.008 to 1.010.

The specific gravity is proportional both to the *number* of solute particles present and to the *weight* of the solute particles present. It is therefore different from the more accurate measurement of *urine osmolality*, since osmolality is determined only by the number of solute particles present. The relationship between these parameters is relatively predictable in normal subjects in whom the urine primarily contains urea and sodium, potassium, and ammonium salts; for example, a urine osmolality of 300 mOsm/kg—similar to that of the plasma—is equivalent to a specific gravity of 1.008 to 1.010 (Fig. 8.2). However, there is a disproportionate increase in the specific gravity when larger solutes are present, such as glucose (mol wt 180) and radiocontrast media (mol wt approximately 550). In these settings, the urine-specific gravity can exceed from 1.030 to 1.040 even though the urine osmolality may be only 300 mOsm/kg.

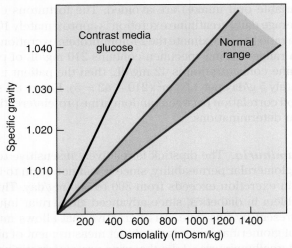

FIGURE 8.2. Relationship between the specific gravity and osmolality in urine from normal subjects. Normal urine contains little glucose or protein (*shaded area*). For comparison, the relationship between specific gravity and osmolality for a pure glucose solution is included.

As described in Chapter 2, the urine osmolality can vary from a low of 50 to 100 mOsm/kg (specific gravity 1.002 to 1.003) after a marked water load and subsequent suppression of ADH release to a high of 1000 to 1400 mOsm/kg (specific gravity 1.030 to 1.040) with dehydration and maximum ADH effect. Thus, a random value is of little meaning unless correlated with the plasma osmolality or volume status. In the clinical setting, measurement of the urine osmolality is primarily used in the differential diagnosis of hyponatremia, hypernatremia, or polyuria (see Chapter 3). It may also be helpful in distinguishing between prerenal disease (decreased renal perfusion) and acute tubular necrosis as the cause of acute kidney injury (see Chapter 11).

Examination of Urine Sediment

The sediment should first be inspected under a low-power objective with reduced light. The high, dry objective ($40\times$) can then be used to identify the casts and cells that might be present.

Casts

Casts represent precipitated proteins and cells that form within the tubular lumen. As a result, they have a cylindrical shape and regular margins to conform to the shape of the tubular lumen. These characteristic findings distinguish casts from irregular clumps of cells or debris.

All casts have an organic matrix comprised primarily of Tamm–Horsfall mucoprotein (THMP or uromodulin). The chemical characteristics of this protein determine the conditions in which cast formation is likely to occur, a process that has been likened to the setting of gelatin. Casts generally form in the collecting tubules, the site at which the urine is most concentrated and most acidic. Urinary stasis, as in poorly functioning nephrons with low flow, also promotes cast formation.

When the lumen is free of cells, the cast will be composed almost entirely of matrix. These casts are called *hyaline* casts and are of no diagnostic significance. However, cellular casts can occur if there are cells (white cells, red cells, epithelial cells) in the lumen as THMP precipitates. This finding is important clinically, since it *identifies the kidney as the source of the cells* (see Table 8.2). For example, white cells can enter the urine at any site in the urinary tract, from the kidney to the bladder to the urethra. However, the presence of casts containing white cells (called white cell casts) indicates inflammation in the kidney.

Granular and Waxy Casts. Granular and waxy casts are thought to represent successive stages in the degeneration of cellular casts as they flow through the nephron. In addition to representing cellular debris, the granules in granular casts can also represent aggregated plasma proteins. Thus, granular casts can form in any proteinuric condition.

TABLE 8.2

Correlation between Characteristic Urinary Findings and Some Major Causes of Acute and Chronic Renal Disease

Urinary Findings	Etiology
Hematuria with red cell casts, proteinuria (>3.5g/day), and lipiduria (as seen in the nephrotic syndrome)	Any of these findings, singly or in combination, is virtually diagnostic of glomerular disease or vasculitis. Why some patients have an active urine sediment with hematuria and red cell casts while others have only proteinuria is discussed in Chapter 9. In addition, the absence of these findings does not exclude mild glomerular disease, which may present with only a few red cells or low-grade proteinuria.
Renal tubular epithelial cells with granular and epithelial cell casts	Seen in acute renal failure and, suggestive of acute tubular necrosis. However, some patients with this disorder lack these findings and have a relatively normal urinalysis.
Pyuria with white cell and granular casts with no or mild proteinuria (<1.5 g/day) and variable hematuria	Suggestive of some form of tubulointerstitial disease or obstruction. Can be seen with acute interstitial nephritis, a disorder in which eosinophiluria may be seen. Can also occur with urinary tract infection due to common bacteria or tuberculosis.
Normal or near normal—few cells with few or no casts and little or no proteinuria; hyaline casts are not an abnormal finding	**Acute**: May be found in prerenal disease, urinary tract obstruction, and tubular diseases such as hypercalcemia, multiple myeloma,* or some cases of acute tubular necrosis. **Chronic**: May be seen in prerenal disease, urinary tract obstruction, benign hypertensive nephrosclerosis, and tubular or interstitial diseases.

*The urinalysis is typically negative in myeloma kidney since the dipstick detects albumin, but not the immunoglobulin light chains responsible for the disease both by precipitating and obstructing nephrons and by directly damaging the tubular cells (see Chapter 11).

Red Cells

As with white cells, red cells can enter the urine (called hematuria) at any site in the urinary tract. The bleeding may be microscopic (seen only under the microscope) or grossly visible. As little as 1 mL of blood in 1 L of urine can induce a visible color change.

The most common causes of hematuria in an adult are *extrarenal*, including kidney stones, trauma, prostatic disease, and, particularly in men over the age of 50, cancer of the prostate, bladder, or kidney. As a result, older patients usually undergo an extensive radiologic and urologic evaluation (including insertion of a cystoscope into the bladder) to exclude malignancy. Although less common, glomerular bleeding is important to identify since it can be associated with acute kidney injury, and obviates the need for these diagnostic procedures. The following findings can be used to distinguish glomerular from extraglomerular bleeding:

- **Red cell casts**—Red cell casts (in which red cells are contained within casts) are virtually diagnostic of some form of glomerulonephritis or vasculitis. However, the absence of red cell casts does not exclude glomerular disease.
- **Red cell morphology**—Glomerular bleeding is typically associated with fragmentation of the red cells, leading to a dysmorphic appearance manifested by blebs, budding, and segmental loss of membrane. Both mechanical trauma as the red cells pass through rents in the glomerular capillary wall and osmotic trauma as the red cells pass through the different nephron segments are thought to contribute to the red cell damage. In comparison, red cells that are round and uniform in size and shape (as in a normal peripheral blood smear) are more likely to have an extrarenal origin in the pelvis, ureter, bladder, prostate, or urethra.
- **Proteinuria**—Protein excretion above 500 mg/day is highly suggestive of intrarenal abnormalities and can be seen with both glomerular and tubular lesions. Proteinuria in excess of 3000 mg/d is virtually diagnositic for a glomerular lesion.
- **Blood clots**—Blood clots, if present in a patient with grossly visible hematuria, are almost always extrarenal in origin. Clots are rarely seen with glomerular bleeding, perhaps due to the presence of thrombolytic factors, such as urokinase and tissue-type plasminogen activators in the glomeruli and in the tubules.

White Cells

White cells are larger than red cells (about twofold) and can be identified by their granular cytoplasm and multilobed nuclei. Urinary white cells (pyuria) are usually indicative of infection or inflammation at some site in the urinary tract. White cell casts locate the lesion to the kidney as with acute pyelonephritis (an infection of the renal parenchyma) or a

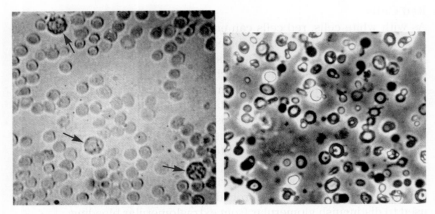

PLATE 8.1.   Red and white cells in the urine sediment (*left panel*). White cells are about twofold larger and have a granular cytoplasm and multilobed nucleus (*red arrows*). Red blood cells are smaller and have no nucleus. For comparison (*right panel*), dysmorphic red blood cells seen in a patient with acute glomerulonephritis. Note the abnormal blebbing, irregular shape, and varied sizes that result from red blood cells traversing the glomerular basement membrane and from passaging through hypertonic medullary interstitium.

tubulointerstitial disease such as acute interstitial nephritis (see Chapter 11). Pyuria can also be seen with glomerular inflammation, but hematuria and proteinuria are usually more prominent in this setting.

Neutrophils are usually the predominant white cell in the urine. However, other white cells can be seen, with eosinophils having the greatest potential diagnostic significance. Eosinophiluria is a frequent finding in allergic, generally drug-induced acute interstitial nephritis, although it is not pathognomonic of this condition. Conversely, the absence of eosinophiluria does not exclude an acute allergic interstial nephritis as other types of white blood cells may predominate (neutrophils, lymphocytes). Eosinophiluria can be detected by the use of special stains (such as Hansel's stain) on the urine sediment.

Epithelial Cells and Lipiduria
Renal tubular epithelial cells are from 1.5 to 3 times the size of a white cell with a round, large nucleus. Although epithelial cells from the lower urinary tract tend to be much larger with a small nucleus, the only way to be certain of their renal origin is if the cells are contained within a cast.

Occasional renal epithelial cells are excreted in the urine, a probable reflection of normal cell turnover. Increased numbers of epithelial cells may be shed into the urine in a variety of renal diseases, including tubulointerstitial disorders and glomerular diseases associated with proteinuria. In the latter setting, the tubular cells may undergo fatty degeneration with fat droplets appearing in the cytosol; these fat-laden cells are called oval fat bodies. The fat droplets may also be free in the urine, where they are of the same size as or smaller than red cells. They can be identified by viewing the urine under polarized light. Fat is doubly refractile and shows a characteristic "Maltese cross" appearance (Plates 8.2).

The fat within the epithelial cells is probably derived from the filtration and subsequent cellular uptake of lipoprotein-bound cholesterol. This sequence will occur only when glomerular disease leads to the filtration of normally nonfiltered macromolecules. Thus, lipiduria is essentially diagnostic of glomerular disease and the nephrotic syndrome. In addition to intracellular droplets, both free fat droplets and fatty casts may be seen.

Crystals

A variety of crystals can be seen in the urine sediment depending upon the urine composition, concentration, and pH (Plate 8.3). For example, uric acid tends to precipitate in an acidic urine (pH <5.5), while phosphate salts precipitate in an alkaline urine (pH >7.0). In comparison, the solubility of calcium oxalate is pH independent.

Urinary crystals can be seen in normal subjects and are generally of no diagnostic importance. One major exception is the presence of cystine crystals with their characteristic hexagonal shape. These crystals are essentially seen only in patients with cystinuria, a hereditary disorder characterized by mutations in two genes that encode a protein responsible for cystine and diabasic acid transport or an amino acid transporter. Mutations lead to impaired proximal cystine reabsorption, increased cystine excretion, and the formation of cystine stones.

Normal Urine Sediment

In addition to a small amount of protein, normal urine contains up to 1 million red cells, 3 million white and epithelial cells, and 10,000 casts (almost all hyaline) per day. When a random urine specimen is examined, these observations translate into 0 to 4 white cells and 0 to 2 red cells per high-power field. Occasional calcium oxalate, uric acid, or phosphate crystals also may be seen, depending upon the urine pH.

Although the excretion of more protein, cells, or casts may be indicative of underlying renal disease, it is important to appreciate that a variety of conditions (including extreme exercise and fever) can induce transient changes in the urine in normal subjects. How this occurs is not clear, but alterations in renal hemodynamics may play a contributory role.

The frequency of transient urinary abnormalities was illustrated in a study of 1000 young men who had yearly urinalyses between the ages of 18 and 33. Hematuria was seen in 39% on at least one occasion and in

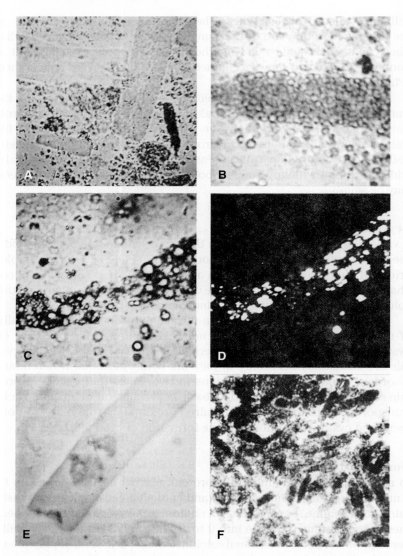

PLATE 8.2. Casts in the urine sediments. **A.** Hyaline cast, which is only slightly more refractile than the surrounding fluid. These can normally be seen in the urine. **B.** Red blood
cell cast. Although this cast contains tightly packed red cells, it is more common to see
fewer red cells trapped within a hyaline or granular cast. **C.** Fatty cast. The fat droplets
within this cast can be differentiated from red cells by their dark outlines and variable
size. **D.** Under polarized light, the fat droplets within this cast show the characteristic
"Maltese cross" appearance and are characteristically seen in diseases associated with
the nephrotic syndrome. **E.** Waxy cast, which represents a degenerative granular cast.
F. Muddy brown casts. These casts are named for the pigment giving rise to the typical
color of these casts seen in the urine sediment. They are characteristically seen in
patients with acute tubular necrosis; they contain necrotic debris and degenerated
epithelial cells.

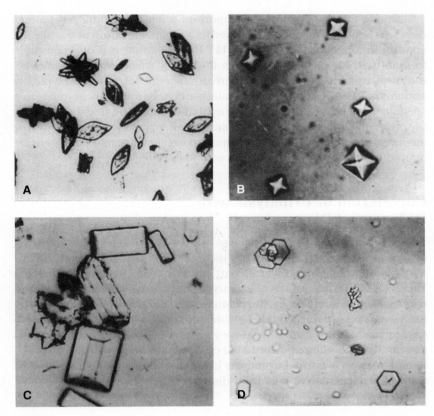

PLATE 8.3. Crystals in the urine sediment. **A.** Uric acid crystals are yellow or reddish-brown and are seen only in urine with an acid pH. These crystals are pleomorphic, most often appearing as rhombic plates or rosettes. **B.** Calcium oxalate crystals with the characteristic "envelope" appearance; these crystals may also assume a dumbbell shape. **C.** "Coffin-lid" ammonium magnesium phosphate crystals only form in urine with alkaline pH. **D.** Cystine crystals have a characteristic hexagonal shape.

16% on two or more occasions in the absence of any known disease in almost all subjects.

Acute versus Chronic Renal Disease

In addition to the urinary findings, knowledge of the duration of the renal disease (acute versus chronic) also may be diagnostically important. This can be done most accurately if previous information is available. As an example, gross hematuria following an upper respiratory infection in a patient with a previously normal urinalysis is indicative of acute disease. In comparison, a progressive rise in the plasma creatinine concentration over several years is clearly indicative of chronic renal failure.

Timing may be particularly important when a hospitalized patient develops acute kidney injury (defined as a recent elevation in the plasma creatinine concentration; Chapter 11). In this setting, it is often possible to identify the exact day on which the injury was sustained, since serial measurements of the plasma creatinine concentration are typically obtained. A rise in the plasma creatinine concentration beginning on a specific day may be due to renal injury that occurred on that day (such as the onset of hypotension or the administration or radiocontrast media) or due to the cumulative effect of a renal toxin (such as an aminoglycoside antibiotic) or excess fluid removal with a diuretic.

Correlation of Urinalysis with Differential Diagnosis

The different types of renal disease will be reviewed in the following chapters. However, it is useful at this time to briefly review how the urinary findings can point toward a particular disease. As can be seen from Table 8.2, different patterns of urinary findings are associated with different diseases; in some cases, the changes seen may be virtually diagnostic for a single disorder. Examples include red cell casts for glomerular disease or vasculitis and, in acute kidney injury, renal tubular epithelial cells and multiple granular and epithelial cell casts for acute tubular necrosis. Even a relatively normal urinalysis is helpful by excluding a number of disorders, particularly glomerular diseases.

Urine Sodium Excretion

Estimation of the rate of sodium excretion is used in a variety of clinical settings, including the differential diagnosis of hyponatremia (see Chapter 3) and distinguishing between prerenal disease and acute tubular necrosis as the cause of acute kidney injury (see Chapter 11). The basic principle is that with intact tubular function, sodium retention is the appropriate renal response to decreased systemic and renal perfusion. As a result, the rate of sodium excretion should be low (usually less than 25 mEq/day) with effective volume depletion causing hyponatremia or acute kidney injury. In comparison, sodium excretion is normal (equal to intake) or even elevated when the patient is normovolemic (as with hyponatremia due to the syndrome of inappropriate ADH secretion) or when renal tubular function is impaired (as with acute kidney injury due to acute tubular necrosis or with diuretic therapy).

Two different methods are used to estimate sodium excretion from a random urine specimen: measurement of the urine sodium concentration, or calculation of the fractional excretion of sodium (FENa).

Urine Sodium Concentration

The urine sodium concentration is usually below 25 mEq/L with volume depletion and above 40 mEq/L with normovolemia or acute tubular necrosis. There is, however, substantial overlap, particularly at values between 25 and 40 mEq/L.

 At a given rate of sodium excretion, what additional factor will influence the urine sodium concentration?

Fractional Excretion of Sodium

Calculation of the FENa allows sodium handling to be looked at directly without the confounding effect of the rate of water reabsorption. The FENa reflects the percent of the filtered sodium load that is excreted:

$$FENa \ (percent) = \frac{Quantity \ of \ sodium \ excreted}{Quantity \ of \ sodium \ filtered} \times 100$$

Sodium excretion is equal to the product of the urine sodium concentration and the urine flow rate (V), while the quantity of sodium filtered is equal to the product of the glomerular filtration rate (estimated from the creatinine clearance) and the plasma sodium concentration:

$$FENa \ (percent) = \frac{UNa \times V}{PNa \times (UCr \times V/PCr)} \times 100$$

$$= \frac{UNa \times PCr}{PNa \times UCr} \times 100 \qquad \text{(Eq. 1)}$$

Patients with prerenal disease and acute kidney injury generally have a FENa that is less than 1%, indicating that the patient is sodium avid with over 99% of the filtered sodium being reabsorbed. In comparison, the FENa is generally above 2% when tubular reabsorption is impaired in acute tubular necrosis. The overlap is much less than that seen with the urine sodium concentration alone, since the latter is also influenced by the rate of water reabsorption (see Chapter 11).

 A patient with acute kidney injury has a plasma creatinine concentration that is continuously rising due to the fall in GFR and is now 3.2 mg/dL. The following additional values are obtained: Urine sodium concentration is 35 mEq/L, plasma sodium concentration is 140 mEq/L, and the urine creatinine concentration is 160 mEq/L. Calculate the FENa.

There is, however, an important potential problem with using the FENa in patients with normal GFR. Both the FENa and the urine sodium concentration are generally obtained in an effort to determine if a patient is effectively volume depleted. A urine sodium concentration below 25 mEq/L is usually indicative of hypovolemia at any level of renal function; as noted above, however, somewhat higher values do not exclude this diagnosis since there may also be a high rate of water reabsorption. In comparison, there is *no absolute value* for the FENa in volume depletion because this parameter is greatly influenced by the filtered sodium load, which in turn is dependent upon the GFR. This principle is illustrated in the following example.

QUESTION 4   **A patient with hyponatremia and normal renal function is evaluated. The patient is taking no medications. The urine sodium concentration is 67 mEq/L and the urine volume is approximately 1500 mL on the first day. The plasma sodium concentration is 120 mEq/L, the plasma creatinine concentration is 1.0 mg/dL, and the urine creatinine concentration is 67 mg/dL. Calculate the FENa. From the urinary findings, is the patient volume depleted or normovolemic?**

Urine Volume

The urine volume is variable in patients with renal disease and is generally of little diagnostic importance. Although the GFR may be reduced, the urine volume is determined not by the GFR alone but by the difference between the GFR and the amount of water reabsorbed. Thus, the urine output often remains normal (equal to water intake) in patients with advanced chronic renal disease because tubular reabsorption can be decreased to balance the reduction in filtered load. In numerical terms, a normal subject with a GFR of 180 L/day must reabsorb 179 L (more than 99% of that filtered) to excrete 1 L. A patient with severe renal disease and a GFR as low as 10 L/day (7 mL/min) can also excrete 1 L if only 9 L is reabsorbed (90% of that filtered). The ability to make this compensation is frequently impaired in acute renal failure, where the urine output is often less than intake leading to progressive fluid retention.

One setting in which the urine volume is important diagnostically is when there is virtually no output (<50 mL/day), a finding that is called anuria. Anuria is primarily seen only in certain forms of acute kidney injury, particularly complete bilateral obstruction and marked renal hypoperfusion in shock. Less often, severe glomerulonephritis or bilateral vascular occlusion (as in the hemolytic–uremic syndrome or a dissecting aneurysm) may be responsible. In comparison, patients with acute tubular necrosis often have a reduced urine output (oliguria <400 mL/day) but are rarely anuric.

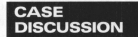 **CASE DISCUSSION**   The patient presented at the beginning of the chapter has severe kidney injury associated with renal failure as manifested by marked elevations in the BUN and plasma creatinine concentration. The normal plasma creatinine concentration 3 months previously suggests that this process is relatively acute. Easy fatigability, anorexia, weight loss, and anemia can be induced by the

renal failure. However, the concurrent presence of persistent back pain raises the question of an underlying malignancy. As described in the chapter, a protein/creatinine ration or sulfosalicylic acid test should be performed when there is unexplained renal failure and a negative dipstick, looking for the possible presence of immunoglobulin light chains. This patient had a 4+ sulfosalicylic acid test and was found to have multiple myeloma.

Other possible causes of acute renal failure with a bland urine sediment include prerenal disease, urinary tract obstruction (which is associated with dilatation of the collecting systems that can be detected by ultrasonography), and hypercalcemia (Table 8.2). Both urinary tract obstruction and hypercalcemia may be induced by an underlying malignancy, and hypercalcemia can contribute to the decline in renal function in multiple myeloma (see Chapter 11).

ANSWERS TO QUESTIONS

1 The urine albumin concentration is proportional to the urine volume as well as the quantity of albumin present. For example, drinking a large volume of fluid will dilute the urinary protein concentration and reduce the intensity of the finding on the urine dipstick. Likewise, the urinary creatinine excretion will be reduced to a similar degree allowing variability in urine volume to be ignored in the estimation of daily protein excretion when both the urine protein and creatinine are measured on the same sample and expressed as the urine protein/creatinine ratio.

2 The urine sodium concentration is affected by the rate of water excretion as well as by the rate of sodium excretion. For example, the urine sodium concentration will be 60 mEq/L in a patient ingesting 60 mEq of sodium and 1 L of water. If, however, water intake and excretion were increased to 2.5 L, the urine sodium concentration would fall to 24 mEq/L even though there had been no change in sodium excretion.

3 The FENa equals 0.5% [(35 × 3.2 × 100) ÷ (140 × 160)], suggesting that the patient has prerenal disease with intact tubular function.

4 The FENa is 0.83% [(67 × 1.0 × 100) ÷ (120 × 67)]. Although this might suggest volume depletion, note that the patient is excreting a total of 100 mEq of sodium per day (67 mEq/L × 1.5 L/day) and is therefore likely to be normovolemic. The apparent discrepancy relates to the effect of the filtered sodium load (determined primarily by the GFR) on the level of FENa that is indicative of volume depletion. A value below 1% applies to advanced renal failure when the filtered sodium load is relatively low. If, for example, the GFR is markedly reduced at 20 L/day (14 mL/min) and the plasma water sodium concentration is 150 mEq/L, then the filtered sodium load is 3000 mEq/day. To reduce sodium excretion to less than 20 mEq/day with volume depletion requires a FENa below 1%.

The results are quite different when the GFR is relatively normal. At a GFR of 180 L/day (125 mL/min) and a plasma water sodium concentration of 150 mEq/L, the filtered sodium load is much greater at **27,000** mEq/day. A FENa of 1% in this setting represents the excretion of 270 mEq/day, which is greater than the average sodium intake of 80 to 250 mEq/day. Thus, almost all normal subjects have a FENa below 1% as in the patient described. To reduce sodium excretion to less than 20 mEq/day requires a FENa below 0.1%. As the GFR falls in patients with renal disease, the *FENa indicative of volume depletion* (i.e., the FENa associated with sodium excretion below 20 mEq/day) gradually rises from 0.1% to, as noted above, almost 1% in near end-stage renal disease.

These examples illustrate that the difficulty is using the FENa in settings other than advanced renal failure. Unless the FENa is very low (less than 0.1% to 0.2%), the approximate GFR must be known to determine if sodium is being appropriately conserved.

SUGGESTED READINGS

Ginsberg JM, Chang BS, Matarese RA, et al. Use of single voided urine samples to estimate quantitative proteinuria. NEJM 1983;309:1543–1546.

Greenberg, A. Urinalysis. In: Greenberg A (ed.). Primer on Kidney Diseases, 2nd Ed. New York: National Kidney Foundation, 1998:27–35.

Rose BD, Post, TW. Clinical Physiology of Acid Base and Electrolyte Disorders. New York: McGraw-Hill, 2001:405–414.

Steiner RW. Interpreting the fractional excretion of sodium. Am J Med 1984;77:699.

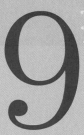

9

PATHOGENESIS OF MAJOR GLOMERULAR AND VASCULAR DISEASES

CASE PRESENTATION

Case 1

A 27-year-old man consults his family physician because of the recent onset of edema. He has no other relevant history and the physical examination is remarkable only for significant pitting edema in the lower extremities. His blood pressure is 135/80.

The blood and urine tests reveal the following:

BUN	= 15 mg/dL
Creatinine	= 0.9 mg/dL
Albumin	= 1.7 g/dL (normal = 3.5 to 5 g/dL)
Urinalysis	= 4+ protein (by dipstick)
Sediment	= oval fat bodies, occasional hyaline casts, rare red cells

The total protein-to-creatinine ratio is 10.8, suggesting that daily protein excretion is approximately 10.8 g/day per 1.73 m^2 body surface area (normal equals less than 150 mg/day; see Chapter 8). The kidney biopsy findings are illustrated in Figure 9.1.

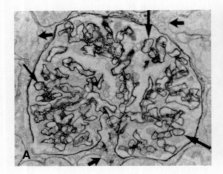
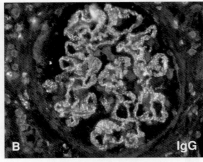
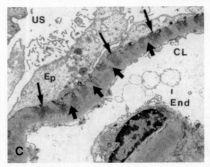

FIGURE 9.1. Membranous glomerulopathy, a noninflammatory immune complex–mediated disease. **A.** The light microscopic examination of the periodic acid-Schiff–stained section shows open capillary loops without inflammation. The glomerular basement membranes appear distinctly thickened (*long arrows*), especially when compared to the tubular basement membranes (*small arrows*). **B.** The presence of immunoglobulins within the thickened capillary wall is demonstrated in this immunofluorescence micrograph; a frozen section of the kidney cortex was incubated with fluorescein-tagged rabbit antibody to human gamma heavy chains (IgG). The distribution of the IgG-containing immune complexes is diffuse and granular and follows the glomerular basement membrane. Small amounts of complement are also detected in a similar distribution (not illustrated). **C.** This electron micrograph shows the characteristic subepithelial electron-dense deposits (*long arrows*), which appear on the outer aspect of the glomerular basement membrane (GBM). Adjacent immune deposits are separated by extensions of the basement membrane, or "spikes"; this additional basement membrane material surrounds the deposits like a calyx and imparts to the GBM the thickened appearance. Note an intact delicate fenestrated endothelial layer (End) separating the basement membrane from the capillary lumen (CL) and complete absence of inflammation. The visceral epithelial cell (Ep) has lost its interdigitating foot processes, which now are replaced by a continuous epithelium. Numerous microvillous cell surface extensions reach into the urinary space (US). This pattern of injury is characteristic for membranous nephropathy, one of the conditions in humans associated with nephrotic syndrome.

Case 2

A 16-year-old girl notes the sudden onset of periorbital edema and dark maroon urine. This is a rather frightening experience for the patient and her parents, and it prompts an immediate visit to the emergency ward.

The patient had been in good health until 2 weeks prior to consultation, when she developed a sore throat in connection with an upper respiratory tract infection. This was accompanied by persistent fever, forcing her to miss school for 3 days. The fever and the respiratory symptoms resolved spontaneously.

Physical examination revealed an elevated blood pressure of 150/105 mm Hg, edema of the face, and only minimal inflammation of the pharynx.

The blood and urine tests reveal the following:

BUN   = 32 mg/dL
Creatinine   = 2.1 mg/dL
Albumin   = 3.7 g/dL
Urinalysis   = 1+ protein, many red cells (by dipstick)
Sediment   = multiple red cells (most of which have a dysmorphic appearance) and occasional red cell casts and granular casts

The total protein-to-creatinine ratio is 1:1.

A kidney biopsy was performed on the third day when she developed pulmonary infiltrates. The biopsy findings are illustrated in Figure 9.2.

OBJECTIVES

By the end of this section, you should have an understanding of each of the following issues:

■ The major glomerular syndromes—nephrotic (Case 1) and nephritic (Case 2)—and their clinical presentation.
■ The mechanisms responsible for the different immune-mediated forms of glomerular injury.
■ The factors responsible for the different expression of immune complex–mediated diseases.
■ The basic structural patterns of glomerular injury and their underlying mechanisms.
■ The mechanisms by which the vasculature in the kidney can be damaged.

Introduction

The kidney is similar to other organs in that it has only a limited number of ways to respond to injury. It is therefore useful to begin by reviewing

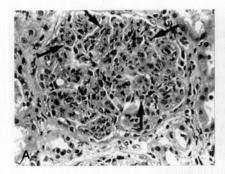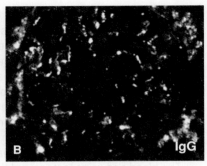

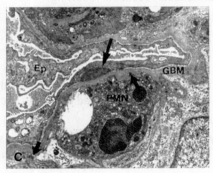

FIGURE 9.2. Diffuse proliferative glomerulonephritis, an inflammatory immune complex–mediated disease. **A.** This light micrograph shows prominent hypercellularity of the glomerular tuft due to infiltration and occlusion of the capillaries by polymorphonuclear and mononuclear leukocytes (*arrows*). This pattern of injury usually affects all glomeruli, resulting in a marked reduction of the glomerular filtration rate and oliguria. Some of the capillaries are destroyed, resulting in the extravasation of red blood cells into the urine (hematuria and red blood cell casts). **B.** The immunofluorescence microscopy illustrated in this figure shows few discrete IgG-containing deposits along the capillary wall; complement components can also be found in a similar distribution. **C.** This electron micrograph shows the details of the inflammatory injury of the capillary wall. A polymorphonuclear neutrophil (PMN) occupies the lumen of the capillary, which has lost its endothelial lining. The inflammatory cell is in close apposition with the glomerular basement membrane. Electron-dense deposits are present on both sides of the lamina densa of the glomerular basement membrane (GBM): The subepithelial deposit with a prominent hump-like appearance (*long arrow*) is not likely to contribute significantly to the pathogenesis of the active inflammation, while the smaller subendothelial immune deposits (*small arrows*) are likely to trigger an active recruitment of inflammatory cells. These latter deposits are likely to be short lived, since they are efficiently removed by the "professional" leukocytes. This pattern of injury is characteristic of acute postinfectious glomerulonephritides that present with the nephritic syndrome and an active urinary sediment. The visceral epithelial cell (Ep) shows focal simplification of foot processes.

the basic definitions that describe the histologic findings that may be seen:

- **Focal**—Involving less than 50% of the glomeruli on light microscopy. This limitation to light microscopy is important because most glomerular diseases involve almost all of the glomeruli if the latter are examined by electron or immunofluorescence microscopy.
- **Diffuse**—Involving more than 50% of the glomeruli on light microscopy.
- **Segmental**—Involving part of the glomerular tuft, usually in a focal manner.
- **Global**—Involving the entire glomerular tuft; can be seen with either focal or diffuse disease.
- **Membranous**—Thickening of the glomerular capillary wall, usually with distinctive basement membrane "spikes."
- **Proliferative**—An increased number of cells in the glomerulus; these cells can be either proliferating glomerular cells or infiltrating circulating inflammatory cells. The term *exudative* is also used when there is prominent infiltration by neutrophils.
- **Membranoproliferative**—The presence of thickening of the glomerular capillary wall with distinctive double contours or "tram tracks" and proliferative changes in the glomeruli.
- **Crescent**—An accumulation of cells (mostly mononuclear cells derived from the circulation and proliferated parietal epithelial cells) within Bowman's space; crescents often compress the capillary tuft and are associated with more severe disease.
- **Glomerulosclerosis**—Segmental or global capillary collapse or obsolescence with closure of the capillary lumens; it is presumed that there is little if any filtration across sclerotic areas.
- **Glomerulonephritis**—Any condition associated with inflammation in the glomerular tuft.

Nephrotic versus Nephritic Syndromes

The two cases presented at the beginning of the chapter illustrate the characteristic clinical manifestations of the two major glomerular syndromes: *nephrotic* and *nephritic*. Case 1 represents a nephrotic state in which the major clinical finding is proteinuria with a urine sediment that is relatively inactive, containing few cells or casts. Some patients present with asymptomatic proteinuria that is discovered on routine examination, while others, such as this patient, have the full-blown nephrotic syndrome. The latter consists of heavy proteinuria (typically exceeding 3.5 g/day), hypoalbuminemia (due in part to the urinary losses that are not matched by increased hepatic albumin synthesis), edema [due mostly to retention of sodium by the kidney rather than to hypoalbuminemia (see Chapter 4)], lipiduria (see Chapter 8), and hyperlipidemia. The last abnormality primarily reflects increased hepatic lipoprotein synthesis and decreased catabolism induced in an unknown manner by the fall in plasma oncotic pressure (which is primarily determined by the plasma albumin concentration).

One of the primary concepts that must be appreciated is the difference between the *clinical manifestations* and the *structural expression* of the disease as observed on histologic examination of tissue that is usually obtained by percutaneous kidney biopsy (Table 9.1). For example, the nephrotic presentation generally reflects *noninflammatory* injury to the glomerular capillary wall that can be induced by one of three basic mechanisms:

■ Injury to the glomerular epithelial cells in minimal change disease or primary focal glomerulosclerosis; cytokines released by mononuclear cells may be responsible for the epithelial cell damage in this setting.
■ Immune complex formation and subsequent complement activation in the subepithelial space, as in membranous nephropathy; over time, the epithelial cells lay down additional basement membrane matrix around the deposits, which results in thickening of the glomerular basement membrane (GBM) and the membranous pattern of injury (why the subepithelial localization of the deposits is important for the manifestation of the disease will be discussed in the section "Mechanisms of Glomerular Disease").
■ Deposition diseases affecting the glomerular capillary wall (GCW), such as AL-amyloidosis and light chain deposition disease (in which abnormal circulating proteins, such as monoclonal immunoglobulin light chains, are deposited) and diabetic nephropathy (in which there is dysfunction of all cells within the glomerular tuft that results ultimately in an increased synthesis of basement membrane–like material).

The lack of glomerular inflammation and therefore of severe acute tissue injury explains two other aspects of the clinical presentation of the nephrotic syndrome: The urine sediment is relatively inactive, containing few cells or cellular casts, and the plasma creatinine concentration is usually normal or only mildly elevated at presentation. The common structural finding in all nephrotic conditions is prominent and extensive damage of the glomerular visceral epithelial cells manifested by diffuse simplification or effacement of foot processes, also commonly referred to as "fusion" of foot processes.

Nephritic Syndrome

Although heavy proteinuria can also occur in nephritic states, the characteristic clinical finding is an active urine sediment containing red cells

TABLE 9.1

Clinical Manifestations, Structural Patterns of Injury, and Mechanism of Glomerular Diseases

Clinical Manifestation	Structural Pattern of Injury	Mechanism(s)
Nephrotic syndrome	1. Diffuse glomerular epithelial cell injury 2. Focal and segmental glomerulosclerosis 3. Membranous nephropathy	1. and 2. Direct cytokine effect; experimentally, direct effect of toxins or following antibody binding to the visceral epithelial cells 3. In situ formation of IC in subepithelial space of the GBM and antibody-directed and complement-mediated injury of visceral epithelial cells
Acute nephritic syndrome	4. Diffuse proliferative glomerulonephritis 5. Membranoproliferative glomerulonephritis	4. and 5. Entrapment of circulating IC and in situ formation of IC in the subendothelial space of the GBM and in the mesangium
Rapidly progressive glomerulo-nephritis	6. Focal proliferative and necrotizing glomerulonephritis 7. Crescentic glomerulonephritis	6. and 7. Antibody- dependent cell cytotoxicity (ADCC); or T-cell dependent injury
Hematuria/ proteinuria	8. Mesangioproliferative glomerulonephritis 9. Glomerular basement membrane abnormalities	8. Entrapment of circulating IC in the mesangium; abnormal glycosylation of IgA 9. Genetic defects of basement membrane collagens
Chronic kidney failure	10. Diffuse and global glomerulosclerosis	10. Obsolescence of glomeruli; tubular atrophy; interstitial fibrosis due to primary glomerular, tubulointerstitial, or vascular disease

GBM, glomerular basement membrane; IC, immune complexes.

(sometimes with gross hematuria), white cells, and cellular and granular casts, as in Case 2. The prominent urinary abnormalities in this setting reflect the influx of circulating inflammatory cells including neutrophils, macrophages, monocytes, and perhaps lymphocytes.

The type and severity of the glomerular inflammation determines the level of the kidney dysfunction and associated clinical manifestations (Table 9.1). Patients with severe glomerular injury involving most or all of the glomeruli with active inflammation present with a variable and usually sudden elevation in the plasma creatinine concentration. The fall in glomerular filtration rate (GFR) in this setting reflects a decrease in the surface area available for filtration due to partial or complete closure of the capillary lumens by the inflammatory cells or by proliferating glomerular cells within the tuft. The sudden reduction in the rate of glomerular filtration in diseases with diffuse involvement of glomeruli can also induce sodium retention, leading sequentially to extracellular fluid volume expansion, edema, and hypertension. These patients usually present with a constellation of signs and symptoms that constitute the acute nephritic syndrome. Other inflammatory diseases result mostly in a focal necrotizing and/or crescentic pattern of glomerular injury. Also, these patients present with an active urinary sediment; however, since the inflammatory process takes longer to get established, the elevation of the serum creatinine is noticed over the course of several days or few weeks, usually without the hemodynamic consequences of volume retention; in general, these patients do not develop edema or systemic hypertension. This syndrome is called rapidly progressive glomerulonephritis to differentiate it from the more sudden acute nephritic syndrome; the symptoms in the latter are usually noticed overnight.

Another group of diseases presents only with focal and usually segmental inflammation of the glomeruli; such processes typically present with asymptomatic hematuria, mild or even no proteinuria, and a normal plasma creatinine concentration and systemic blood pressure. Another noninflammatory mechanism of isolated hematuria in some patients is a genetically determined fragility of the GBMs.

A fifth glomerular syndrome, chronic kidney failure, is characterized by slowly progressive loss of function over many months or years, often associated with increasing proteinuria and variable hematuria; advanced glomerular, tubulointerstitial, vascular, and systemic diseases with kidney damage can result in this constellation of signs and symptoms, often also referred to as end-stage kidney disease.

There are three primary mechanisms by which the glomerular inflammatory process and the nephritic state can be induced; these are *different* from the mechanisms responsible for the nephrotic presentation:

■ Immune complex formation and complement activation in the subendothelial space or in the mesangium as occurs in poststreptococcal glomerulonephritis, other postinfectious glomerulonephritides, IgA nephropathy, and in some patients with lupus nephritis.

■ Circulating antibodies directed against the GBM as in anti-GBM antibody disease; this disorder is usually quite severe and presents with rapidly progressive kidney failure and sometimes with the pulmonary–renal syndrome.

■ Circulating antibodies directed against neutrophil cytoplasm antigens (ANCA) as seen in most systemic polyangiitides; antibody-induced leukocyte activation leads to necrotizing injury and inflammation of the vascular and GCWs.

The common structural finding in all nephritic conditions is injury of the endothelium that results in active inflammation due to antibody-mediated binding in close proximity to this cell or immune complex formation and deposition in the subendothelial and mesangial areas. The possible role of cell-mediated immunity remains uncertain in most glomerular and vascular diseases; however, this mechanism is clearly responsible for some interstitial nephritides and allograft rejection.

The remainder of this chapter will discuss these mechanisms of glomerular and vascular disease (with the exception of the deposition diseases). It is useful, however, to begin with a brief review of glomerular structure and function, which helps to explain how proteinuria might occur and the sites at which immune deposits are likely to form. These sites are an important determinant of the type of disease that will ensue; as noted previously, subepithelial immune deposits lead to epithelial cell injury and a nephrotic presentation, while mesangial or subendothelial immune deposits typically lead to inflammation of the glomerulus and a nephritic presentation.

Structure and Function of the Glomerular Microcirculation

The glomerular microvasculature is structurally distinct from other peripheral capillaries (Fig. 9.3A and B). The innermost aspect of the GCW, which is in contact with the vascular space, is covered by a *fenestrated endothelium*; individual fenestra measure between 70 and 100 nm or between one and two orders of magnitude larger than most plasma proteins. Nevertheless, the endothelial cells can act as part of the barrier to the filtration of anionic macromolecules (such as albumin) because they are covered by negatively charged compounds, including sialoproteins and glycosaminoglycans such as heparan sulfate.

The endothelial cells are attached to the GBM, which is a continuous porous feltwork of various extracellular *matrix proteins*, including type IV collagen, laminin, fibronectin, entactin, and other negatively charged glycoproteins and sulfated glycosaminoglycans. The central portion of

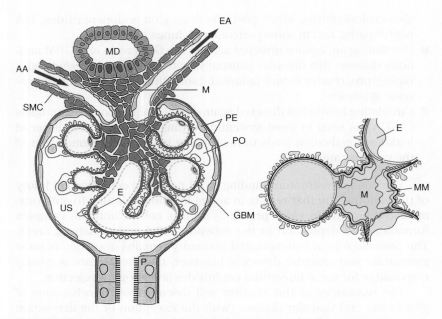

FIGURE 9.3. Schematic representation of a glomerulus. **Left:** At the vascular pole, the afferent arteriole (AA) enters the capillary network and the efferent arteriole (EA) leaves the tuft. The wall of the arterioles contains smooth muscle cells (SMCs). The capillaries are lined internally by the fenestrated endothelium (E). The continuous glomerular basement membrane (GBM) anchors the endothelium and the epithelium. The peripheral segment of the capillary wall is covered by the visceral epithelial cells or podocytes (PO) with their numerous extensions, the foot processes. The primary ultrafiltrate reaches the urinary space (US), or Bowman's space, which is continuous with the lumen of the proximal tubule (P). At the level of the vascular pole, the GBM continues to form the basement membrane of Bowman's capsule, which is lined by the parietal epithelial cells (PE). **Right:** Schematic diagram of a glomerular capillary. Note the relationships of the mesangial cell (M) and its mesangial matrix (MM) to the endothelium (E) and the GBM. The mesangial cell connects to the GBM by means of fibrillary elements. In this diagram, the artist has chosen to place the body of the endothelial cells (E) with their nuclei facing the mesangium. This is not always the case. Note that the capillary lumen is separated from the mesangium only by the fenestrated endothelium without an interposed GBM proper.

the GBM is known as the lamina densa, while the more peripheral layers are the lamina rara interna (on the endothelial side) and externa (on the epithelial side). These less electron-dense aspects of the GBM serve as attachment sites for the endothelial cells and visceral epithelial cells and, as will be seen, they are often the site of formation or entrapment of immune complexes in glomerular diseases. In addition to α-1 and α-2 collagen IV present in all basement membranes, the lamina densa of the GBM includes unique peptides encoded by autosomal and X-linked genes:

α-3, α-4, and α-5 collagen IV. It is believed that these additional collagens contribute to increased tensile strength of the GBM; defects in these genes result in molecular defects and structurally abnormal basement membranes. These genetic conditions result in increased fragility of the GBM and are associated with persistent, often familial hematuria.

The outermost layer of the capillary wall is made up of the *visceral epithelial cells* or *podocytes*. These are complex terminal cells with numerous primary, secondary, and tertiary extensions, called foot processes or pedicels (Fig. 9.3). Adjacent foot processes are derived from different epithelial cells and are connected to each other by modified desmosomes known as the filtration slit diaphragms. Several key proteins are part of these structures, including nephrin, podocin, NEPH1, p-cadherin, and FAT1, that connect the cell membrane to the cytoskeleton, which includes myosin, actin, and α-actinin 4. Defects in the genes that encode for some of these proteins result in epithelial cell dysfunction and simplification of the foot processes and nephrotic syndrome at birth (congenital nephrotic syndrome), steroid-resistant nephrotic syndrome in early childhood, or familial focal and segmental glomerulosclerosis.

The glomerular capillary network is attached and organized around a central zone, the *mesangium*. This glomerular compartment includes an extracellular matrix and the mesangial cells. The mesangial matrix is similar in composition to the GBM but less well organized and less electron dense. There are two types of cells in the mesangium. The first type is an *intrinsic glomerular cell*, the true mesangial cell, with smooth muscle cell-like phenotype. This cell connects to the GBM through specialized fibrillary structures at the site of transition from the peripheral capillary wall to paramesangial basement membrane (Fig. 9.3). Failure of these complex connecting structures through increased intracapillary pressure or injury of the mesangial cell leads to the formation of microaneurysms and loss of the capillary integrity. The second cell type has phenotypic characteristics of monocytes and can probably be considered the equivalent of *tissue macrophages or histiocytes*. Experimental studies suggest that both types of mesangial cells may contribute to the development of immune-mediated glomerular disease by secreting and by responding to a variety of cytokines (such as transforming growth factor-β), which may result in increased accumulation of matrix material and proliferation or recruitment of inflammatory cells in the mesangial space.

The intraglomerular mesangium is continuous with the extraglomerular lacis, which is the hilar area that occupies the space between the afferent glomerular arteriole, the macula densa of the distal tubule, and the efferent glomerular arteriole. Lacis cells in the vascular pole of the glomerular tuft (also called juxtaglomerular cells) produce and secrete renin, which is stored in electron-dense granules.

One important characteristic of the glomerular capillary with relevance for immune complex–mediated injury is that the GBM *does not completely surround* the entire circumference of the capillary. The endothelium facing the mesangial area attaches directly to the mesangial matrix, without an intervening basement membrane (Fig. 9.3). Hence, the GBM extends from one peripheral GCW into an adjacent capillary, passing over the mesangium that holds them together. Thus, circulating immune complexes have direct access to the mesangium and to the subendothelial space without having to cross the size-selective barrier represented by the GBM.

The factors that regulate the GFR, primarily via alterations in arteriolar resistance, have been reviewed in Chapter 1. The unique structural features of the GCW with its fenestrated endothelium, a continuous basement membrane with hydrated spaces delimited by unique cross-linked basement membrane collagens, and the interdigitating foot processes of the podocytes linked by complex filtration slit diaphragms all contribute to the very high specific hydraulic conductivity (i.e., permeability to water and small solutes) of these capillaries, which is between 100 and 100,000 times higher in the glomerulus than in any other microvessel (the relatively open hepatic sinusoid is a notable exception).

Glomerulus as a Size-Selective and Charge-Selective Barrier

In spite of the extraordinarily high permeability to water, the glomerular capillary is able to prevent virtually all but the smallest plasma proteins from entering the urinary space.

QUESTION
1

A normal subject has a GFR of 180 L/day (125 mL/min), a plasma albumin concentration of 4 g/dL, and an albumin excretion rate of 20 mg. If we assume that albumin is not reabsorbed and therefore that all the urinary albumin is derived from glomerular filtration, calculate the quantity of albumin delivered to the glomeruli each day and the fraction that is filtered. The patient in Case 1 has the nephrotic syndrome with the same GFR, a plasma albumin concentration of 1.7 g/dL, and a markedly elevated albumin excretion rate of 7.6 g/day (globulins account for most of the remaining proteins being excreted). Calculate the fractional filtration of albumin in this setting.

The ultrafiltration path is entirely extracellular and includes the endothelial fenestrae, the spaces between the cross-linked components of the GBM, and the spaces between adjacent foot processes—the filtration slits, which are bridged by the filtration slit diaphragms. This entire pathway can be envisioned as a cross-linked feltwork with hydrated spaces. The GCW can therefore be compared in its diffusion characteristics to a negatively charged chromatographic gel that interacts with circulating macromolecules by virtue of their *size* and *charge* characteristics:

- Larger molecules are restricted more than smaller molecules.
- Anionic molecules are restricted more than neutral or cationic molecules.
- Cross-linked molecules with a speroidal shape are restricted more than elongated rigid or flexible molecules, especially under conditions of convective transport.

These size-selective and charge-selective characteristics are illustrated in Figure 9.4, which depicts experiments in which dextran macromolecules of different sizes and charges were infused into rats. Additional ultrastructural studies using labeled tracer proteins have shown that the lamina densa of the GBM and the filtration slit diaphragms represent the major areas of size selectivity in the GCW, since large macromolecules aggregate proximally to these sites. It has been estimated that the effective glomerular pore radius for spherical molecules is about 42 Å. In comparison, the anionic charges in the fenestrated endothelium and in the lamina rara interna are the primary sites of charge selectivity, at which the filtration of anionic macromolecules is restricted.

We can use these principles to understand why the filtration of albumin is so markedly restricted. Albumin has an approximate effective

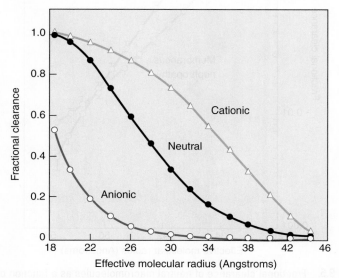

FIGURE 9.4. Fractional clearances (the ratio of the filtration of a substance to that of a substance that is freely filtered such as inulin) of anionic, neutral, and cationic dextrans as a function of effective molecular radius. Both molecular size and molecular charge are clearly important, as smaller or cationic dextrans are more easily filtered.

molecular radius of 36 Å and is highly anionic, with a net negative charge of roughly 14 mEq/L and a plasma albumin concentration of 4 g/dL. Thus, both size and charge contribute to the prevention of albumin filtration.

Mechanisms of Glomerular Proteinuria

Studies in humans with glomerular diseases have demonstrated that proteinuria due to increased glomerular permeability to macromolecules can involve both size-selective and charge-selective defects. The latter may result from injury to the glomerular cells that are responsible for the production of the glomerular polyanions such as sialoglycoproteins and heparan sulfate.

Figure 9.5 shows the results of infusing neutral macromolecules of differing sizes in normal subjects and in patients with the nephrotic

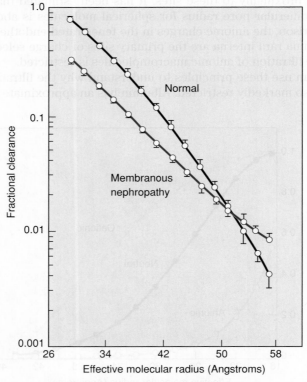

FIGURE 9.5. Fractional clearance of neutral macromolecules as a function of effective molecular radius in normal patients (*black line*) and in patients with the nephrotic syndrome due to membranous nephropathy (*red line*). There is a selective increase in clearance of molecules with a radius above 52 Å, indicative of a defect in the size-selective properties of the glomerular capillary wall.

syndrome due to membranous nephropathy. When compared to normal patients, nephrotic patients excrete fewer smaller molecules (radius <44 Å), a reflection of the loss of filtration surface area (i.e., in the number of smaller pores) induced by the glomerular disease. However, there is enhanced filtration of larger molecules with an effective radius above 52 Å, suggesting the presence of an increased number of large pores. These studies do not preclude an additional contribution from an impairment of the charge barrier. However, infusion of highly charged macromolecules to evaluate the charge barrier is contraindicated in humans because of potential allergic reactions and disturbances in coagulation.

In addition to albumin, the excretion of IgG is also typically enhanced in the nephrotic syndrome. Circulating IgG is primarily neutral; therefore, the increase in its excretion in glomerular disease largely reflects a size-selective rather than a charge-selective defect. In view of the importance of the filtration slit diaphragms in the size-selective properties of the GCW, it is generally felt that epithelial cell injury plays an important role in the associated proteinuria. For example, distortion of the slit diaphragms and focal detachments of the epithelial cells from the GBM can be identified in most nephrotic patients. A schematic representation of the normal GCW and the diffuse epithelial cell injury in nephrotic states is given in Figure 9.6.

QUESTION 2 Considering that the glomerulus contains both small and large pores, how would you explain the combination of a reduction in GFR (indicating less filtration of small solutes and water) and increased filtration of albumin and other large plasma proteins?

The amount of protein that reaches the Bowman's space through convective flow across the larger, non–size-selective pores is a direct function of the intraglomerular pressure. This relationship assumes clinical importance because a fall in protein excretion (that can exceed 50%) may be a useful marker for reduced intraglomerular pressure in patients with chronic kidney disease who are treated with antihypertensive agents or dietary protein restriction. Animal and human studies suggest that such a change in glomerular hemodynamics may slow the rate of progressive glomerular injury independent of the activity of the underlying disease. These principles are discussed in detail in Chapter 12.

Mechanisms of Glomerular Disease

Many of the mechanisms underlying kidney diseases are immune in nature. It is therefore pertinent to review briefly the basic steps involved in these processes. The four traditionally accepted types of immunologic

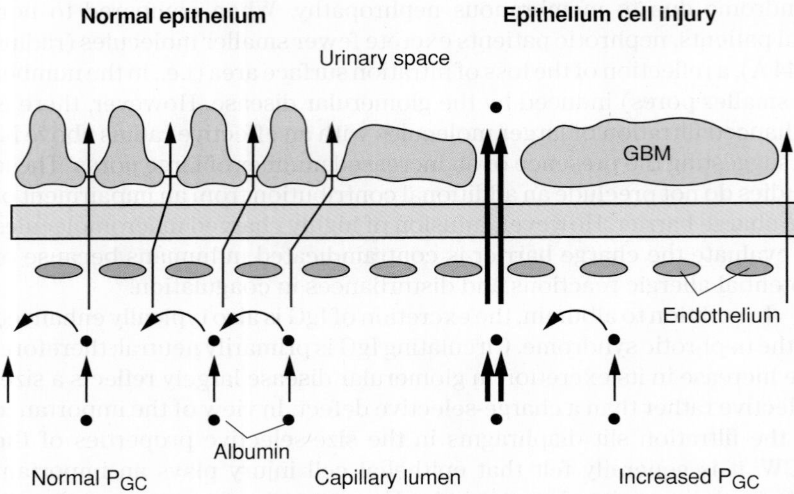

FIGURE 9.6. Schematic representation of the glomerular capillary wall (GCW) under normal conditions with preserved epithelium and in proteinuric states due to epithelial cell injury. The imbalance of hydrostatic and colloid oncotic pressure differences across the GCW, two of the determinants of ultrafiltration, results in flow of fluid from the capillary lumen to the urinary space, represented here by the long single arrows (*left side of the diagram*). In a normal glomerulus, the pathway for ultrafiltration includes the endothelial fenestrae filled with negatively charged glycoproteins and sulfated glycosaminoglycans, the negatively charged glomerular basement membrane (GBM), and the spaces between adjacent foot processes of the visceral epithelial cell with their filtration slit diaphragm. All these layers offer a certain resistance to the flow of fluid, the sum of which is another key determinant of the ultrafiltration process. These numerous pathways represent the small pore system of the physiologists. Under these normal conditions of ultrafiltration, the negatively charged elements of the proximal layers of the GCW are effective in reflecting back into the circulation negatively charged proteins, such as serum albumin (represented by the *black dots*). When there is damage of the epithelium (*right side of the diagram*), the cell responds with retraction or "fusion" of foot processes, which results in loss of filtration surface and a corresponding loss of hydraulic conductivity. At the same time, defects of the epithelial layer appear, represented by segments of the capillary wall denuded of epithelium and filtration slit diaphragms. Such areas can be expected to have a higher hydraulic conductivity since the last resistor of the GCW is lost. Hence, the flow through these abnormal channels is increased (represented by the *double arrows*), also in part driven by the increased intracapillary hydrostatic pressure (P_{GC}), a hemodynamic response seen in all proteinuric conditions due to a relative efferent arteriolar vasoconstriction; these latter changes represent a means to restore the glomerular filtration rate and counteract the loss of hydraulic conductivity due to the "fusion" of foot processes elsewhere. Under these abnormal filtration conditions, the negative charges in the proximal layers of the GCW become insufficient in their function to reflect back negatively charged and eventually all types of proteins. These abnormal large "pores" allow protein to escape into Bowman's space and into the tubules. In diffuse conditions, every nephron contributes to proteinuria, resulting in sodium chloride and water retention and the nephrotic syndrome.

diseases and some classical examples of the diseases caused by them are listed in Table 9.2:

- Type I, immediate or anaphylactic hypersensitivity, is not known to play a direct role in kidney diseases. This type of reaction is triggered when a divalent hapten or allergen cross-links IgE bound to specialized receptors for this immunoglobulin class on the surface of mast cells. While a direct role of IgE in kidney diseases is not known, patients with asthma can develop an ANCA-associated crescentic glomerulonephritis (Churg–Strauss syndrome), and allergic reactions to drugs can be accompanied by an acute interstitial nephritis, believed to be T-cell mediated.
- Type II, antibody-mediated processes, includes three groups of diseases: (1) abnormalities in cell, receptor, or enzyme function induced by direct antibody binding; (2) the traditional antibody-directed and complement-mediated lysis or damage of target cells; and (3) the antibody-dependent cell cytotoxicity reactions.
- Type III, or immune complex–mediated processes, is well represented among the glomerular diseases; the classical paradigm for this group is serum sickness. Immune complexes form in circulation elsewhere and then get trapped in the glomeruli, triggering active inflammation and eventually repair processes.
- Type IV, or T-cell-mediated diseases, is also relevant to the pathology of the kidney, especially to allograft rejection and interstitial nephritis.

Visceral Epithelial Cell Injury

Minimal change disease and primary focal glomerulosclerosis (FGS) are two common causes of the nephrotic syndrome that are thought to represent a similar pathogenetic process of differing severity. Light microscopy in minimal change disease is essentially normal or may reveal a mild mesangial hypercellularity. Immunofluorescence microscopy (in which fluorescein-labeled antibodies directed against the different human immunoglobulins and other plasma proteins of interest are incubated with the kidney tissue) usually reveals no immunoglobulin deposition. The characteristic finding in this disorder is seen on electron microscopy, which demonstrates diffuse simplification or "fusion" of the epithelial cell foot processes (Fig. 9.7), often with some detachment of the epithelial cells from the GBM.

The changes in primary or idiopathic FGS are similar except that light microscopy reveals segmental areas of capillary collapse with obliteration of the capillary lumens, entrapment of hyaline material in some capillaries, and adhesion of the tuft to Bowman's capsule; this lesion is called segmental glomerulosclerosis with hyalinosis (Fig. 9.8). For a definition of these terms, see the beginning of this chapter.

TABLE 9.2

Classification of Immune-Mediated Disorders

Type	Mechanism of Tissue Injury	Postulated Diseases
I. Immediate hypersensitivity	IgE antibodies—immediate release of vasoactive amines, lipid mediators, cytokines from mast cells—recruitment of inflammatory cells	Allergic rhinitis (hay fever), asthma, atopy, anaphylactic shock; no known kidney diseases
II. Antibody mediated	IgG, IgM antibodies; binding to target cell or matrix component:	
	A. Direct loss or enhancement of an enzyme, receptor, or cell function	A. Myasthenia gravis, hyperthyroidism, sporadic TTP, antiphospholipid syndrome; minimal change disease and idiopathic FGS, MPGN type II or dense deposits disease
	B. Lysis of target cell via complement activation	B. Autoimmune hemolytic anemia, erythroblastosis fetalis, membranous nephropathy, congenital membranous nephropathy, humoral graft rejection
	C. Antibody-dependent cell cytotoxicity (NK and ADCC cells)	C. Bullous pemphigoid, several forms of thyroiditis, rheumatic fever, autoimmune adrenalitis (Addison disease), hypoparathyroidism, type I diabetes mellitus; anti-GBM disease, ANCA-associated polyangiitis, and pauci-immune crescentic glomerulonephritis

III. Immune complex mediated	Antigen–antibody complexes in circulation—C- and Fc receptor–mediated recruitment of neutrophils—release of lysosomal enzymes and other toxic mediators	Serum sickness; systemic lupus erythematosus and various forms of lupus nephritis; postinfectious glomerulonephritis, including poststreptococcal glomerulonephritis and hepatitis B– and C–associated glomerulonephritis; cryoglobulinemia
IV. T-cell mediated	CD4+ T cells—macrophage activation—cytokines—inflammation	Hashimoto thyroiditis, insulitis in type I diabetes mellitus, rheumatoid arthritis, contact dermatitis, sarcoidosis, vasculitides (Takayasu aortitis; temporal arteritis), dermatomyositis, systemic sclerosis, inflammatory bowel disease, primary biliary cirrhosis, multiple sclerosis, autoimmune orchitis; crescentic glomerulonephritis
	CD8+ T cells—direct cytotoxicity—cytokines—inflammation	Acute (drug-induced) interstitial nephritis, allograft rejection; several forms of thyroiditis, autoimmune adrenalitis (Addison disease), hypoparathyroidism, insulitis in type I diabetes mellitus, Sjögren syndrome, polymyositis, myocarditis following Coxsackievirus B infection, inflammatory bowel disease, allograft rejectioncrescentic glomerulonephritis

ANCA, antineutrophil cytoplasm antibody; FGS, focal glomerulosclerosis; GBM, glomerular basement membrane; MPGN, membranoproliferative glomerulonephritis; TTP, thrombotic thrombocytopenic purpura.

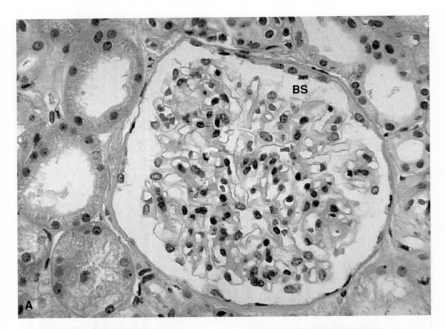

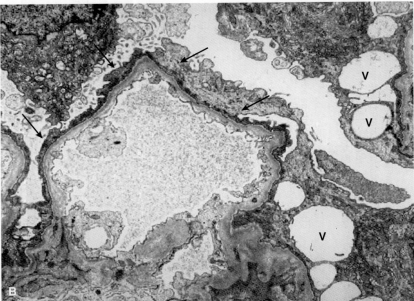

FIGURE 9.7. Diffuse epithelial cell injury, as in minimal change disease. **A.** The light microscopy shows normal-appearing glomeruli. Note open capillary lumen, open Bowman's space (BS), normal cellularity without inflammatory elements, and delicate basement membranes and mesangial matrix. **B.** The electron microscopy reveals marked degenerative changes of the glomerular visceral epithelial cell, with diffuse retraction and effacement of foot processes, often referred to as "fusion" (*arrows*), microvillous degeneration of the cell surface (best seen in left upper segment), and presence of vacuoles (V) in the cytoplasm. The immunofluorescence microscopy does not show immunoglobulin or complement deposition.

Two findings suggest that minimal change disease and primary FGS result from a primary epithelial cell injury. First, only the epithelial cells appear abnormal on electron microscopy. Second, similar changes can be induced in experimental animals by the administration of toxins such as puromycin or Adriamycin, which affect predominantly the glomerular epithelial cells, or by antibodies specific for various cell surface components of the visceral epithelium. It has been suggested that primary

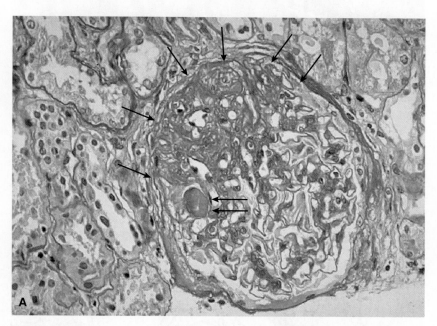

FIGURE 9.8. Focal and segmental glomerulosclerosis (FGS), a pattern of injury seen very frequently. **A.** The glomerulus shows segmental sclerosis of the tuft with disappearance of the capillary lumens, adhesion between the obsolescent part of the tuft and Bowman's capsule (*arrows*), and hyaline accumulation in isolated capillaries (*double arrow*). **B.** The electron microscopy in primary or idiopathic FGS shows diffuse effacement ("fusion" of foot processes (*large arrows*) and early hyaline deposition; this amorphous, granular material, marked by the *thin arrows,* is expanding the subendothelial space of the capillary wall that has lost focally its epithelial cell cover; note the denuded basement membrane with missing epithelium, marked by the *arrowheads.* **C.** Secondary FGS in a patient with unilateral kidney agenesis and obesity is indistinguishable from primary FGS by light microscopy, except for enlargement of the tuft. **D.** Secondary FGS; the foot processes of the visceral epithelial cells are largely preserved (*arrows*). **E.** Focal and segmental glomerular scarring in a patient with ANCA-associated polyangiitis. This type of lesion represents the healed stage of a focal necrotizing and crescentic glomerulonephritis. The scar (S) is only weakly periodic acid-Schiff positive, the remnants of the basement membrane matrix of the collapsed and fragmented tuft stain slightly stronger (*arrows*). CL, capillary lumen; Ep, parietal epithelial cell; US, urinary space.

(continued on next page)

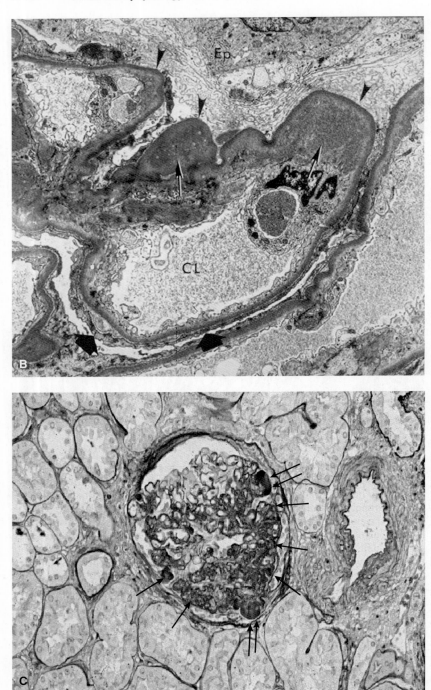

FIGURE 9.8. *(Continued)*

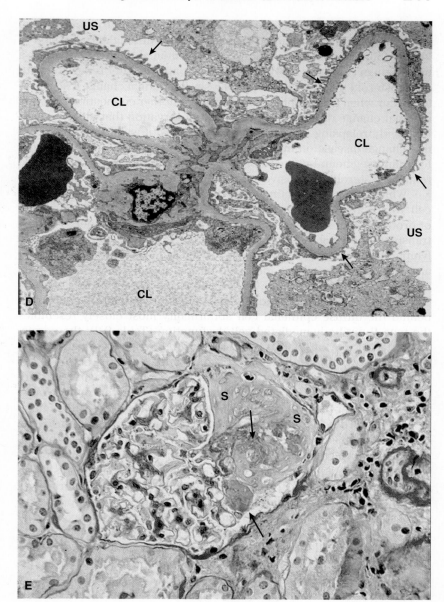

FIGURE 9.8.   *(Continued)*

FGS represents a more severe and/or prolonged insult to the epithelial cell than is present in minimal change disease. Although progression to kidney failure is not uncommon in FGS, minimal change disease is a more benign condition in which almost all patients enter remission with corticosteroid therapy. However, relapses in minimal change disease often occur when treatment is discontinued. Another connection between minimal change disease and FGS is the observation that children with frequently relapsing steroid-responsive nephrotic syndrome and minimal change disease on initial examination of the kidney often develop focal and segmental glomerulosclerosis on subsequent biopsies, while remaining steroid responsive or steroid dependent.

What remains unclear in human disease is the nature of the epithelial cell "toxin," also known as the "permeability factor." The rapid recurrence of proteinuria in some patients with primary FGS who undergo kidney transplantation suggests that a circulating factor is involved, perhaps a lymphokine released from thymus-derived lymphocytes. While unique antibodies have not been identified as the specific cause of minimal change disease and primary FGS in humans and a precise identity of the circulating permeability factor remains elusive, the overall mechanism behind the diffuse epithelial cell abnormality most closely resembles the type II antibody-mediated cell dysfunction (Table 9.2); the permeability factor may alternatively interfere with a receptor or cell surface antigen involved in transduction of signals initiated in the extracellular compartment. It is known, for example, that patients with end-stage kidney disease secondary to steroid-resistant nephrotic syndrome develop proteinuria after receiving a kidney allograft; these patients with familial disease have a defect in the gene that encodes for podocin, and during the posttransplant period they develop antibodies directed against this epithelial cell surface protein associated with the filtration slit diaphragm. The interaction between podocin and antipodocin antibodies results in abnormalities of the visceral epithelial cells that cause proteinuria.

Similar diffuse epithelial cell damage with "fusion" of foot processes can also be induced during the formation of immune complexes in the lamina rara externa (or subepithelial space), which is in close proximity to the epithelial cell membrane. This form of injury known as membranous glomerulopathy, however, is clearly complement mediated, as discussed below. These three processes—minimal change disease, primary FGS, and membranous nephropathy—have in common diffuse damage to the glomerular visceral epithelial cells, resulting in proteinuria. These diseases are diffuse, and we can expect that every nephron is excreting abnormal levels of proteins, which in turn leads to sodium retention, edema, and ultimately the full nephrotic syndrome. In contrast, diseases with only focal damage of the visceral epithelial cells (as in secondary FGS) also result in significant proteinuria, but these processes are usually not accompanied by edema, at least in the early phases of the disease, since most nephrons are not excreting abnormal levels of protein and hence do not contribute to sodium retention (see Chapter 4).

Secondary Focal Glomerulosclerosis

It is important to appreciate that the light microscopic finding of focal and segmental sclerosis is relatively nonspecific. In addition to primary FGS, similar changes can be seen in two other settings:

- As a consequence of hemodynamically mediated glomerular injury following nephron loss or functional adaptations related to the metabolic syndrome (see Chapter 12)
- During the healing phase of any focal inflammatory, necrotizing, or ischemic glomerular injury as might occur in IgA nephropathy, lupus nephritis, or systemic vasculitis

There is one histologic and one clinical finding that may allow primary and secondary FGS to be distinguished. The foot process fusion is diffuse in primary FGS, but tends to be seen only in damaged glomeruli in secondary disease. In addition, primary FGS typically presents with the acute onset of the nephrotic syndrome (similar to minimal change disease) while secondary FGS is a chronic disorder characterized by slowly increasing proteinuria over a period of years, usually without hypoalbuminemia or edema. The lack of edema can be explained by the focal nature of the epithelial cell abnormality, which results in elevated levels of protein excretion and hence abnormal sodium retention only in some but not all nephrons.

Immune Complex Formation

The glomerulus is highly susceptible to the entrapment or formation of immune complexes. The high plasma flow rate (20% of the cardiac output), high intraglomerular pressure, and high glomerular hydraulic conductivity that are required to promote filtration also increase the propensity for the deposition of antigens, antibodies, or antigen–antibody complexes. The subsequent growth of an immune complex lattice can be detected as electron-dense aggregates by electron microscopy or as fine or coarse granules by immunohistochemistry (immunofluorescence microscopy or immune-enzymatic techniques) using antibodies against human immunoglobulin light and heavy chains. These immune techniques also allow us to detect in the tissue other proteins of the complement and coagulation systems or their breakdown products.

The type of injury that is induced and the ensuing clinical manifestations critically hinge on the location of the complexes within the GCW (Fig. 9.9). It is therefore important to review the factors that determine the site of immune complex formation and the structural and functional (nephrotic or nephritic) abnormalities that may ensue (Table 9.3).

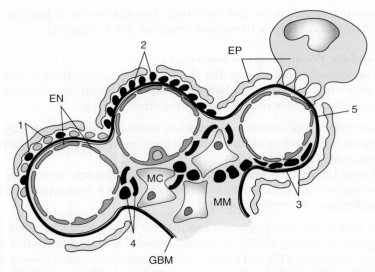

FIGURE 9.9. Schematic representation of three glomerular capillaries depicting the sites of immune complex formation. Subepithelial deposits are seen in postinfectious glomerulonephritis (1) and membranous nephropathy (2) and are likely to be assembled locally by an in situ mechanism. Subendothelial deposits (3) and mesangial deposits (4) may also form locally but are more often the result of passive entrapment of preformed circulating immune complexes. Antiglomerular basement membrane (anti-GBM) antibodies bind in a linear pattern to the GBM (5), and since the specific antigen is part of the heavily cross-linked basement membrane, electron-dense deposits at the ultrastructural level are missing. EN, endothelial cell; EP, visceral epithelial cell or podocyte; MC, mesangial cell; MM, mesangial matrix.

Immune Complex Formation in the Lamina Rara Externa (or Subepithelial Space)

Subepithelial deposits are virtually always assembled locally by the interaction of local or deposited antigen with filtered antibodies. This process has been called in situ immune complex formation. Deposition of circulating intact immune complexes in the subepithelial space is prevented by the inability of these large complexes to pass through the GBM. As will be described below, intact circulating complexes can deposit in the mesangium and lamina rara interna.

Experimental studies have suggested two models for the in situ formation of subepithelial deposits:

■ A circulating cationic antigen, which can more easily enter the GCW and pass through the GBM (Fig. 9.4), is deposited in the subepithelial space, where its filtration into the urinary space is limited by size-restrictive properties of epithelial cell slit diaphragms. Some time later, specific antibodies directed against this entrapped antigen pass through the GBM and an immune lattice gradually accumulates. Such a

TABLE 9.3

Major Causes of Immune Complex–Mediated Glomerular Disease According to Site of Complex Formation and Clinical Presentation

I. Subepithelial dense deposits that are typically associated with a nephrotic picture
   A. Membranous nephropathy—idiopathic and due to systemic disorders such as systemic lupus erythematosus, hepatitis B virus infection, and certain drugs including gold and penicillamine
   B. Postinfectious glomerulonephritis—the nephrotic syndrome is seen late in the course of the disease after subendothelial and mesangial deposits have been removed and the inflammation has abated

II. Subendothelial and mesangial dense deposits, which are associated with a nephritic picture
   A. Focal or diffuse proliferative lupus nephritis
   B. Postinfectious glomerulonephritis, early phase
   C. IgA nephropathy—in which prominent IgA-containing deposits accumulate in the mesangium

III. Antiglomerular basement membrane antibody disease, which is associated with a rapidly progressive glomerulonephritis and typically prominent crescent formation

mechanism is likely to operate in poststreptococcal glomerulonephritis; in this case, the glomerular deposition of appropriate IgG antibodies generally occurs from 10 to 14 days after the onset of a group A, β-hemolytic streptococcal infection. There is reasonable evidence that cationic proteins produced by the bacteria reach the GCW via the systemic circulation, deposit in the capillary wall, and represent the target antigens for an in situ formation of immune complexes in this condition. The candidate proteins are endostreptosin and NSAP, or *nephritis strain–associated protein.*

■ Alternatively, subepithelial deposits can result from the interaction between a filtered *autoantibody* and a locally generated endogenous antigen; such antigen may be a protein or glycoprotein expressed on the podocyte cell membrane that faces the GBM. The experimental model for this process is called *Heymann nephritis.* Genetically susceptible rats are immunized with a proximal tubule brush border cell membrane preparation in complete adjuvant. Although autoantibodies are developed against many brush border components, the major antigen involved in the formation of subepithelial deposits was initially characterized as a 330-kD cell membrane glycoprotein called gp330 or megalin. Circulating antibodies filter in small amounts and initiate the formation of antigen–antibody complexes in the lamina rara externa, in close proximity to the epithelial cell membrane; these complexes are then shed into the subepithelial space. Growth of the immune lattice occurs by the interaction between newly expressed cell surface gp330 and continuously filtered anti-gp330 antibodies.

Regardless of the mechanism, the growing complexes appear to stimulate the production of basement membrane components at sites where the epithelium remains attached to its basement membrane. These newly formed matrix components appear as characteristic "spikes" on electron microscopy (Fig. 9.1) and on histologic preparations stained by silver impregnation.

Two common examples of subepithelial deposits in humans are the formation of characteristic semilunar subepithelial "humps" in postinfectious glomerulonephritis (most often due to a streptococcal infection; see Fig. 9.2) and the more amorphous subepithelial deposits in membranous nephropathy (Fig. 9.1). The name of the latter disease is a reflection of the thickening of the GBM induced by new basement membrane formation around the immune deposits.

As mentioned previously, it has been proposed that a cationic antigen is responsible for the subepithelial deposits in postinfectious glomerulonephritis. In contrast, membranous nephropathy may be a more heterogeneous disease, with several potential target antigens on the epithelial cell surface. The membranous nephropathy in humans may be viewed as a limited autoimmune disease similar to Heymann nephritis in rats in which autoantibodies are formed against a local epithelial cell antigen; one such epithelial cell target antigen has recently been identified in patients with idiopathic membranous nephropathy as M-type phospholipase A2 receptor, a 185 kDa transmembrane glycoprotein of the mannose receptor family. Another target antigen on the epithelial cell is a neutral endopeptidase responsible for a congenital form of membranous glomerulopathy; this disease is caused in the newborn by passive transplacental immunization of the fetus by antibodies from the mother who lacks this particular enzyme. The pathogenesis of the membranous nephropathy in the newborn therefore bears striking similarities to the hemolytic disease due to Rh blood group incompatibility. Membranous nephropathy in systemic diseases such as systemic lupus erythematosus (SLE), hepatitis B virus, and other chronic infections may be initiated by the deposition or planting in the lamina rara externa of a circulating cationic antigen. Alternatively, the autoantibodies produced in SLE may be directed at specific cell surface antigens similar in nature to gp330, the receptor for phospholipase A2, or the neutral endopeptidase. Chronic infections in susceptible hosts may also trigger the production of a limited number of autoantibodies directed against these or similar epithelial cell antigens.

Subepithelial deposits are associated with injury to the epithelial cell that is characterized by retraction and effacement (or fusion) of foot processes. This process is clearly complement dependent, being mediated by the generation of the membrane attack complex (C5b-9). Intermediary chemotactic fragments (C3a and C5a) generated during complement activation at the level of the immune complexes in the lamina rara externa cannot establish a concentration gradient against the ultrafiltration flux and are filtered into the urinary space and probably further processed by the tubules without inducing an inflammatory response.

Clinical Manifestations. Patients who have only subepithelial deposits (as in membranous nephropathy) typically present with a nephrotic picture. Proteinuria in this setting results from complement-induced epithelial cell damage (leading to distortion of the slit diaphragms), but an inflammatory response leading to an active urine sediment does not occur because complement is activated *across the GBM at a site that is not in contact with circulating inflammatory cells* (Fig. 9.9). The lack of inflammatory (or phagocytic) cell infiltration accounts for the second clinical characteristic of this disorder: Once the underlying disease is controlled, as demonstrated for drug-induced membranous nephropathy, removal of the subepithelial deposits and therefore resolution of the proteinuria are very slow, taking months or even 1 to 2 years in some cases.

Immune Complex Formation in the Lamina Rara Interna (or Subendothelial Space) and the Mesangium

An in situ mechanism of immune complex formation may also be responsible for the development of subendothelial and mesangial deposits. In this setting, the targets for circulating antibodies are endogenous or exogenous antigens (such as DNA in lupus nephritis) that are planted at these sites by virtue of their size, charge, and/or affinity characteristics. As an example, larger or weakly anionic antigens are more likely to be involved, since they will be less able to cross the GBM and enter the subepithelial space.

However, subendothelial and mesangial deposits can also result from the entrapment of circulating intact immune complexes. Examples include lupus nephritis and postinfectious glomerulonephritis, disorders in which subepithelial deposits can also be formed by mechanisms described previously. Thus, a given disorder can lead to a spectrum of clinical disease depending on the nature of the antigens that are involved and the site of the immune complex deposition. Complexes located in the subendothelial space or the mesangium have access to the systemic circulation, since they are proximal to the GBM (Fig. 9.9). Thus, C3a and C5a generated from complement activation can attract neutrophils, monocytes, and macrophages, leading to a potentially marked inflammatory response (Fig. 9.2). Alternatively, immune complex formation in close proximity to the endothelium may result in upregulation of adhesion molecules as discussed below. Other mediators of this type of damage of the capillary wall include platelets and the coagulation system, triggered by the generation of Hageman factor and loss of thromboresistance of the damaged endothelium.

Recent studies also support the notion of the damaged endothelium as an active participant and regulator of the inflammatory process. Locally released cytokines and autocoids together with activated fragments of complement components have been shown to upregulate the expression of adhesion molecules both on the endothelium and on circulating inflammatory cells. Cytokines such as tumor necrosis factor and interleukin-1 activate the endothelial cells, while C5a, leukotrienes, and other cytokines act on the inflammatory cells. The net effect is an enhanced local inflammatory response that results in a diffuse proliferative glomerulonephritis and the acute nephritic syndrome.

When the conditions for subendothelial immune complex deposition continue due to persistent or episodic antigenemia (as in chronic serum sickness, SLE, and chronic infections), the disease process in the glomerulus results in the membranoproliferative pattern of injury (Fig. 9.10) and persistence of the hematuric condition. This pattern of glomerular injury is characterized by hypercellularity of the tuft, mostly due to an increase in mononuclear cells within the expanded mesangium and within the lumen of the capillaries, and capillary wall changes that result in double contours of the GBM or a "tram-track" appearance. The second additional basement membrane is formed by the endothelium, displaced by the presence of subendothelial immune deposits and cell projections derived from the damaged endothelium and potentially infiltrating macrophages. For a long time, it has been erroneously believed that these cellular elements entrapped between the two tracks of basement membrane represent mesangial cells that would have been "enticed" by unknown mysterious forces to move out into the peripheral capillary wall to "participate in the clean-up operation." True mesangial cells do not have macrophagic capacity, but monocyte-derived cells do; these cells populate the mesangium and infiltrate the tuft in various disease conditions, especially in diseases that result in the membranoproliferative pattern of injury.

It is worth mentioning at this point that the membranoproliferative pattern of injury is not exclusively the result of persistent subendothelial deposition of immune complexes. Other forms of endothelial cell damage followed by repair can also result in the formation of double contours and hypercellularity of the mesangium. These other conditions fall into three general categories:

■ Defects in complement-regulatory proteins resulting in a condition called dense deposit disease and other related glomerulopathies.

■ Chronic thrombotic angiopathies (described later in this chapter).
■ Glomerular diseases that result from entrapment of paraproteins.

Dense deposits disease, also known as MPGN type II or hypocomplementemic glomerulonephritis of childhood, and the related glomerulonephritis C3 represent examples of inflammatory conditions of the kidney brought about by an uncontrolled activity of the C3 convertase of the alternative pathway (C3bBb). These unusual glomerulopathies are associated either with autoantibodies directed against the alternative complement pathway convertase (the C3 nephritic factor or C3NeF) that render the C3bBb less susceptible to enzymatic degradation or to particular and usually homozygous defects in complement-regulatory proteins,

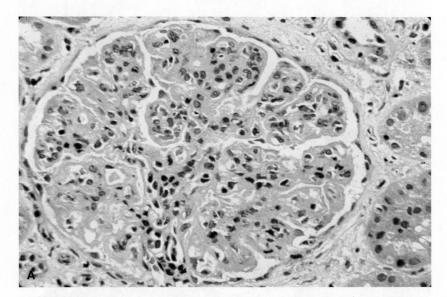

FIGURE 9.10.   The membranoproliferative pattern of injury due to a disease with circulating immune complexes. **A.** By light microscopy, there is hypercellularity of the tuft due to increase in mononuclear cells, predominantly infiltrating the expanded mesangium; there is also thickening of the glomerular capillary wall, best visualized in panel B, with frequent double contours or basement membranes with "tram track" appearance (*arrows*). The immunofluorescence microscopy (not illustrated) shows coarse granular deposits of IgG and C3. **C.** The electron microscopy shows a greatly distorted and thickened capillary wall. The peripheral capillary wall shows, from bottom to top, the endothelial cell with its nucleus (End), a newly synthesized thin basement membrane (*arrows*), a broad layer with subendothelial electron-dense deposits (D) mixed with cell projection (C) of mononuclear inflammatory cells and endothelial cells (in most textbooks, this is called "mesangial cell interposition") and basement membrane-like matrix and cell debris between cell projections and deposits, and, finally, the original basement membrane (*double arrows*) with the distorted foot processes of the visceral epithelial cells on the top of the illustration. CL, capillary lumen; US, urinary space.

(continued on next page)

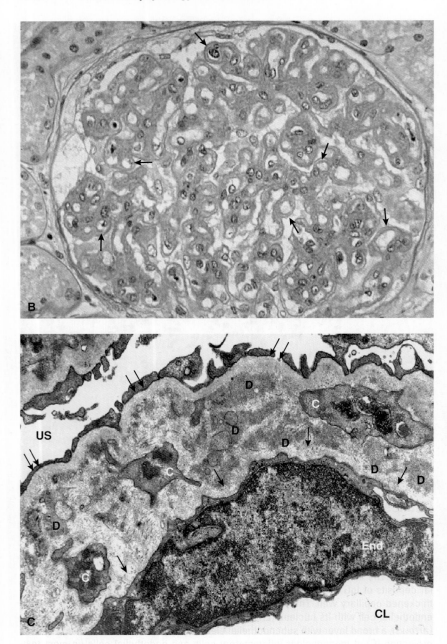

FIGURE 9.10. *(Continued)*

in particular complement Factor H (see also section on HUS later in this chapter). The precise composition and nature of the dense deposits in type II MPGN and the role played by the C3 nephritic factor in the formation of the dense deposits along the basement membranes seen by electron microscopy are poorly understood.

Paraproteins are most often but not invariably overproduced in the course of B-cell lymphoproliferative disorders, plasma cell dyscrasias, or multiple myeloma; these paraproteins include variably modified and sometimes truncated monoclonal immunoglobulins, some of them with cryoglobulin characteristics, macroglobulins (monoclonal IgM), or isolated heavy chains or light chains. Some of these paraproteins possess unique but poorly defined physicochemical characteristics that result in protein aggregates and unusual dense deposits within the extracellular matrix of the kidney. These deposits can trigger an inflammatory response, often via complement activation, or induce an overproduction of basement membrane and mesangial matrix components by unknown mechanisms. This results in the formation of mesangial nodules and thickening of the basement membranes that can be confused with the changes seen in patients with advanced diabetic nephropathy. The paraproteins are usually identified as the cause of this process by their restricted staining for heavy and light chains on immunofluorescence microscopy. Other paraproteins not derived from B cells that can also deposit in the subendothelial space are the result of genetically encoded abnormal cell products (i.e., a defective α-1 antitrypsin) or of unknown origin (fibrillary glomerulonephritis).

A unique set of pathogenetic mechanisms are believed to operate in a group of diseases characterized by IgA-containing immune complexes that get deposited predominantly in the mesangium and less frequently along the peripheral capillary wall. These diseases include IgA nephropathy, the kidney-limited variant, and Henoch–Schönlein purpura, a form of systemic vasculitis. IgA nephropathy can also occur as a complication of rheumatic diseases (ankylosing spondylitis), skin conditions (dermatitis herpetiformis), and gastrointestinal and liver diseases (celiac disease, inflammatory bowel disease, and cirrhosis). These IgA-mediated processes are usually triggered by an infection of the upper respiratory tract or the gastrointestinal system. The mucosal immune system responds by producing an IgA_1 with a defective level of glycosylation; the cause for this defective process is currently poorly understood. Immune complexes form in the circulation and these macromolecular aggregates get trapped in the mesangium, where they interact with specific receptors on the mesangial cells. Under certain conditions, this interaction results in episodic focal and segmental proliferative or necrotizing glomerulitis (Fig. 9.11) and asymptomatic hematuria, or a more diffuse proliferative and sometimes crescentic glomerulonephritis with a more acute nephritic or rapidly progressive clinical course. The episode of

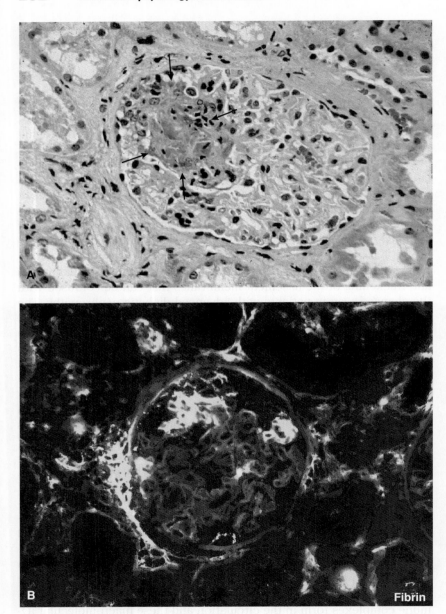

FIGURE 9.11. Focal necrotizing glomerulonephritis. **A.** The glomerulus depicted here shows a segmental necrotizing lesion, with prominent karyorrhexis (nuclear fragmentation) and fibrinoid necrosis of the tuft (*arrows*). This lesion often antedates by few days the formation of cellular crescents (see also Fig. 9.13). This pattern can be seen in association with immune complex deposition, including IgA nephropathy, and in patients with ANCA-associated glomerulonephritis or polyangiitis. **B.** The immunofluorescence microscopy shows fibrin deposits in the segments affected by necrosis and inflammation and focally in the periglomerular space.

nephritis in IgA nephropathy usually occurs shortly within 1 to 2 days following an infection (hence the term synpharyngitic hematuria as opposed to poststreptococcal glomerulonephritis, which has an incubation time of 10 to 14 days). The long-term response in IgA nephropathy also includes activation of the mesangial cell, production of growth factors, proliferation of these cells, and overproduction of matrix; the result of all these processes is a mesangioproliferative pattern of glomerular injury (Fig. 9.12).

Clinical Manifestations. The clinical manifestations associated with subendothelial and mesangial deposits are markedly different from the nephrotic pattern seen with subepithelial deposits. The local inflammatory and proliferative response in this setting results in a *nephritic* picture characterized by an active urine sediment (as described previously) and, depending upon disease severity, a GFR that can range from normal to markedly reduced (compare Cases 1 and 2 at the beginning of this chapter). If, however, the underlying disease can be controlled (as in poststreptococcal glomerulonephritis), the recovery is more rapid than

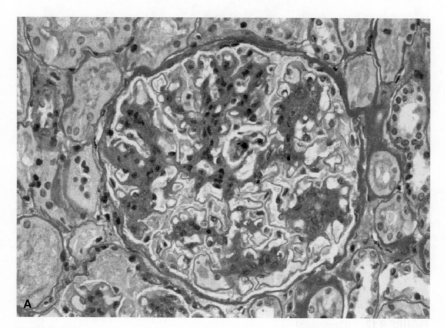

FIGURE 9.12. Mesangioproliferative glomerulonephritis. **A.** The mesangium is expanded by excess matrix and infiltrating and/or proliferated cells. **B.** Often this pattern of injury is associated with electron-dense immune complexes deposited predominantly in the mesangial areas (*arrows*). **C.** The immunofluorescence microscopy shows prominent mesangial IgA deposits in patients with IgA nephropathy and Henoch–Schönlein purpura. CL, capillary lumen; Ep, epithelial cells; US, urinary space.

(continued on next page)

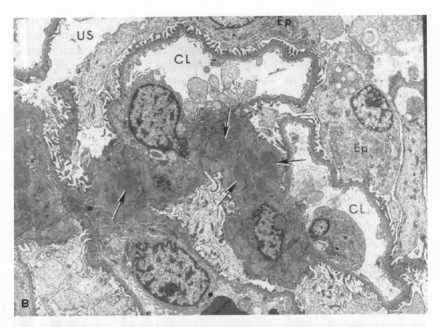

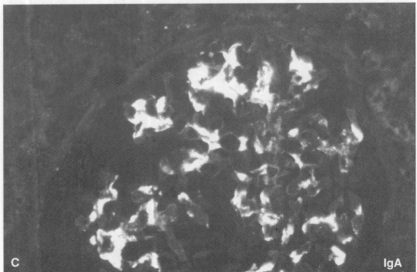

FIGURE 9.12.   *(Continued)*

with subepithelial deposits. The inflammatory cells can remove by phago-cytosis the subendothelial deposits, which are readily accessible from the circulation. However, severe inflammation can also be deleterious, producing irreversible cell injury that leads to the development of glomerulosclerosis.

Antibodies Directed against Glomerular Basement Membrane Antigens

Some patients develop a usually severe form of glomerulonephritis that is initiated by the generation of autoantibodies directed against the GBM. The target antigen in this disorder appears to represent a single, well-defined epitope on the noncollagenous portion of the α-3 chain of type IV collagen. In addition to the activation of complement and the other mediators described previously for subendothelial and mesangial deposits, anti-GBM antibody disease is also characterized by focal glomerular necrosis and prominent crescent formation (Figs. 9.11 and 9.13) that are responsible for the often rapid development of kidney failure, hence the clinical presentation as a rapidly progressive glomerulonephritis.

The pathogenesis of this disorder is confirmed by immunofluorescence microscopy, although circulating anti-GBM antibody levels can

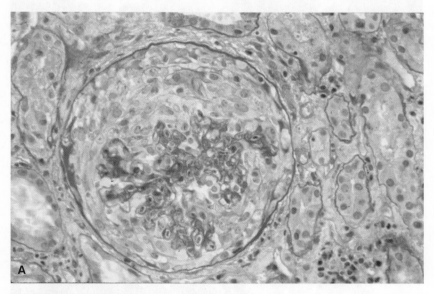

FIGURE 9.13. Crescentic glomerulonephritis due to antiglomerular basement membrane (anti-GBM) disease. **A.** By light microscopy, this pattern of injury is characterized by inflammation and influx of mononuclear cells into the Bowman's space; the cellular lesion adopts the shape of a crescent moon. This lesion is also known as extracapillary cell proliferation. **B.** The immunofluorescence microscopy reveals characteristic linear or ribbon-like deposition of IgG. The cellular crescents are usually reactive for fibrin, as is the rule for acute inflammatory processes in general. **C.** The electron microscopy fails to reveal electron-dense deposits in anti-GBM disease, as shown here, but other immune complex–mediated diseases that develop crescents show electron-dense deposits, usually along the peripheral capillary walls or in the mesangium. A third group of diseases with glomerular crescents is pauci-immune; many of these diseases are ANCA associated. There is fibrin (F) in the urinary space (US) and in the capillary lumen (CL).

(continued on next page)

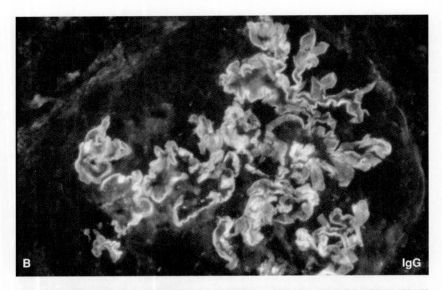

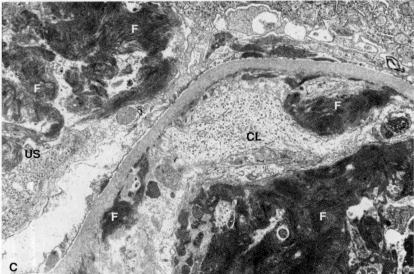

FIGURE 9.13. *(Continued)*

also be documented and measured by sensitive and specific enzyme-linked immunosorbent assay (ELISA) and Western blot techniques to establish the diagnosis and to monitor the course of disease activity. The anti-GBM antibodies, usually of the IgG class, bind in a relatively uniform manner to the cross-linked and relatively immobile GBM antigens, leading to a characteristic *linear* or *ribbon-like* appearance on immunofluorescence microscopy. In contrast, the immune complex–mediated diseases described earlier in this chapter are formed by antibodies and relatively soluble or movable cell-associated antigens; this results in discrete electron-dense deposits assembled in either lamina rara or mesangium by formation of a discontinuous immune lattice, leading to a *granular* appearance on immunofluorescence microscopy.

Crescent Formation and Cell-Mediated Immunity

Crescents refer to the accumulation and proliferation of cells outside the glomerular tuft in an extracapillary location; this inflammatory process, if marked, can compress the glomerular tuft and produce relatively rapid progression to severe kidney failure. By convention, the presence of crescents in more than 50% of glomeruli on light microscopy is called diffuse crescentic glomerulonephritis. These disorders are typically associated with progressive kidney failure that ensues over a period of weeks to several months and known as *rapidly progressive glomerulonephritis*. The early stages of crescentic glomerulonephritis are often characterized by segmental proliferative and necrotizing lesions of the glomerular tuft; the formation of cellular crescents usually follows in few days. Eventually, the necrotic segments of the glomerular tuft and the cells within the cellular crescents organize into scar tissue rich in type I collagen. This process eventually culminates in focal and segmental scarring of the tuft and fibrocellular and fibrous crescents.

The pathogenesis of crescent formation remains elusive. The primary event appears to be damage to the capillary wall severe enough to produce necrosis and rents in the GBM, thereby allowing red blood cells, fibrinogen, and other plasma constituents to enter Bowman's space. Thus, any severe glomerular disease (almost always one of the nephritic conditions in Table 9.1) can lead to crescent formation, although anti-GBM antibody disease or one of the ANCA-associated disorders (see below) is more often responsible for a focal necrotizing and crescentic glomerulonephritis.

The early necrotizing lesions of the glomerulus are often preceded in experimental models by infiltration of mononuclear cells, probably large granular lymphocytes that may in part represent NK cells. The crescentic lesions that ensue are composed of both fairly aggressive mononuclear cells, such as lymphocytes and activated macrophages, and proliferating parietal epithelial cells that normally line Bowman's capsule. Epithelioid and multinucleated giant cells derived from circulating monocytes may also be present in the crescent, suggesting a similarity to a granulomatous disease. It is therefore likely that crescents are an expression of either an antibody-dependent cell cytotoxicity, a delayed-type hypersensitivity reaction (cell-mediated immune injury), or a combination of these immune processes (Table 9.2). The occurrence of crescentic variants in virtually all immune complex–mediated and antibody-dependent diseases with a nephritic presentation suggest a variable participation of a unique mediator or effector system dependent on antibody binding; such a mediator system in these aggressive glomerulonephritides might just be the NK and ADCC cells.

Basement Membrane Abnormalities

This pattern of glomerular injury is not a reflection of an immune mechanism but results from defects in the genes that encode for basement membrane collagens, or type IV molecules, and potentially other matrix components. Defects in these genes result in various hereditary syndromes. Heterozygous defects in the genes that encode for α-4 and α-3 collagen IV result in attenuated GBMs about half the thickness of a normal basement membrane (Fig. 9.14). Such defects are associated with

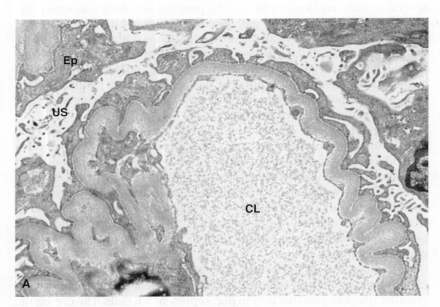

FIGURE 9.14. Basement membrane abnormalities. This pattern of injury is usually the expression of an inherited abnormality of basement membrane collagens. **A.** Normal thickness glomerular basement membrane (GBM). **B.** This panel shows a capillary wall with an attenuated lamina densa of the basement membrane, roughly half the thickness of the normal GBM. This patient had familial persistent microscopic hematuria but no proteinuria and normal glomerular filtration rate. **C.** The GBMs in patients with X-linked Alport syndrome show fragmentation or "splintering" of the lamina densa; this lesion is usually seen in patients with increasing proteinuria and progressive kidney failure. CL, capillary lumen, End, endothelium; Ep, epithelial cell; US, urinary space.

(continued on next page)

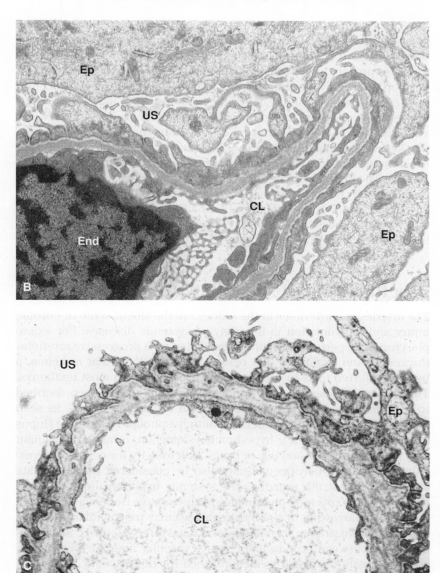

FIGURE 9.14. *(Continued)*

asymptomatic and often familial hematuria with a benign clinical course and known as thin GBM disease. Homozygous or compound heterozygous defects in these genes result in a condition also characterized by persistent hematuria but with a progressive clinical course that results in kidney failure, usually between the third and fifth decade of life (autosomal recessive hereditary nephritis).

The gene that encodes for α-5 collagen IV is located on the X chromosome. Heterozygous female carriers of defects in this gene often have benign hematuria and thin basement membranes. Affected hemizygous men also present with persistent hematuria in childhood; however, they develop progressive proteinuria and kidney failure during adolescence, with end-stage occurring usually in their 20s or early 30s. The biopsies of these patients show, in addition, more disruptive changes of the GBM, with dissolution and "splintering" of the lamina densa that results in a "basket weave" appearance (Fig. 9.14). These patients also suffer from sensorineural hearing loss, lens abnormalities, and sometimes platelet defects. The familial conditions that result in hematuria and kidney failure are usually referred to as hereditary nephritis, either autosomal recessive (defects in α-3 or α-4 collagen IV) or X linked (defects in α-5 collagen IV). When deafness is part of the clinical presentation, the condition is usually known as Alport syndrome.

Mechanisms of Vascular Injury

The arteries and arterioles in the kidney are the site of acute or chronic injury and inflammation in a variety of systemic diseases. For example, chronic hypertension is often associated with progressive arteriolar thickening and hyalinosis that results in distal glomerular ischemia, a process referred to as hypertensive nephrosclerosis in most textbooks. These vascular lesions in the kidney have traditionally been ascribed to hypertension; however, a primary form of vascular injury, as seen in systemic sclerosis (scleroderma), antiphospholipid syndrome (lupus anticoagulant syndrome), hyperhomocysteinemia, other procoagulant states, cocaine abuse and use of drugs with toxicity for cells of the vascular wall, and hyperuricemia may also be considered the immediate cause of the vascular scarring. The systemic hypertension could then be seen as an expected consequence of the relative ischemia of the kidney due to narrowing of the intrarenal vascular tree, similar in nature to the pathophysiology seen in bilateral renal artery stenosis. Such a relationship between procoagulant states, vascular injury, hypertension, and end-organ damage is well established for the placenta and the fetus in women who present clinically with severe complications in late pregnancy.

From the viewpoint of mechanisms of disease, it is useful to review the pathogenesis of two types of vascular disorders: inflammation of the blood vessels in the various forms of systemic vasculitis or polyangiitis and a loss of thromboresistance in the thrombotic angiopathies. Both of these groups of diseases have a frequent and very damaging expression in the kidney.

Systemic Vasculitis and Antineutrophil Cytoplasmic Antibodies

Inflammatory processes of the arteries can involve vessels of varying sizes, ranging from those of large caliber to the smaller arterioles. The renal manifestations of this systemic process vary with the type of vessel affected:

- The large vessel arteritides, such as the classic form of polyarteritis nodosa, often result in kidney infarcts and distal glomerular ischemia, producing a decline in kidney function that may be associated with a normal or near-normal urinalysis since there is no glomerular inflammation.

- A completely different pattern occurs when the glomerular tuft is directly affected by a small vessel vasculitis, such as in various microscopic polyangiitides, formerly known as the microscopic form of polyarteritis nodosa, Wegener granulomatosis, and Churg–Strauss syndrome. These disorders are characterized on biopsy by focal necrotizing glomerular lesions and frequent crescent formation, and clinically by an active nephritic urine sediment in the setting of a rapidly progressive kidney failure. Unlike anti-GBM disease that shows linear IgG binding and the crescentic variants of various immune complex–mediated glomerulopathies that reveal granular immunoglobulin deposits, an ANCA-associated crescentic glomerulonephritis does not show significant immunoglobulin deposition in the glomerulus, hence the term pauci-immune crescentic glomerulonephritis.

The presence of vasculitis is usually suspected from the combination of a rapidly progressive glomerulonephritis and extrarenal findings, such as arthritis, arthralgias, myalgias, and fatigue. In some cases, however, there is no evident extrarenal involvement. Most of these patients have circulating autoantibodies—*antineutrophil cytoplasm antibodies*, or ANCA. These autoantibodies were first detected by indirect immunofluorescence microscopy using neutrophils as the target cells, but the more specific and quantitative ELISA technique is now preferred. The immunofluorescence microscopy reveals two distinct patterns that reflect antibodies to different neutrophil antigens:

- Antibodies with a diffuse cytoplasmic reactivity, or C-ANCA; these antibodies are directed against a cytoplasmic serine protease called proteinase 3 or PR3-ANCA.
- Antibodies with a perinuclear reactivity, or P-ANCA; these antibodies are usually directed against a lysosomal myeloperoxidase, or MPO-ANCA.

Patients with Wegener granulomatosis usually test positive for PR3-ANCA, whereas those with microscopic polyangiitis or renal limited pauci-immune crescentic glomerulonephritis can present with either C-ANCA or P-ANCA. There seems to be very little ANCA positivity in other renal or extrarenal diseases; a notable exception is patients with anti-GBM disease—30% of them are also positive for ANCA. Low levels of P-ANCA can also be detected in some patients with SLE, while a different nonmyeloperoxidase form of P-ANCA (anti-elastase and others) has been detected in patients with sclerosing cholangitis, ulcerative colitis, and Crohn disease.

The plasma ANCA titers do not always parallel the activity of the disease, yet ANCA is a useful serologic marker of a group of diseases. It also seems clear now that these antibodies directly mediate the vascular injury. Target antigens for ANCA are expressed on the cell surface of neutrophils and monocytes when these leukocytes are stimulated by cytokines. In vitro studies in which neutrophils were incubated with ANCA obtained from patients with active Wegener granulomatosis have shown that these cells undergo a respiratory burst, release oxygen-free radicals, undergo a degranulation reaction, and then adhere to cultured endothelial cells and cause direct injury and cell death. This process involves both Fc and FAB'2 interaction. This reaction is greatly enhanced after priming of the neutrophils with tumor necrosis factor, a possible explanation for exacerbations of systemic vasculitis following acute infections.

Thrombotic Angiopathies

A completely different response is elicited in other disease processes collectively referred to as the thrombotic angiopathies or microangiopathies. The basic problem in these disorders occurs at the level of the endothelium or the platelet. For reasons that are not always completely understood, the injured endothelial cell loses its natural thromboresistance, leading sequentially to platelet activation and the deposition of platelet and, to a lesser degree, fibrin thrombi in the lumen of the affected vessels (Fig. 9.15); if there is fibrinoid necrosis of the wall of an artery or arterioles, fibrin deposition will be seen in the subintima and media.

A classical clinical syndrome develops when the process is systemic and widespread. The primary features include thrombocytopenia due to increased consumption of platelets, signs of a microangiopathic hemolytic anemia (hemolysis with schistocytes and other fragmented cells in the peripheral smear), and a variable decline in kidney function. This triad has been called the hemolytic–uremic syndrome (HUS) and sometimes follows an infection by bacteria that produce a shiga-like toxin (epidemic HUS). Some patients also have fever and neurologic dysfunction in addition to thrombocytopenia, hemolysis, and

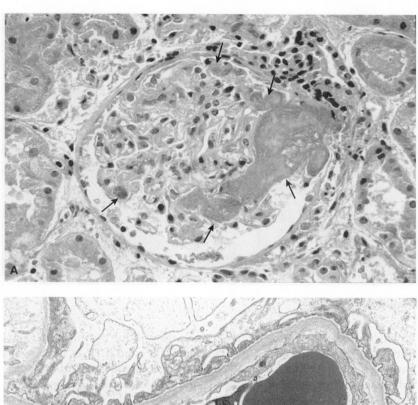

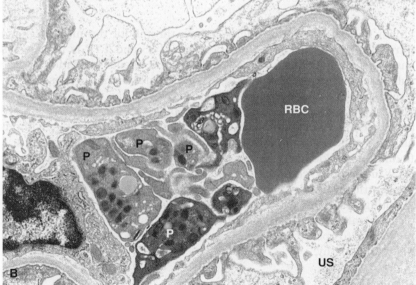

FIGURE 9.15.   Acute thrombotic angiopathy. **A.** The light microscopy reveals glomerular capillaries occluded by eosinophilic thrombi and entrapped red blood cells (*arrows*). **B.** The electron microscopy reveals a capillary occluded by aggregated and partially degranulated platelets (P) and a dysmorphic red blood cell (RBC). **C.** This immunofluorescence micrograph shows fibrin within the capillaries in two glomeruli. US, urinary space.

(continued on next page)

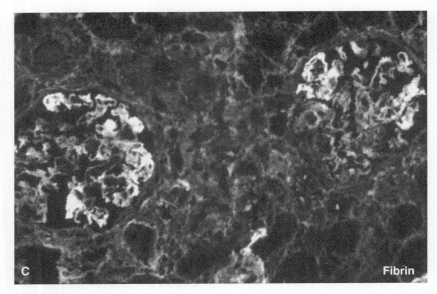

FIGURE 9.15. *(Continued)*

kidney failure, and are considered to have thrombotic thrombocytopenic purpura (TTP). The distinction between HUS and TTP is not always easy to make (see also below), and physical agents (radiation), toxic substances (chemotherapeutic agents), and autoimmune processes (systemic sclerosis and antiphospholipid syndrome) can result in identical clinical and pathologic manifestations. Some patients will have a more protracted and indolent clinical course over weeks or months, without an overt episode of microangiopathic hemolytic anemia; the structural findings in the kidney in such cases will show signs of remodeling of the GCW and "double contours" and sclerosis of arteries and arterioles with concentric layers of connective tissue alternating with cellular elements, resulting in a vessel with an "onionskin" appearance (Fig. 9.16).

Several different pathogenetic mechanisms have been shown or are postulated to operate in the various conditions that result in a thrombotic microangiopathy.

Direct Injury to the Endothelium
One of the common causes of the HUS is a diarrheal illness in infants, children, or adults infected with verotoxin-producing *Escherichia coli* or other microorganisms that produce a shiga-like toxin; these toxins are known to interfere with protein synthesis that results in damage of the endothelial cells. Non-diarrheal-associated HUS or atypical and often recurrent or familial HUS is attributable to certain defects in the genes that encode for complement-regulatory proteins, in particular

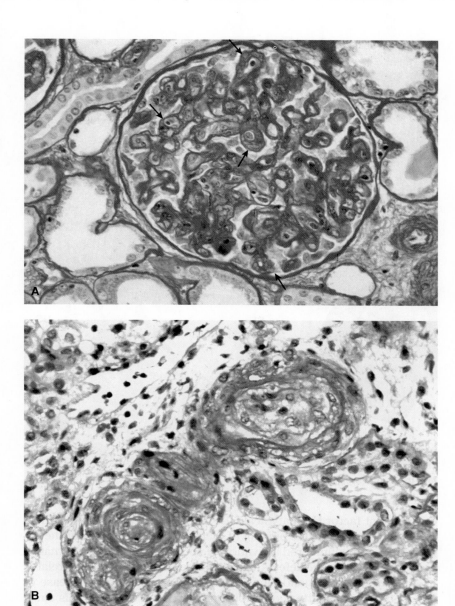

FIGURE 9.16. Chronic thrombotic angiopathy. **A.** This glomerulus shows only slight hypercellularity of the tuft but prominent thickening of the capillary walls, often with duplicated basement membranes or "double contours" (*arrows*). **B.** Small arteries and arterioles show an occluded lumen by swollen cells and fibrin and the media reveal concentric layers of basement membrane material and cells, in a classical "onionskin" pattern. **C.** The ultrastructural changes in a healed or chronic thrombotic angiopathy include thickening of the capillary wall, with widening of the subendothelial space by electron-lucent debris, duplication of the basement membrane (*arrows*) under the endothelium (End), and cell fragments (C) embedded in this matrix; there are no electron-dense deposits in the glomerular capillary wall in these disorders. Ep, visceral epithelial cell; US, urinary space.

(continued on next page)

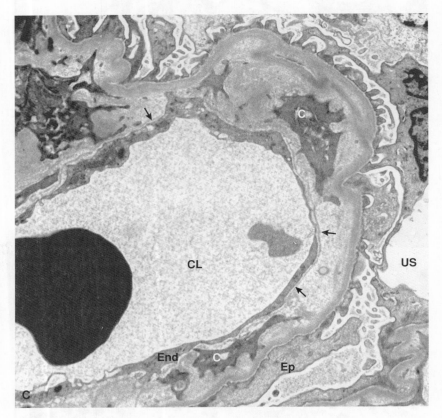

FIGURE 9.16. *(Continued)*

complement factor H. In atypical HUS, the damage to the endothelium occurs through defective binding of factor H to anionic sites of the endothelium and unhindered activation of complement via the alternative pathway. Other genetic defects in factor H are associated with age-related macular degeneration and familial forms of dense deposits disease or MPGN type II; this latter condition was discussed earlier in this chapter. A similar toxic damage to the endothelium can occur with a number of medications, including the immunosuppressive calcineurin inhibitors; with certain chemotherapeutic agents, such as gemcitabine and the combination of bleomycin and cisplatin; and with ionizing radiation used to treat malignancies or to prepare a patient for bone marrow transplantation. It is not clear if these agents always act independently or in the setting of predisposing factors, such as hereditary procoagulant states. Such a "two-hit" situation is well established for other forms of vascular injury, such as deep vein thrombosis and pulmonary embolism, and severe pregnancy-related complications, including preeclampsia, abruptio placentae, some forms of stillbirth, and postpartum acute kidney failure.

Direct Activation of Platelets

There is also evidence that primary activation of platelets may be responsible for intravascular platelet aggregation and thrombus formation, even if the endothelium is intact. In many cases, an increased level of unusually large von Willebrand factor multimers can be identified in the circulation and might directly enhance platelet aggregation. A genetic deficiency of von Willebrand factor–cleaving protease (ADAMTS13) leads to familial TTP, while patients with autoantibodies against this protease develop sporadic or autoimmune TTP. This latter condition can be viewed as a type II immune disease with direct antibody-mediated loss of enzyme function. In TTP, the persistence in circulation of uncleaved multimers of von Willebrand factor released by the injured endothelium results in more persistent platelet aggregation. On the other hand, an autoantibody directed against naturally occurring inhibitors of platelet aggregation has been described in patients with the lupus anticoagulant who may present with arterial and/or venous thrombosis.

Antibody-Mediated Endothelial Injury

Cytotoxic antiendothelial antibodies are responsible for the intravascular and intraglomerular thrombus formation that is characteristically seen in hyperacute and accelerated kidney allograft rejection and other forms of antibody or "humoral" rejection. Some of these allograft recipients have a blood group incompatibility and preexisting natural antibodies, or they develop antibodies against class I or II histocompatibility molecules or other endothelial-specific antigens by prior antigen exposure during pregnancy, blood transfusions, or prior organ transplantation. A similar situation with antibody-induced endothelial injury may occur in some children with the HUS and perhaps in other forms of autoimmune vascular injury such as scleroderma and overlap syndrome.

All these vascular disorders differ fundamentally in their pathogenesis from disseminated intravascular coagulation (DIC), as seen following amniotic fluid embolism or as a consequence of snake bites, since these latter processes are brought about by activation of the clotting cascade usually by an exogenous protease; this leads to prolongation of the prothrombin time (PT) and partial thromboplastin time (PTT), reductions in the circulating levels of fibrinogen and factors V and VIII due to sudden consumption, very high levels of circulating fibrin split products, and a "consumption coagulopathy" manifested by a bleeding diathesis. In comparison, the clotting factor levels tend to be normal in the thrombotic angiopathies, which are characterized by primary platelet consumption; these patients present with thrombocytopenia and suffer from a thrombotic diathesis.

ANSWERS TO QUESTIONS

1 The normal subject presents 7200 g [180 L/day × 40 g/L (note the conversion from g/dL to g/L)] of albumin to the glomerular filter. An excretion rate of 0.02 g/day (20 mg/day) represents a fractional excretion of 0.00028%. The patient with "heavy" proteinuria presents 3060 g/day of albumin to the glomeruli, and an excretion of 7.6 g/day reflects a fractional excretion of 0.25%. Thus, even in a disease in which glomerular permeability appears to be markedly increased clinically, virtually all of the circulating albumin remains unfiltered.

2 The fall in GFR in glomerular disease reflects a reduction in the filtering surface area and therefore in the total number of small pores. A very small increase in the number of large pores will allow the passage of normally nonfiltered macromolecules as in Question 1. However, the percentage of large pores as a function of the total number of pores is still very low; therefore, the large pores do not appreciably contribute to the filtration of water and small solutes.

SUGGESTED READINGS

Feehally J, Floege J, Johnson RJ. Comprehensive Clinical Nephrology, 3rd Ed. Philadelphia: Mosby Elsevier, 2007.

Greenberg A, Cheung AK, Falk RJ, et al. Primer on Kidney Diseases, 4th Ed. Philadelphia: Elsevier Saunders, 2005.

Kumar V, Abbas AK, Fausto N. Robbins & Cotran Pathologic Basis of Disease, 7th Ed. Philadelphia: Elsevier Saunders, 2005.

10

TUBULOINTERSTITIAL DISEASES

CASE PRESENTATION

Case 1

A 62-year-old woman has a history of benign hypertension, atherosclerotic cardiovascular disease, and bilateral cerebrovascular accidents, resulting in expressive aphasia. The patient also had a neurogenic bladder, requiring a chronic indwelling bladder catheter for urinary drainage. The patient has been cared for at home by her family. She now presents with 2 to 3 days of malaise and fever up to 105°F. She is hypotensive on physical examination, and the following laboratory data are obtained:

BUN   = 45 mg/dL
Creatinine   = 4.4 mg/dL (baseline value is 2.0 mg/dL)
WBC count   = 16,900/mm^3
Urinalysis   = 40 to 50 white cells and Gram-negative rods in the sediment

She is treated with intravenous hydration and antibiotics and slowly returns to her previous baseline state (Fig. 10.1).

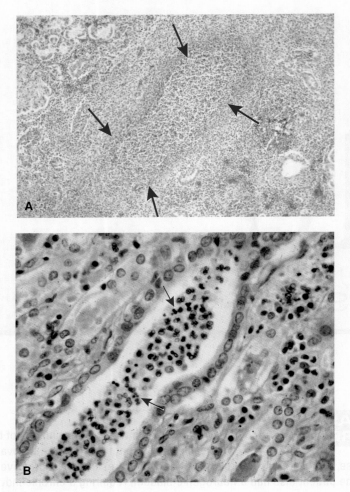

FIGURE 10.1.   Acute pyelonephritis. **A.** There is destruction of the normal cortical elements by an inflammatory process that has resulted in early abscess formation (*arrows*). **B.** The inner medulla also reveals interstitial inflammation and a collection of neutrophils in the lumen of a collecting duct (*arrows*). These aggregates of degenerating neutrophils form pus casts.

Case 2

An 18-year-old woman is admitted to the hospital for elective removal of a small, nonfunctioning left kidney. Her past medical history is remarkable for repeated episodes of urinary tract infection during infancy, and, more recently, a single episode of acute pyelonephritis. A voiding cystoureterogram showed bilateral vesicoureteral reflux and segmental scars in both kidneys. The left kidney is much smaller than the right.

Her preoperative laboratory tests reveal the following:

BUN = 21 mg/dL
Creatinine = 1.6 mg/dL
Urinalysis = 3+ protein, 5 to 10 white cells/high power field (hpf),
occasional hyaline casts
24-h urine = 3.2 g of protein

The findings of the nephrectomy specimen are depicted in Figure 10.2.

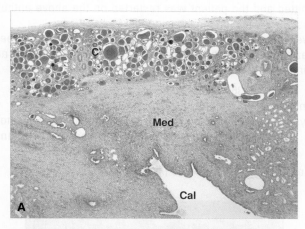

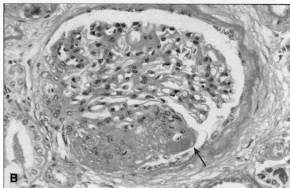

FIGURE 10.2. Chronic pyelonephritis and reflux nephropathy. **A.** This low-power magnification micrograph depicts the classical findings of chronic pyelonephritis. The cortex (C) shows marked atrophy of the tubules, with extensive cast formation (periodic acid–Schiff–positive hyaline casts), that results in an appearance that resembles the normal follicular architecture of the thyroid (thyroidization). The medulla (Med) shows marked scarring and loss of tubular elements; note the missing protruding tip of the papilla. The calix (Cal), incompletely shown here, is deformed and distended. **B.** Secondary focal glomerulosclerosis (FGS). The cortical areas not affected by atrophy usually show enlarged glomeruli, glomeruli with segmental sclerosis and hyalinosis (*arrow*) as depicted in this micrograph, hypertrophied tubules, and variable arterial and arteriolar sclerosis.

Case 3

A 42-year-old man is admitted to the hospital for general malaise and a rapidly rising plasma creatinine concentration. His past medical history is remarkable for pulmonary tuberculosis, treated 1 year ago with rifampin and isoniazid. He discontinued the drugs 6 months previously. He was seen as an outpatient 2 weeks ago for persistent productive cough, low-grade fever, and night sweats. A chest x-ray showed focal consolidations in the right upper lobe with two 2.5-cm cavitations. A presumptive diagnosis of active tuberculosis was made; cultures were submitted and the patient was restarted on the above antituberculous medications. His kidney function was normal.

Two weeks later, routine laboratory tests are obtained to screen for possible isoniazid hepatotoxicity. Although his liver function tests are normal, the following findings are noted:

BUN   = 36 mg/dL
Creatinine   = 3.8 mg/dL
Urinalysis   = 20 to 30 white cells (some of which are eosinophils),
               three to six red cells, occasional white cell and
               granular casts in the urine sediment

A kidney biopsy was performed (Fig. 10.3).

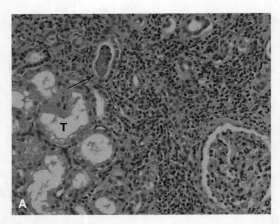

FIGURE 10.3.   Acute interstitial nephritis, drug-induced. **A.** There is marked infiltration of the cortical interstitium by an inflammatory infiltrate that separates tubules (T) and glomeruli (G). Tubules often contain white blood cell casts or cellular debris (*arrow*). The inflammation spares the glomeruli. **B.** At higher magnification, the polymorphic nature of the infiltrate becomes apparent. Mononuclear cells dominate the process; often eosinophils are a prominent component of the inflammatory infiltrate. Inflammatory cells insinuate themselves between epithelial cells of the tubule (*arrows*); this process is referred to as "tubulitis." **C.** The infiltrate in this biopsy includes multinucleated giant cells (*arrows*), resulting in a granulomatous inflammation that suggests a T cell–dependent delayed type hypersensitivity reaction.

(continued on next page)

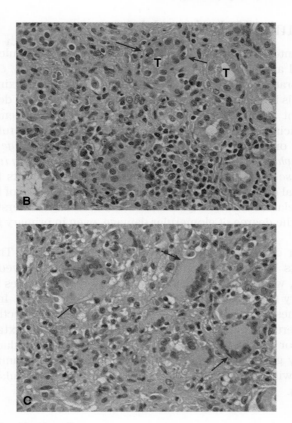

FIGURE 10.3. *(Continued)*

OBJECTIVES

Tubulointerstitial diseases also share common pathogenetic mechanisms and morphologic expressions; however, these mechanisms are different from those that are responsible for the glomerular diseases. The primary involvement is of the tubules and/or the interstitium. The previously mentioned three patients represent examples of three different underlying disorders. By the end of this section, you should have an understanding of the following issues:

■ The clinical manifestations that may be induced by these disorders, including those that are directly related to preferential tubular injury.

■ The mechanisms by which tubular and interstitial injury can occur.

■ How cyst formation might occur and how it can lead to progressive kidney failure in polycystic kidney disease.

Anatomic Relationships

The renal interstitium is the narrow space between the tubules that contains small amounts of connective tissue elements, a few cells, and a very elaborate network of capillaries that is in close proximity to the tubules. It is important to recall that this capillary network derives from the efferent arterioles; furthermore, the capillaries that emerge from the superficial and mid cortical glomeruli supply cortical tubules from more than one nephron. As a result, there may be *damage to several nephrons when a single glomerulus or the vessel supplying it succumbs to a disease process.* This relationship probably accounts for a common clinical observation on kidney biopsy: The prognosis of kidney diseases correlates more closely with the severity of tubulointerstitial injury than with the degree of glomerular damage, even in primary glomerular diseases.

Similar considerations apply to the kidney medulla. The medulla receives its blood supply entirely from capillaries derived from the vasa recta, which in turn come from the efferent arterioles of the juxtamedullary nephrons near the corticomedullary junction. In the outer medulla, these capillaries perfuse loops of Henle and collecting tubules from glomeruli throughout the cortex. Thus, injury to the juxtamedullary glomeruli or vasculature can lead to dysfunction of tubular segments from many glomeruli; if these tubules are irreversibly damaged, their glomeruli will ultimately fail to contribute to the glomerular filtration rate (GFR).

Clinical Manifestations

As with other forms of kidney disease discussed in preceding chapters, tubulointerstitial disorders have a variable clinical course. In some, the onset of the disease is rapid (as with acute tubular necrosis or acute interstitial nephritis), resulting in acute or subacute renal failure that is usually reversible. In comparison, more chronic disorders (such as reflux nephropathy or polycystic kidney disease) are characterized by continued damage occurring over a period of months or years and a progressive decline in kidney function.

The urinary findings, although variable, are of diagnostic importance because they reflect the pathogenesis of the underlying disease (see also Chapter 8):

■ The urine sediment is active in disorders characterized by acute inflammation, such as acute interstitial nephritis or acute pyelonephritis. The primary findings are pyuria (including neutrophils, mononuclear cells, and, in some cases, eosinophils), white cell casts, and, with infection, bacteriuria. White cell casts, if present, are important diagnostically, because they indicate that the white cells are derived from the kidney rather than some other site in the urinary tract. Marked hematuria and red cell casts, which are commonly seen in glomerulonephritis and vasculitis, are rare in tubulointerstitial disorders.

■ Acute toxic tubulopathies, as occurs with aminoglycoside-induced acute kidney failure, are characterized by degeneration and desquamation of tubular cells, leading to the appearance of epithelial cells and epithelial cell and granular casts in the urine sediment. The lack of interstitial inflammation explains the absence of pyuria and white cell casts.

■ The urine sediment is typically inactive in patients with chronic tubulointerstitial disease [such as reflux nephropathy, chronic exposure to toxic levels of lithium, or analgesic (phenacetin) abuse nephropathy], containing a few white cells and few casts. The bland urinary findings reflect the interstitial fibrosis and tubular atrophy that are seen on kidney biopsy. Increased excretion of low molecular weight proteins (such as amino acids and small peptides or proteins such as β_2-microglobulin) also may be seen, since these smaller proteins are filtered but, due to proximal tubular injury, may not be normally reabsorbed. This type of proteinuria cannot be detected by the dipstick for protein, which is relatively specific for albumin (see Chapter 8).

■ One additional finding that may be seen in chronic progressive and more advanced tubulointerstitial diseases is increasing glomerular proteinuria, which can exceed 4 g/day. Proteinuria in this setting reflects the development of secondary or adaptive focal glomerulosclerosis induced by nephron loss. As described in Chapter 12, nephron loss leads to hypertrophy of the tuft and hyperfiltration (mediated in part by intraglomerular hypertension) in the remaining more normal nephrons. Although this response is initially adaptive in that it maximizes the total GFR, it is maladaptive over the long term, leading to progressive glomerular scarring and proteinuria, even though the glomeruli are not the initial target of the disease.

Tubulointerstitial diseases may also be associated with well-defined syndromes that reflect dysfunction in particular nephron segments. Proximal tubular injury, for example, can lead to type 2 renal tubular acidosis due to impaired bicarbonate reabsorption and to signs of a more generalized defect in proximal reabsorption, resulting in hypophosphatemia, hypouricemia, renal glucosuria (glucose excretion in the urine despite a normal plasma glucose concentration), and aminoaciduria (Fanconi syndrome).

The manifestations are different with collecting tubule dysfunction. Patients with this problem can present with type 1 renal tubular acidosis due to impaired hydrogen secretory capacity and decreased concentrating ability and perhaps polyuria and isosthenuria resulting from a decreased responsiveness to antidiuretic hormone.

 Suppose a patient had primary injury to the kidney medulla, resulting in impaired function in the loop of Henle. Considering the functions of sodium chloride reabsorption in this segment, what would you expect the primary clinical manifestations to be?

Mechanisms of Tubulointerstitial Injury

A variety of different mechanisms can lead to tubulointerstitial injury. The remainder of this chapter will review the pathogenesis of bacterial infection, drug-induced hypersensitivity and toxic reactions, intratubular obstruction, urinary tract obstruction, and cyst formation in polycystic and acquired cystic kidney diseases.

Bacterial Infection

Bacterial infection in the urinary tract is a relatively common clinical problem. Bacteria can reach the kidney parenchyma and cause an infection within the kidney (pyelonephritis) via the blood stream (*hematogenous* spread) or, much more commonly, via *ascending* infection from the bladder.

Pathogenesis

Hematogenous pyelonephritis occurs during the bacteremic phase of a systemic infection by a relatively virulent microorganism such as *Staphylococcus aureus*. Studies in experimental animals have shown that, in the absence of an underlying renal lesion, it is difficult to induce renal infection by inoculation of bacteria into the blood stream. The factors responsible for the resistance of the kidney to bacterial invasion are not known. However, the susceptibility to colonization and infection is increased if there are focal areas of hypoperfusion or incomplete obstruction of the urinary tract.

In comparison, *ascending* infection is caused by organisms of relatively low virulence (such as Gram-negative bacteria), which are present in the patient's normal fecal flora. The normal urinary tract is sterile and ascending infections begin with the movement of these bacteria from the periurethral area into the urethra and then into the bladder. In the absence of an anatomic lesion (such as prostatic hypertrophy), bladder infections (cystitis) occur primarily in women. The enhanced susceptibility of women is due to three factors:

■ The presence of a vaginal reservoir of bacteria, such as *Escherichia coli*, derived from the fecal flora

■ The short female urethra, which promotes growth of colonies and movement of bacteria into the bladder, particularly during intercourse
■ The lack of prostatic fluid with antibacterial properties

The net effect is that the incidence of urinary tract infection is 3% to 5% in normal women during the reproductive age, approximately 50 times higher than that in normal young men. Urinary tract infections are more common in elderly patients and almost as likely to occur in men as in women in this age group. Prostatic disease is an important risk factor in older men, since the prostate can act as a nidus of infection and incomplete emptying due to partial urethral obstruction can prevent bacterial elimination by voiding.

In addition to gender, both bacterial and host factors are important determinants of infection by *increasing adhesion of bacteria* to the uroepithelial cells; in the absence of adhesion, bacterial excretion during urination is likely to occur. As an example, almost all bacteria that cause acute pyelonephritis in otherwise healthy women have Gal–Gal pili that attach to digalactoside receptors contained in glycolipids on the surface of uroepithelial cells; these glycolipids are part of the P blood group antigen. (These pili are not required for infection in abnormal urinary tracts, as with urinary tract obstruction or vesicoureteral reflux.)

Studies in women who have recurrent urinary tract infections have shown increased adhesion of bacteria to their mucosal cells. This response is in part genetically determined, as the cell surface glycolipids from these patients more avidly bind *E. coli* than those from women without recurrent infections.

Once bladder infection has occurred, *vesicoureteral reflux* plays a central role in the development of ascending pyelonephritis. Under normal circumstances, the most distal portion of the ureter is located within the bladder wall and traverses it at an angle. This intramural segment of the ureter is compressed when the pressure inside the bladder increases during micturition, resulting in an effective valve-like mechanism that prevents the retrograde flux of urine. This protective response is lost when the vesicoureteral junction is distorted due to bladder infection or a congenital malformation often associated with a shortened intramural segment. In this setting, increased bladder pressure during urination results in the movement of infected urine into the ureter and the renal pelvis.

The development of pyelonephritis requires an additional step: *intrarenal reflux* of infected urine into the kidney parenchyma. During embryonic development in higher mammals, several lobes of parenchyma can fuse, resulting in compound papillae; this is most likely to occur at the upper and lower poles. Approximately two-thirds of the kidney papillae are compound in humans. The ducts of Bellini that end at the concave portion of a compound papilla do so through circular,

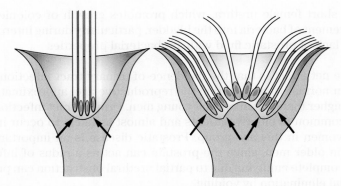

FIGURE 10.4. Mechanisms of intrarenal reflux. On a simple conical papilla, shown on the *left side of the diagram*, the ducts of Bellini have slender slit-like openings. This is a nonrefluxing papilla. On a compound papilla, shown on the *right side of the diagram*, an increase in pressure (as occurs during micturition in patients with vesicoureteral reflux) results in forces perpendicular to the surface of the papilla; orifices on the convex surface act as valves and tend to close while those that open on the concave portion are distended, a process that allows urine and bacteria to be propelled into the kidney parenchyma.

relatively open orifices, particularly in children under age 7. Thus, increased intrapelvic pressure transmitted upstream by vesicoureteral reflux generates a force that promotes reflux of urine into the parenchyma at these sites. In contrast, simple conical papillae are nonrefluxing, since the forces generated on the convex surface will tend to compress and close off the slit-like ductal orifices (Fig. 10.4).

Symptoms
Urinary tract infections may be asymptomatic or symptomatic. The site of infection primarily determines the symptoms that can be seen. Involvement of the lower urinary tract (urethra and bladder) is confined mostly to the superficial layers of the mucosa and significant tissue invasion does not usually occur. As a result, the primary symptoms are local discomfort on urination (dysuria) and urinary frequency and urgency; signs of systemic infection, such as fever and malaise, are absent. Examination of the urine sediment typically shows bacteria and white cells (pyuria). White cell casts are not seen, since there is no involvement of the kidney.

   In comparison, pyelonephritis is a parenchymal process. Thus, affected patients typically complain of pain and tenderness over the kidney, fever, and chills. Bacteriuria and pyuria are again present (unless there is infection behind a completely obstructed kidney); white cell casts, if seen, confirm kidney involvement.

QUESTION 2 Given the differing pathogeneses of hematogenous and ascending pyelonephritis, the presence or absence of which symptoms might help to distinguish clinically between these disorders?

Pathology

The distribution of lesions within the kidney in acute pyelonephritis is somewhat unpredictable, although the upper and lower poles with compound papillae are more frequently involved in ascending infection. The initial lesion is characterized by interstitial edema and neutrophilic infiltration. The inflammatory process in hematogenous pyelonephritis soon involves the tubules and spreads into the medullary segments of the nephron, where large collections of neutrophils can be seen filling the collecting ducts. These collections of cells may form white cell casts that can be seen in the urine sediment (Fig. 10.1). In the presence of severe infection or delayed antimicrobial therapy, there is eventual destruction of the kidney parenchyma and the formation of irregular abscesses and eventually scars. The glomeruli are usually unaffected.

More severe injury can be seen when complicating factors are present. For example, diabetic vascular disease or the increased intrarenal pressure induced by urinary tract obstruction can lead to a critical reduction in medullary blood flow that, in the presence of infection, can induce papillary necrosis.

Healing in the kidney after resolution of the infection occurs through transformation of the neutrophil-rich exudate into active granulation tissue. The final development is a scar. Scarring is more prominent and more easily detected by radiologic procedures (such as intravenous pyelography) in children with congenital vesicoureteral reflux who, as noted above, are also more likely to have intrarenal reflux due to open orifices of the ducts of Bellini present in the compound papillae.

It is not always easy on radiologic examination to distinguish pyelonephritic scars from ischemic lesions or healed infarcts. One important difference is that ischemic scars are randomly distributed, whereas those due to prior infection characteristically affect the poles and are located over calyces that have also been distorted by the infectious process (Fig. 10.5).

Reflux Nephropathy

Infants with vesicoureteral reflux may have repeated episodes of infection in which diagnosis and therapy are delayed or even missed because the infant cannot express the characteristic symptoms described previously. These infections can lead to significant loss of functioning parenchyma, resulting in the picture of *chronic pyelonephritis*.

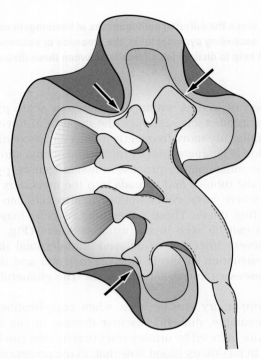

FIGURE 10.5. Pyelonephritic scars characteristically affect the renal poles where compound papillae occur. There is atrophy of the cortical elements, which results in an irregular indentation of the surface of the kidney (*arrows*). The underlying tissue is scarred and the calix that drains such a papilla is deformed.

At the histologic level, areas of tubular atrophy and interstitial fibrosis characterize chronic pyelonephritis, with persistence of mononuclear cell inflammation and initially intact glomeruli. Older lesions are characterized by thinning of the cortex due to tubular atrophy, extensive cast formation (which gives a thyroid-like appearance to the kidney parenchyma), and the virtual absence of glomeruli (Fig. 10.2). These findings are not diagnostic, however, since they can be seen with any form of chronic tubulointerstitial injury, including vascular scars. The diagnosis of chronic pyelonephritis is made from the characteristic radiologic findings noted previously and the deformities of the pelvis and calyces; active infection is often absent at the time of diagnosis.

Even if the vesicoureteral reflux disappears (spontaneously or after corrective surgery) and recurrent infection is prevented, some children develop progressive kidney failure, hypertension (that is induced by the chronic kidney disease), and proteinuria over a period of many years. These findings reflect injury to areas of the cortex that were *not affected* by the previous infections. The most prominent histologic changes are compensatory enlargement of glomeruli, focal global and segmental glomerulosclerosis, and vascular disease (arterial and arteriolar sclerosis). The glomerular injury is a reflection of the functional and structural adaptations (intraglomerular hypertension and glomerular hypertrophy) that occur in response to nephron loss; this process, as described in Chapter 12, is independent of the activity of the underlying disease.

Acute Drug-Induced Interstitial Nephritis

Acute interstitial nephritis is one of the more common causes of acute kidney failure. Acute inflammation of the interstitium has been recognized for almost 100 years as an occasional complication of severe systemic streptococcal, staphylococcal, or diphtherial infections (Councilman nephritis); a similar process has more recently been recognized in legionnaire's disease and in necrotizing fasciitis. At the present time, however, acute interstitial nephritis is almost always a process unrelated to sepsis that reflects a drug-induced hypersensitivity-type reaction. Many drugs can cause this problem but the most common are the penicillins, sulfonamide drugs, and nonsteroidal anti-inflammatory drugs.

Patients with drug-induced acute interstitial nephritis (AIN) typically develop kidney failure in 1 to 2 weeks after being exposed to the offending drug; preexposure to the drug can accelerate this process. Other signs of an allergic reaction, such as fever, skin rash, and eosinophilia, may also be present, but are often absent. The urine sediment contains white cells, white cell casts, occasional red cells, and, in some cases, eosinophils, which can be detected by special stains. Proteinuria, if present, is usually mild (less than 1 g/day) but heavy proteinuria and overt nephrotic syndrome have been described, particularly with the nonsteroidal anti-inflammatory drugs. These patients have a superimposed glomerulopathy that is indistinguishable from idiopathic minimal change disease in addition to the tubulointerstitial inflammation.

Pathogenesis
The involvement of the immune system in AIN has long been suspected but not conclusively proven. The latent period between exposure to the drug and clinical onset of the disease, the accompanying eosinophilia and rash, the type of inflammatory reaction in the kidney, and the recurrence of the disease following reexposure to the offending drug all suggest an immune-mediated reaction. In almost all cases, however, there is no evidence for the participation of antibodies in the pathogenesis of this disorder. In contrast, the nature of the inflammatory infiltrate (which is primarily composed of T lymphocytes) and, in selected patients, a positive skin test to the drug strongly suggests a *cell-mediated immune reaction*.

Several in vitro studies with cells isolated from various segments of the nephron have shown that glomerular and tubular cells have the capacity to process and present complex antigens to T cells when properly stimulated with interferon-γ. Although it is as yet unproven that this occurs in the intact animal, in vivo studies have demonstrated that exposure to simple haptens directly delivered to the kidney of presensitized animals results in a lymphocytic or granulomatous inflammation in the interstitium in the absence of significant antibody production. These observations plus the prominence of T cells in the interstitial infiltrate are consistent with a cell-mediated process. Cytokines released from the invading T cells are thought to be responsible for the development of the minimal change disease-like picture, originally described in AIN due to nonsteroidal anti-inflammatory drugs.

Pathology

The kidneys appear enlarged and edematous on gross examination in AIN. Histologically, there is a patchy or diffuse interstitial inflammatory infiltrate composed predominantly of lymphocytes, monocytes, macrophages, and, in some cases, eosinophils or neutrophils. The inflammatory cells can actively infiltrate between epithelial cells of the tubules, often resulting in significant injury to or frank necrosis of isolated cells or tubular segments. The tubular involvement can also result in the formation of intratubular casts containing intact and degenerating inflammatory cells and cellular debris. The inflammatory process typically spares the glomeruli.

Clinical Course

Discontinuation of the offending drug usually leads to virtually complete resolution of the kidney disease over a period of weeks to months. Patients with relatively advanced kidney failure may recover the function more quickly and more completely if they are also given a short course of corticosteroids. Irreversible chronic kidney failure is rare unless the offending drug is inadvertently administered for a longer period of time.

Drug-Induced Tubular Injury

The kidney is vulnerable to pharmacologic, environmental, and industrial toxins because of its high perfusion rate and solute transport functions. With aminoglycoside antibiotics, for example, filtration and subsequent reabsorption leads to marked accumulation of the aminoglycoside in lysosomes in the proximal tubule cells; if the exposure is sufficient, tubular injury and necrosis can occur (see Chapter 11). The reabsorption of 98% to 99% of the filtered water also can contribute to nephrotoxicity, since water-soluble drugs and chemicals can reach concentrations in the tubular lumen far above those in the plasma and other organs.

In addition to attaining high concentrations within the kidney, some nephrotoxins act via the generation of highly reactive metabolites, a process requiring activation by enzyme systems in the tubular cells. These enzyme systems include the cytochrome P450 mixed-function oxidases, xanthine oxidase, and prostaglandin endoperoxide synthetase. Superoxide and hydroxyl radicals and singlet oxygen generated by these systems can react chemically with cytoplasmic macromolecules (proteins and nucleic acids) and induce injury by covalent binding. Reactive species also damage the cell membrane and the membranes of cytoplasmic organelles via lipid peroxidation. Superoxide dismutase and catalase can minimize this damage, while known scavengers such as reduced glutathione, ascorbic acid, and vitamin E can neutralize peroxide and other free radicals.

A number of drugs can induce acute or chronic kidney failure via one or more of the above mechanisms. Among the common causes of acute kidney failure are antimicrobial or antiviral agents (such as the aminoglycosides, pentamidine, foscarnet, and amphotericin B) and antineoplastic platinum-based compounds. On the other hand, chronic kidney failure can result from prolonged exposure to phenacetin-containing analgesics, lithium, or aristolochic acid included sometimes in Chinese herbs.

Analgesic Abuse Nephropathy

Analgesic abuse nephropathy is a form of chronic interstitial nephritis that results from excessive consumption of analgesic mixtures containing phenacetin and aspirin. This complication is not known to occur with monotherapy with aspirin or other nonsteroidal anti-inflammatory drugs.

The etiologic link between analgesic abuse and chronic interstitial nephritis was first described in workers in watch factories in Switzerland and shortly after the influenza pandemia of 1918 in a community in Sweden in which the ingestion of phenacetin-containing medications became part of the everyday routine for many individuals. The nephrotoxicity of phenacetin-containing analgesics is dose dependent. Decreased concentrating ability or a mild reduction in GFR can be seen after cumulative phenacetin intake of 1 kg. In comparison, clinically evident kidney disease requires a minimum intake of 2 to 3 kg each of phenacetin and aspirin. This will take from 6 to 8 years in a patient ingesting six to eight tablets (or about 1 g) of phenacetin per day.

At its peak, estimates suggested that analgesic nephropathy was a major public health problem, being responsible for 1% to 3% of cases of end-stage kidney disease in the United States as a whole, up to 10% in areas of North Carolina, and 13% to 20% in Australia and some countries in Europe (such as Belgium). The incidence of analgesic nephropathy has fallen markedly in recent years as its recognition led to the removal of phenacetin from most over-the-counter pain medications.

However, an important question that remains unresolved is the renal risk of monotherapy with *acetaminophen* (Tylenol and others), which is the primary metabolite of phenacetin and which is now widely used as a minor analgesic. Two recent studies suggested that acetaminophen alone may be nephrotoxic; however, this was not confirmed in a third trial.

Pathology

The earliest lesions in analgesic nephropathy affect the vasa recta and capillaries in the kidney medulla and the small vessels in the submucosa of the ureters and bladder. These vessels develop a characteristic thickening of the basement membranes, which consists of multiple layers of matrix when viewed under the electron microscope; this lesion closely resembles that seen in chronic thrombotic angiopathies. At a later stage, the medulla shows focal areas of necrosis with fibrosis and atrophy of tubules, eventually leading to widespread papillary necrosis and calcification. The necrotic papillae can remain in place or can be sloughed into the kidney pelvis, possibly leading to symptoms of urinary tract obstruction. Identical damage to the medulla is seen in patients with hemoglobinopathies (sickle cell disease) and in diabetics with obstruction and acute pyelonephritis; here again, the vascular injury appears to be driving the disease process.

The renal cortex in analgesic nephropathy and other forms of papillary necrosis shows tubular atrophy, interstitial fibrosis, and nonspecific inflammation. The cortical damage is thought to be secondary to nephron injury and obstruction in the medulla. Although the glomeruli are not directly affected, focal and segmental glomerulosclerosis can occur as part of the adaptive response to nephron loss via a mechanism similar to that noted previously in reflux nephropathy.

Pathogenesis

The pathophysiologic mechanisms responsible for analgesic nephropathy are not completely understood. Phenacetin and its metabolites concentrate (as does sodium chloride and urea) in the medullary interstitium, where they induce the generation of reactive metabolites. These free radicals cause cell injury by direct covalent binding and oxidative damage. They also appear to be carcinogenic, as affected patients are at increased risk for transitional cell carcinomas of the urinary tract and for renal cell cancer.

Aspirin appears to potentiate the toxicity of phenacetin via one or both of two mechanisms. First, aspirin inhibits the production of vasodilator prostaglandins, which will lower the rate of medullary blood flow and predispose to further ischemic injury. Second, aspirin inhibits the hexose monophosphate shunt, which normally generates reduced glutathione, a scavenger of free radicals.

Course

The course of analgesic nephropathy depends upon whether analgesics are discontinued and upon the severity of the disease at diagnosis. Patients with relatively mild disease who discontinue therapy have stable or even improved kidney function. In contrast, progressive kidney failure is common in patients who continue analgesic therapy or in those who have suffered sufficient nephron loss to lead to secondary hemodynamic and structural injury (see Chapter 12).

Urinary Tract and Intratubular Obstruction

Obstruction to the flow of urine can occur in the tubules or in the collecting system (renal pelvis, ureter, or bladder). Regardless of the site of obstruction, a characteristic sequence of events is initiated that, if uncorrected, can lead to irreversible kidney injury and tubular atrophy. The onset of obstruction is associated with an initial increase in pressure proximal to the obstruction due to continued glomerular filtration. This rise in pressure is eventually responsible for the dilation of the collecting system and the nephron segments that can be detected by renal ultrasonography or computed tomography (CT) scanning and on biopsy, respectively.

The elevation in pressure is also transmitted back to the proximal tubule, thereby lowering the GFR by counteracting the high intraglomerular pressure that normally drives glomerular filtration. However, the rise in intratubular pressure induces secondary renal vasoconstriction and an often marked reduction in glomerular blood flow. This response is regulated *locally* by individual obstructed nephrons and is mediated in part by the release of angiotensin II and thromboxane. It can be viewed as an *appropriate* physiologic adaptation, since the increase in local glomerular resistance shunts blood flow away from obstructed nonfunctioning nephrons. However, total kidney perfusion will be diminished if all nephrons are obstructed due to disease affecting the collecting system.

The parenchyma in chronic severe urinary tract obstruction is often reduced to a thin rim of compressed and atrophic tissue. The tubular atrophy is induced in part by ischemia due to the persistent hypoperfusion. In addition, obstructed tubules appear to release a lipid that is chemotactic for monocytes and macrophages. These infiltrating cells can then release proteases and oxygen-free radicals that can contribute to the tubular injury.

Intratubular Obstruction and Myeloma Kidney

Intratubular obstruction can result from sloughed tubular cells and debris in acute tubular necrosis (see Chapter 11) or from the precipitation of a filtered solute in the tubular lumen. Examples of the latter problem include monoclonal immunoglobulin light chains (called Bence Jones proteins) in multiple myeloma, uric acid in the tumor lysis syndrome when excess tissue breakdown leads to a marked increase in uric acid production, and the administration of certain drugs, such as methotrexate, sulfonamide antibiotics, or acyclovir. These drugs are relatively insoluble in urine and intratubular precipitation is promoted by the increase in concentration induced by the reabsorption of almost all of the filtered water.

Acute or chronic kidney failure due to the toxicity of filtered light chains is called *myeloma kidney*. Light chains have a molecular weight of approximately 22,000. They are freely filtered across the glomerulus and then largely reabsorbed by the proximal tubular cells. The normal rate of light chain excretion is less than 30 mg/day. However, reabsorptive capacity can be exceeded due to overproduction in multiple myeloma, resulting in an increase in light chain excretion that can range from 100 mg to more than 20 g per day.

The mechanism by which urinary light chains lead to kidney failure is incompletely understood. Two factors are likely to be of primary importance: intratubular cast formation and direct tubular toxicity. Light chains can precipitate in the tubules, leading to obstructing, dense, intratubular casts in the distal and collecting tubules. In addition to precipitated light chains, these casts contain other filtered proteins and Tamm–Horsfall mucoprotein, which is a protein that is normally secreted by the cells of the thick ascending limb of the loop of Henle and that constitutes the matrix of all urinary casts. The limitation of obstructing casts to the distal nephron may reflect both the lower urinary flow rate in the distal nephron and the requirement for excreted light chains to aggregate with Tamm–Horsfall mucoprotein derived from the loop of Henle.

Excess urinary light chains can also induce tubular injury, particularly in the proximal tubule. This complication presumably results from the reabsorption of some of the filtered light chains into the tubular cell, where their accumulation can interfere with lysosomal function. Some light chains can also induce the formation of crystalline structures inside the tubule cells, and not infrequently will patients with light chain proteinuria present with proximal tubule dysfunctions, including the Fanconi syndrome.

 How might proximal tubular dysfunction increase the tendency to light chain precipitation and cast formation in the distal nephron?

Different monoclonal light chains have *variable nephrotoxic potential*. Thus, some patients develop kidney failure while others with an equivalent rate of light chain excretion maintain normal kidney function.

Why this occurs is not well understood but the biochemical characteristics of the individual light chain appear to be important. For example, infusion of light chains from individual patients into mice produces the same form of kidney disease (or lack of disease) as was seen in the patient.

One determinant of nephrotoxicity may be the isoelectric point (pI) of the light chain. Those Bence Jones proteins with a value above 5.1 (i.e., above the tubular fluid pH in the distal nephron) will have a net positive charge, a characteristic that may promote binding via charge interaction to anionic Tamm–Horsfall mucoprotein (pI = 3.2) and subsequent cast formation. Urinary alkalinization might therefore be beneficial, since the light chains will become less cationic or even anionic, thereby decreasing the interaction with Tamm–Horsfall mucoprotein. Dehydration, hypercalcemia, and the administration of certain contrast solutions are known risk factors for myeloma kidney.

Obstruction in the Collecting Systems

Partial or complete obstruction in the collecting systems is a relatively common problem. The major causes in adults are calculi in the renal pelvis or ureter, retroperitoneal malignancies affecting the ureters, cancer of the bladder or prostate affecting the site at which the ureters insert into the bladder, and urethral obstruction due to prostatic hypertrophy.

The clinical findings vary with the site, rate, and completeness of obstruction. Consider, for example, the symptom of pain due to distension of the bladder, collecting system, or renal capsule. Pain is typically minimal or absent with partial or slowly developing obstruction (as with a pelvic tumor). In comparison, severe pain can be seen with acute complete obstruction (as with a ureteral calculus). The site of obstruction determines the location of pain. Upper ureteral or renal pelvic lesions lead to flank pain and/or tenderness; lower ureteral obstruction causes pain that typically radiates to the ipsilateral testicle or labia; and bladder outlet obstruction is associated with suprapubic pain.

Chronic obstruction does not usually lead to pain and, since there is no inflammation, there is a relatively bland urine sediment with few cells or casts. Thus, affected patients often present with few clues as to the cause of the kidney failure. Urinary tract obstruction should be considered in all such patients. The presence of dilation of the collecting system proximal to the obstruction (hydronephrosis) is essential to establishing the diagnosis radiologically by renal ultrasonography or CT scanning.

Prognosis
Complete or prolonged partial urinary tract obstruction leads to tubular atrophy and eventually irreversible kidney injury. In Europe, for example, it is estimated that acquired obstruction is responsible for 3% to 5% of

TABLE 10.1

Congenital and Inherited Cystic Diseases of the Kidney

Disease	Inheritance	Aberrant Gene	Chromosome	Protein Encoded
Renal dysplasia				
Sporadic	Congenital	None	No	None
Familial syndromes with dysplasia	Variable	Variable	Variable	Variable
Polycystic kidney disease (PKD)				
Autosomal dominant PKD (adult)	AD	*PKD1*	16p13.3	Polycystin-2
	AD	*PKD2*	4q21	Polycystin-1
Autosomal recessive PKD (infantile)	AR	*PKHD1*	6p21-23	Fibrocystin/polyductin
Nephronophthisis (infantile, juvenile, adolescent)				
Juvenile NPHP, RP, Cogan syndrome, Joubert syndrome	AR	*NPHP1*	2q12.3	Nephrocystin-1
Infantile NPHP, situs inversus	AR	*NPHP2*	9q21-22	Nephrocystin-2/inversin
Adolescent NPHP	AR	*NPHP3*	3q22	Nephrocystin-3
Juvenile NPHP, RP, oculomotor apraxia	AR	*NPHP4*	1p36	Nephrocystin-4/nephroretinin
NPHP and RP, Senior Loken syndrome	AR	*NPHP5*	3q21	Nephrocystin-5

Disease	Inheritance	Gene	Locus	Protein
Joubert, Senior Loken, or Meckel–Gruber syndrome, and Leber congenital amaurosis NPHP	AR	NPHP6	12q21	Centrosomal protein
	AR	NPHP7	16p	Kruppel-like zinc finger protein
Joubert or Meckel–Gruber syndrome	AR	NPHP8	16q	Basal body and centrosome protein
NPHP	AR	NPHP9		Nek8 or NIMA-related kinase
Medullary cystic kidney disease type 1	AD	MCKD1	1q21	?
Medullary cystic kidney disease type 2 or Familial juvenile hyperuricemic nephropathy	AD	MCKD2	16p12	Uromodulin or Tamm–Horsfall mucoprotein
Multisystem syndromes with renal cysts				
Tuberous sclerosis	AD	TSC1	9q34	Hamartin
	AD	TSC2	16p13.3	Tuberin
Von Hippel–Lindau syndrome	AD	VHL	3p25	pVHL, an elongin-binding protein

AD, autosomal dominant; AR, autosomal recessive; NPHP, nephronophthisis.

new cases of end-stage kidney disease in patients over the age of 65, due most often to prostatic disease in men.

The renal prognosis after relief of urinary tract obstruction is dependent upon the severity and duration of the obstruction. With acute total ureteral obstruction, for example, relatively complete recovery of GFR can be achieved if the obstruction is relieved within 1 week, while little or no recovery occurs after 12 weeks. As in other settings, however, measurement of the GFR probably overestimates the true degree of recovery. In a rat model in which complete unilateral ureteral obstruction was induced for only 24 hours, approximately 15% of nephrons were nonfunctional as late as 60 days after release, a presumed reflection of irreversible injury. Despite this nephron loss, the total filtration rate returned to normal because of hypertrophy and hyperfiltration in the remaining functional nephrons.

The course of partial obstruction is less predictable, being dependent upon the severity and duration of the obstruction as well as other potential complicating factors, such as hypertension, infection, or preexisting kidney disease. As an example, older men with prostatic hypertrophy and prolonged partial urethral obstruction often present with asymptomatic and moderate to advanced kidney failure. Correction of the obstruction by inserting a catheter into the bladder or by surgery leads to a variable degree of recovery of the kidney function.

Cyst Formation

A number of hereditary diseases, congenital disorders, and acquired conditions result in renal cyst formation. Cysts are enlarged, fluid-filled outpouchings of the nephron or grossly distended tubules that may arise in the cortex and/or the medulla in one or both kidneys (Table 10.1). Simple cysts are most common, occurring in over one-half of subjects over the age of 50. The precise mechanism by which such cysts form is poorly understood; however, we are beginning to get a better understanding of the inherited forms of cystic diseases through molecular genetics and cell biology. Dysplastic kidneys are characterized by the presence of normally occurring tissues and cells but in an abnormal proportion; hence, a dysplastic kidney has excessive connective tissue, sometimes with cartilage and bone tissue, smooth muscle cells around collecting ducts, and variable cyst formation. Most cases are congenital and believed to be the result of obstruction that occurs at various periods during organogenesis. There is also a long list of familial syndromes that also present with renal dysplasia; among these are the Beckwith–Wiedemann syndrome, Ivemark syndrome, several trisomies, and the Zellweger syndrome.

Probably the most important disease state is adult polycystic kidney disease (PKD), which occurs in 1 in every 400 to 1000 live births and is currently one of the major causes of end-stage kidney disease requiring dialysis or kidney transplantation. It has autosomal dominant inheritance. The genetic defect in 86% to 96% of families affects *PKD1*, a gene located on the short arm of chromosome 16 in close proximity to the α-globin gene and adjacent to *TSC2*, one of the genes responsible for tuberous sclerosis, a condition characterized by angiomyolipomas in the kidney, adenoma sebaceum, and also renal cysts in 30% to 46% of patients. *ADPKD1* encodes polycystin-1, an integral protein expressed in plasma membranes and cilium of tubular epithelial cells, hepatic bile ductules, and pancreatic ducts. A different genetic defect is present in most of the remaining patients with autosomal dominant PKD. This defect affects *PKD2*, a gene located on chromosome 4 that encodes polycystin-2, a protein expressed in the cells and cilium of the distal nephron and with homology to voltage-activated Ca–Na channels. Both forms of autosomal dominant PKD are characterized by a progressive increase in the size and number of cysts over a period of many years. The cysts are derived from any segment of the nephron and represent outpouchings that rapidly close off from the tubule of origin. The net effect is markedly enlarged kidneys and progressive destruction of the kidney parenchyma. Cysts can also develop in other organs such as the liver, pancreas, and lung.

The prognosis is different in the two types of autosomal dominant PKD. Patients with the ADPKD2 defect form cysts later in life and have less severe disease. Thus, the mean age at which these patients develop end-stage kidney disease is 69 years, versus 57 years in patients with the ADPKD1 lesion. The net effect is that many patients, particularly those with non-ADPKD1 disease, do not develop end-stage kidney failure during their lifetime.

An autosomal recessive polycystic kidney disease (ARPKD) affects newborns, children, and young adults. The estimated incidence is from 1:10,000 to 1:40,000. It is associated with hepatic cysts, congenital hepatic fibrosis, and portal hypertension. In the newborn variant, with truncating defects in the gene, the disease is characterized by oligohydramnios in the mother, and Potter's facies, lung hypoplasia leading to spontaneous pneumothorax and pneumomediastinum, and lung and kidney failure in the child. Other variants of this condition are associated with missense mutations and present later in infancy or early adulthood with symptoms related to the liver involvement, in particular portal hypertension, and tubular dysfunction such as hyponatremia, and reduced concentrating and acidification capacity. The gene responsible for this disorder, *PKHD1*, encodes fibrocystin or polyductin. The cysts in the kidney in ARPKD represent distended collecting ducts located throughout the cortex and medulla.

Some cystic diseases of the kidney favor medullary segments of the nephron and include nephronophthisis (NPHP) in pediatric patients and medullary cystic kidney disease and familial juvenile hyperuricemic nephropathy in young adults. The various forms of familial nephronophthisis are autosomal recessive and are characterized by cysts restricted to the medulla and associated with a variable degree of tubular atrophy and interstitial fibrosis. Infantile, juvenile, and adolescent clinical variants are described. Mutations in nine genes have been reported (*NPHP1* through *NPHP9*) to date (Table 10.1). They encode for proteins (nephrocystins and others) expressed in cilia, basal bodies, or centromeres. These proteins are believed to interact with other intracellular proteins involved in cell–cell and cell–matrix signaling. These patients present with salt wasting, concentrating defects, polyuria, growth retardation, and progressive kidney failure. Mutations in some of these genes are also expressed in defects in the retina (retinitis pigmentosa or RP) and cerebellar vermis aplasia.

The autosomal dominant medullary cystic disease affects young adults; also, this disease is characterized by salt wasting, polyuria, a bland sediment, minimal proteinuria, and slowly progressive disease that results in end-stage kidney failure between the ages of 20 and 70. The cysts are located in the medulla, and are most often too small to be visualized by standard imaging techniques. In medullary cystic kidney disease type 2 (MCKD2), also known as familial juvenile hyperuricemic nephropathy, the defect involves the gene that encodes for uromodulin or Tamm–Horsfall protein on chromosome 16p12. These patients present with hyperuricemia and gout due to a reduced urate excretion, but no urate deposits in the kidney. The abnormal gene product accumulates in the cells of the thick ascending limb of the loop of Henle. The gene responsible for MCKD1 has not been identified but has been linked to chromosome 1q21. Also these patients present with kidney failure but hyperuricemia and gout are a late finding.

Pathogenesis
The various steps that lead to cyst formation are incompletely understood at present. For ADPKD, it has been postulated that an additional somatic mutation has to occur on the background of the preexisting genetic mutation for cysts to develop (the second hit theory), hence the slowly progressive nature of ADPKD. The proteins encoded by the genes that are defective in PKD are all expressed in the cilium, a cell organelle relevant in mechanosensory calcium signaling, in cell membrane domains that serve as cell-to-cell contact points, and at the interface between cell and matrix. It has been shown that polycystin-1 has extracellular domains that bind various matrix proteins, binding sites for carbohydrates, binding sites for receptor protein tyrosine phosphatases, a low-density lipoprotein-A–related domain, a C-type lectin domain, Ig-like repeats for protein binding, and areas suggestive of sites for protein cleavage. The intracellular portion of the molecule contains several sites suggestive of protein interaction and phosphorylation-signaling sites. Polycystin-2 belongs to the transient receptor potential family of channel proteins

(nonselective Ca channel); it appears to associate with polycystin-1. Fibrocystin is likely to act as a membrane receptor for extracellular proteins and as a signal-transduction element. Nephrocystin probably associates with polycystins to form adhesion complexes for extracellular matrix components.

The current hypothesis for cyst formation in all these disorders suggests that there is an imbalance between cell proliferation and apoptosis and a heightened susceptibility of the cells to the effects of the epidermal growth factor. Other aspects relevant in cyst formation include the loss of polarity of the diseased tubule cells, the reversal of the flow of fluid from net reabsorption to secretion, the abnormal cell–matrix interaction, the defect in ciliary function, and abnormalities in signal transduction that regulates cell proliferation, differentiation, and migration. The loss of cell polarity, for instance, leads to the sodium pump ($Na^+–K^+$-ATPase) being expressed in the apical membrane and the $Na^+–K^+–2Cl^-$ symporter in the basolateral cell membrane; this can be expected to result in reversal of the flow of fluid from reabsorption to secretion. The end result of all these abnormal functions is cyst formation through an uncontrolled cell proliferation, distention of a tubule segment, and eventually remodeling of the tubular basement membrane. Here again, many pathogenetic aspects of cyst formation are still unknown, but we are making progress in our understanding of these processes by learning how these various proteins function and interact under normal and disease conditions.

Acquired Cystic Kidney Disease

A similar stimulation of cell growth may also explain acquired cystic kidney disease, a common disorder that occurs in many patients with advanced kidney disease. Although cyst formation can begin prior to dialysis, the incidence of this disorder rises progressively with increasing time on dialysis, and it is estimated that more than 50% to 80% of patients will be affected after 10 or more years on dialysis. In comparison to the duration of kidney failure, the etiology of the underlying disease is unimportant.

The pathogenesis of acquired cystic disease is also not completely understood. The cysts are limited to the kidney (in comparison to the inherited conditions), suggesting that local intrarenal events play a central role. The following hypothesis has been proposed. As noted in Chapter 12, nephron loss of any cause leads to compensatory hypertrophy in the more normal nephrons. This response is driven by the activation of proto-oncogenes and the release of growth factors (such as epidermal growth factor), which, over a prolonged period of time, can lead to tubular hyperplasia and eventually cyst formation. This primary stimulation of cell growth could also explain the increased risk to develop renal cell carcinoma in patients with end-stage kidney failure.

CASE DISCUSSION

Case 1

The clinical history is classic for acute pyelonephritis. The patient begins with an anatomic abnormality promoting infection, the indwelling bladder catheter, and then develops fever, an elevated white blood cell count, and white cells and bacteria in the urine sediment. The acute decline in kidney function could result from either prerenal disease (due to hypotension) or acute tubular necrosis (due to the combination of hypotension and sepsis). These disorders can be distinguished by measuring urine electrolytes as described in Chapter 11 and by observing the response to rehydration and antibiotics. Rapid improvement suggests prerenal disease. Acute pyelonephritis itself does not usually involve enough of the kidney parenchyma to induce acute kidney failure, unless there is preexisting parenchymal disease.

Case 2

This young woman has the classic presentation of reflux nephropathy: a history of urinary tract infections in early childhood and documented vesicoureteral reflux and segmental renal scars. The excretion of 3.2 g of protein per day suggests the superimposition of hemodynamically mediated glomerulosclerosis induced by the initial nephron loss. Therapy at this time should be directed at minimizing further hemodynamic injury with an angiotensin-converting enzyme inhibitor and angiotensin II blockade (for reasons described in Chapter 12); infection is no longer a major issue in inducing kidney damage.

Case 3

This patient has developed acute kidney failure over a 10-day period after restarting antituberculous therapy with rifampin and isoniazid. The time course is strongly suggestive of a relation between one of the drugs and the kidney disease, since tuberculosis alone does not cause acute kidney failure. The two major mechanisms of drug-induced acute kidney failure are tubular toxicity (acute tubular injury) and AIN. The distinction between these disorders is often made by the urinalysis. A urine sediment showing white cells, eosinophils, red cells, and white cell casts is virtually diagnostic of interstitial nephritis, which has been described with rifampin. Epithelial cells and epithelial cell casts and granular casts would have been the major findings if this had been acute tubular injury.

ANSWERS TO QUESTIONS

1 The loop of Henle performs two major functions: It reabsorbs about one-third of the filtered sodium chloride, and the reabsorption of sodium chloride in excess of water is the primary step in the generation of the

countercurrent gradient that allows a concentrated urine to be excreted. Thus, the clinical manifestations if injury to the loop had occurred would include sodium wasting (which might not become apparent if the damage were not severe and dietary sodium intake were relatively high), hypokalemia and metabolic alkalosis (as some of the excess sodium leaving the loop is reabsorbed in the cortical collecting tubule in exchange for potassium and hydrogen), and polyuria (due to decreased concentrating ability).

2 Ascending urinary tract infection begins in the bladder and almost all affected women have initial symptoms of dysuria (pain on urination) and frequency. These symptoms might be absent or occur after the onset of fever and flank pain with hematogenous pyelonephritis.

3 As with other low molecular weight proteins, filtered light chains are normally reabsorbed in the proximal tubule. If this were impaired, more light chains would be delivered to the distal nephron, thereby promoting intratubular precipitation and cast formation.

SUGGESTED READINGS

Arant BS. Vesicoureteric reflux and renal injury. Am J Kidney Dis 1991;17:491.

Greenberg A, Cheung AK, Falk RJ, et al. Primer on Kidney Diseases, 4th Ed. Philadelphia: Elsevier Saunders, 2005.

Kumar V, Abbas AK, Fausto N. Robbins & Cotran Pathologic Basis of Disease, 7th Ed. Philadelphia: Elsevier Saunders, 2005.

Wilson PD. Polycystic kidney disease. N Eng J Med 2004;350:151–164.

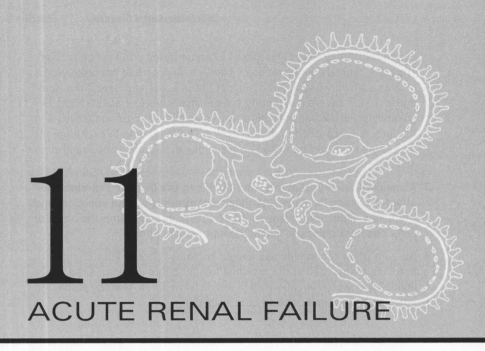

11

ACUTE RENAL FAILURE

Ahya SN, Vescundertura KA, and Flynn JT (eds): The Washington Manual of Nephrology Subspecialty Consult. Lippincott Williams & Wilkins, 2005.

CASE PRESENTATION

A 68-year-old man is admitted for elective removal of an infrarenal abdominal aortic aneurysm. Routine preoperative laboratory findings include a BUN of 20 mg/dL, a plasma creatinine concentration of 1.4 mg/dL, and a normal urinalysis. The surgery is complicated by intermittent periods of hypotension, which are reversed by fluid and blood administration. Postoperatively, the patient is hemodynamically stable but it is noted that the urine output is averaging only 10 mL/h.

The following blood and urine values are noted 6 hours after surgery:

BUN	= 33 mg/dL (9–25)
Creatinine	= 2.5 mg/dL (0.8–1.4)
Urine Na	= 61 mEq/L
Osmolality	= 320 mOsm/kg
FENa	= 3.4%

The urine sediment reveals many muddy-brown granular casts. Intravenous furosemide (a loop diuretic) is begun and the urine output increases to 60 to 80 mL/h.

OBJECTIVES

By the end of this section, you should have an understanding of each of the following issues:

■ Why estimation of the glomerular filtration rate is the primary test used to estimate the degree of renal function.

■ The major causes of acute kidney injury and the diagnostic approach used to establish the correct diagnosis, particularly the distinction between prerenal disease and acute tubular necrosis.

■ The renal response to decreased renal perfusion and the different disorders in which renal ischemia can lead to a reduction in the glomerular filtration rate.

■ The pathogenesis of postischemic and toxic acute tubular necrosis.

■ An appreciation for high-risk clinical situations that can lead to acute kidney injury due to the lack of specific therapies once injury is established.

Definition of Renal Failure

The term *renal failure* (or *renal insufficiency*) is generally applied to an impairment in the glomerular filtration rate (GFR). Renal failure that occurs acutely as the result of injury is generally referred to as acute kidney injury (AKI). Since the GFR is equal to the sum of the filtration rates in all of the functioning nephrons, the total GFR (as estimated from the plasma creatinine concentration or the creatinine clearance) is assumed to be an index of the functioning renal mass (see Chapter 1).

Thus, a fall in GFR with intrinsic renal disease usually reflects disease progression with a reduction in the number of functioning nephrons. However, the GFR can also be reduced and the patient considered to have renal failure if there is a decline in renal perfusion (*prerenal disease*) or if there is obstruction to the flow of urine out of the kidney in the renal pelves, ureters, bladder, or urethra.

The GFR is important because many potential toxins are excreted by glomerular filtration. As a result, worsening renal disease is associated with the gradual retention of a number of substances, some of which are routinely measured [such as blood urea nitrogen (BUN) and plasma creatinine]. However, BUN and creatinine per se are not toxic but rather the elevation in serum levels of these compounds correlates with accumulation and toxicity of unknown *uremic* molecules.

Retention of these toxic substances accounts for many of the signs and symptoms associated with *end-stage renal disease*. Examples of these *uremic* symptoms include pericarditis, altered mental status, and a peripheral neuropathy (see Chapter 13). Inadequate potassium and sodium excretion are also commonly seen, leading to hyperkalemia and edema, respectively. The GFR is typically between less than 15 mL/min at this time (normal equals 90 to 125 mL/min).

The loss of functioning nephrons also impairs the hormonal functions of the kidneys. This may be manifested clinically by bone disease (due in part to decreased calcitriol production) and anemia (due largely to reduced erythropoietin secretion—see Chapter 13).

Early Renal Disease

In addition to reflecting the loss of functioning renal mass, a reduced GFR may be one of the only signs of mild to moderate or even severe renal disease. For example, a patient with a GFR of 40 mL/min (roughly 40% of normal) may have no edema, normal plasma sodium and potassium concentrations, and a normal hematocrit. Only an elevated plasma creatinine concentration and possibly an abnormal urinalysis may point to the presence of underlying renal disease.

 Sodium and potassium balance can be maintained (i.e., urinary excretion equals intake) even in some patients who have a GFR below 20 mL/min. How might these adaptations occur?

For reasons that are not well understood, the intrarenal adaptations that allow the maintenance of fluid and electrolyte homeostasis are more likely to occur with chronic (longstanding) renal disease. At the same reduction in GFR, patients with acute renal failure are more likely to develop edema, hyponatremia, and hyperkalemia due to sodium, water, and potassium retention, respectively. The amount of intake as well as reduced excretion determines the likelihood of these problems being seen.

Acute Renal Failure

The definition of acute renal failure is somewhat arbitrary. The simplest definition is a recent (within the past month) increase in the plasma creatinine concentration of at least 0.5 mg/dL, or an increase of >50% over baseline value of serum creatinine or calculated creatinine clearance. Although a 0.5-mg/dL elevation is numerically small, it usually represents a large fall in GFR when the baseline plasma creatinine concentration is below 2 mg/dL (see Chapter 1 for a discussion of the relationship between the GFR and the plasma creatinine concentration).

In comparison, large increases in the plasma creatinine concentration (above 1 mg/dL) represent relatively small reductions in GFR in patients with advanced renal disease who begin with a low GFR.

QUESTION 2   Consider a patient with underlying renal disease and a baseline plasma creatinine concentration of 4 mg/dL, which reflects a GFR of 20 mL/min. Assuming no change in creatinine secretion, what is the approximate new GFR if the plasma creatinine concentration rises to 6 mg/dL the day after surgery? How are the results different if the plasma creatinine concentration remains at this level for several days?

Diagnostic Approach

The broad categories of acute renal failure are traditionally divided into three broad categories: prerenal, intrinsic, and postrenal (obstruction) causes as summarized in Figure 11.1. Table 11.1 lists the most common causes for each of these categories. The approach to establishing the correct diagnosis was reviewed in Chapter 8 and the clinical characteristics of some of the individual disorders are discussed in Chapters 9 and 10. There is, however, a sequence of steps that should be followed,

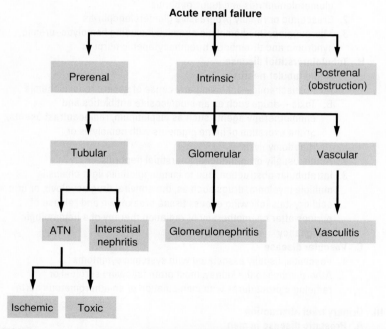

FIGURE 11.1.   Main Categories of Acute Renal Failure. Postrenal (obstuctive etiologies) should be diagnosed early since the etiology and treatment are usually anatomic. About 40% to 50% of patients with acute renal failure in the outpatient setting have prerenal etiologies. Once intrinsic renal disease is established, about 75% to 80% of patients have ATN, ~10% interstitial nephritis, and only about 5% to 10% the result of acute glomerulonephritis or vasculitis.

TABLE 11.1

Major Causes of Acute Renal Failure

I. **Prerenal disease**
   A. True volume depletion due to gastrointestinal, renal, or third-space losses
   B. Congestive heart failure or valvular heart disease
   C. Hepatorenal syndrome in advanced hepatic cirrhosis
   D. Bilateral renal artery stenosis, particularly after the administration of an angiotensin-converting enzyme inhibitor
   E. Drugs that interfere with autoregulation such as nonsteroidal anti-inflammatory drugs (NSAIDS)
   F. Shock due to fluid loss, sepsis, or cardiac failure—frequently progresses to acute tubular necrosis

II. **Intrinsic renal disease**
   A. **Glomerular disease**
      1. Acute glomerulonephritis, including postinfectious glomerulonephritis and lupus nephritis
      2. Crescentic or rapidly progressive glomerulonephritis
      3. Microangiopathic hemolytic anemias including hemolytic–uremic syndrome and thrombotic thrombocytopenic purpura
   B. **Tubulointerstitial disease**
      1. Acute tubular necrosis
         A. Postischemic—following any cause of severe renal ischemia
         B. Toxic—drugs such as aminoglycoside antibiotics and chemotherapy agents such as cisplatinum, radiocontrast agents, or the excretion of heme pigments with hemolysis or rhabdomyolysis
      2. Acute, usually drug-induced, interstitial nephritis
      3. Intratubular obstruction, due to immunoglobulin light chains in multiple myeloma, drugs such as, the antiviral drug acyclovir, or uric acid crystals following excess tissue breakdown and release of purines after chemotherapy or radiation therapy of a hematologic malignancy
   C. **Vascular disease**
      1. Vasculitis, usually associated with systemic symptoms
      2. Atheroemboli to the kidney, most often following surgical or radiologic procedures with manipulation of an atheromatous aorta

III. **Urinary tract obstruction**
   A. Prostatic disease in men
   B. Pelvic or retroperitoneal malignancy

beginning with the history (including timing the onset of the decline in renal function), physical examination, and a careful analysis of the urine.

Time of Onset

In many patients with acute renal failure, the date of onset of the decline in renal function can be identified. This is particularly true when the problem begins in the hospital, since serial routine measurements of the BUN and plasma creatinine concentration are often obtained. Suppose, for example, that the plasma creatinine concentration began to rise on hospital day 8. In this example, some renal injury was sustained in the preceding 24 hours (such as an episode of hypotension, the institution of therapy with an ACE inhibitor or a nonsteroidal anti-inflammatory drug, or the administration of a radiocontrast agent) or the cumulative effect of a toxin became clinically apparent (most often with acute tubular necrosis due to an aminoglycoside antibiotic). *Recall that GFR estimates from the serum creatinine reflect total function, so processes affecting a single kidney (stone, ischemia) may not manifest a noticeable elevation in creatinine concentration.*

We recently evaluated an otherwise healthy patient who had severe herpes zoster infection being treated with acyclovir, a drug that can precipitate in the tubules if an adequate urine flow rate is not maintained. The plasma creatinine concentration began to rise rapidly on day 11; no cause other than acyclovir was apparent even though the patient had been receiving this drug for 9 days. Careful review of the chart revealed that intravenous fluids had been discontinued on day 10. Oral intake and therefore the urine output were relatively low on the ensuing days, thereby creating an environment favoring acyclovir precipitation.

Exclusion of Urinary Tract Obstruction

Unless the diagnosis is clear from the history or urinalysis, urinary tract obstruction should always be ruled out, since it is a relatively common (especially in men) and rapidly reversible cause of acute renal failure. An enlarged bladder can often be palpated with urethral obstruction due to prostatic disease and passage of a catheter into the bladder will both relieve the obstruction and improve renal function.

Obstruction at the level of the bladder or ureters can be detected only by a radiologic procedure such as ultrasonography. This should reveal dilation of the renal pelves and calyces due to obstructing lesion. Again, unilateral obstruction will not manifest with a severe decline in GFR due to compensation from the unobstructed kidney.

A patient with acute renal failure has a urine output of 1500 mL/ day. Does the relatively normal urine output exclude the diagnosis of urinary tract obstruction?

Urinalysis

The urinalysis may reveal findings that are suggestive of a particular type of disease in patients with acute renal failure (see Table 8.3):

- Red cells (particularly if dysmorphic in shape), red cell casts, and proteinuria are virtually diagnostic of glomerulonephritis or vasculitis.
- White cells and white cell casts—with or without some red cells—are highly suggestive of acute pyelonephritis or interstitial nephritis.
- A negative dipstick for protein with a clearly positive sulfosalicylic acid test or positive urine protein/creatinine ratio points toward myeloma kidney, since the immunoglobulin light chains are not detected by the dipstick.
- Many, often muddy-brown granular casts with epithelial cells and epithelial cell casts strongly suggest acute tubular necrosis; the urinary findings in this setting represent cellular debris and desquamation.
- A relatively normal urinalysis is typically seen in prerenal disease, but may also occur in about 10% to 15% of cases of acute tubular necrosis and with urinary tract obstruction.

Distinction between Prerenal Disease and Acute Tubular Necrosis

The different causes of prerenal disease and acute tubular necrosis (ATN) are responsible for approximately 75% of cases of acute renal failure. Distinguishing between these disorders can be difficult, since there is a continuum with the severity and duration of reduced renal perfusion determining whether tubular damage has occurred. The major tool for distinguishing between prerenal disease and ATN is the response to intravenous fluids. An improvement in renal function (over 1 to 2 days) back to the baseline plasma creatinine concentration is considered diagnostic of prerenal disease, while a continued elevation in the plasma creatinine concentration points toward ATN.

In addition, several other blood and urinary findings may be helpful (Table 11.2). These findings largely reflect the difference between intact tubular function in prerenal disease and impaired tubular function in ATN.

Blood Urea Nitrogen to Plasma Creatinine Ratio

In most patients with renal failure, the decline in GFR raises both the BUN and plasma creatinine concentration in proportion. As a result, the ratio between these parameters remains at 10 to 15:1, similar to that seen in normal patients. Prerenal disease represents an exception. Renal ischemia is associated with an appropriate increase in proximal sodium and water reabsorption that are mediated in part by increased release

TABLE 11.2

Laboratory Findings in Prerenal Disease and ATN		
Test	**Favors Prerenal Disease**	**Favors ATN**
BUN-to-PCr ratio	>20:1	10–15:1
Urinalysis	Normal or near normal with few cells or casts; hyaline casts may be seen but are not abnormal	Many granular casts with renal tubular epithelial cells and epithelial cell casts
Urine sodium	<25 mEq/L	>40 mEq/L
FENa	<1%	>2%
Urine osmolality	>500 mOsm/kg	300–350 mOsm/kg

ATN; acute tubular necrosis; BUN; blood urea nitrogen; PCr, plasma creatinine.

of angiotensin II. The reabsorption of water raises the tubular fluid urea concentration, thereby leading to an equivalent elevation in proximal urea reabsorption. The increment in urea reabsorption will raise the BUN out of proportion to any change in GFR, thereby increasing the BUN-to-plasma creatinine ratio.

A ratio above 20:1 is generally indicative of prerenal disease in the absence of a high-protein diet, increased tissue breakdown, or gastrointestinal bleeding all of which raise the BUN independent of the GFR. A normal ratio, however, is less useful. It can be seen with ATN but may also be seen in prerenal disease when urea production is reduced due to decreased protein intake or hepatic disease.

Urine Sodium Concentration and Fractional Excretion of Sodium

Sodium retention is an appropriate response to renal ischemia that is partially impaired in ATN. Thus, the urine sodium concentration is generally below 20 mEq/L in prerenal disease, but above 40 mEq/L in ATN. There is, however, appreciable overlap that is due in part to the urine sodium concentration being influenced by the rate of reabsorption of water as well as that of sodium.

The confounding effect of water transport can be removed and the diagnostic accuracy increased by calculating the FENa, which is a direct measure of the reabsorption of filtered sodium. (The formula for calculating the FENa is derived in Chapter 8.) A FENa below 1% (indicating that more than 99% of the filtered sodium has been reabsorbed) suggests prerenal disease, while a value above 2% is usually due to ATN.

Urine Osmolality

Marked volume depletion is a potent stimulus to the release of antidiuretic hormone. This should result in a highly concentrated urine (osmolality above 500 mOsm/kg) when tubular function is intact, as in prerenal disease. In comparison, concentrating ability is impaired early in ATN because the medullary cells in the thick ascending limb are among the cells that are first damaged by renal ischemia. As a result, the urine is relatively isosmotic to the plasma in ATN, with the urine osmolality being between 300 and 350 mOsm/kg in most cases. There is, however, substantial overlap so that only a high value above 500 mOsm/kg is of diagnostic importance.

Prerenal Disease

Although the response to decreased renal perfusion has been described, there are some important pathophysiologic lessons to be learned by reviewing three of the causes: the hepatorenal syndrome; bilateral renal artery stenosis, particularly after the administration of an angiotensin-converting enzyme (ACE) inhibitor; and the administration of nonsteroidal anti-inflammatory drugs to susceptible subjects.

Hepatorenal Syndrome

The hemodynamic changes occurring in hepatic cirrhosis are discussed in Chapter 4: marked splanchnic vasodilation, leading to reductions in systemic vascular resistance and blood pressure. As in other forms of effective volume depletion, the hypotension in hepatic cirrhosis is associated with progressive elevations in angiotensin II and norepinephrine release, resulting in an increasing degree of renal ischemia. This is manifested by a gradual reduction in GFR as the hepatic disease becomes more severe.

The decline in GFR in hepatic cirrhosis is often masked by reductions in the production of urea (due to the hepatic disease) and creatinine (due mostly to a loss of muscle mass). As a result, the plasma creatinine concentration may remain within the "normal" range of 1.0 to 1.4 mg/dL in patients with a GFR as low as 20 mL/min. Measurement of the creatinine clearance, although not very accurate, should detect the reductions in creatinine production and GFR in this setting.

The *hepatorenal syndrome* is defined as an otherwise unexplained and progressive elevation in the plasma creatinine concentration in a patient with advanced hepatic disease. Although it may appear clinically that this disorder has begun abruptly in a patient with normal renal function, the hepatorenal syndrome represents the end-stage of a process that gradually lowers renal blood flow and GFR (see Fig. 11.5 later in this chapter).

Patient survival is extremely limited in the hepatorenal syndrome unless hepatic function can be improved (as with hepatic transplantation). Mortality in this setting is due to hepatic encephalopathy or variceal bleeding rather than due to renal failure. Reinfusion of the patient's ascites into the internal jugular vein via a *peritoneovenous shunt* can expand the plasma volume and, in many cases, improve renal function. There is, however, no beneficial effect on patient survival, since the hepatic failure persists.

Renal Artery Stenosis and Angiotensin-Converting Enzyme Inhibitors

Narrowing of the renal artery (renal artery stenosis) is associated with a reduction in arterial pressure distal to the obstruction. Despite this fall in pressure perfusing the glomeruli, the GFR can initially be maintained by *autoregulation* (the mechanism of which is discussed in Chapter 1). This phenomenon, depicted in Figure 11.2, shows that the GFR is maintained

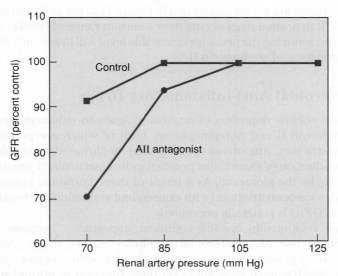

FIGURE 11.2. Effect of reducing renal artery pressure (from a baseline value of approximately 125 mm Hg) on glomerular filtration rate (GFR) in normal dogs (*squares*) and dogs pretreated with an angiotensin II antagonist (*circles*). Autoregulation of GFR was maintained in normal dogs until the renal artery pressure fell to 70 mm Hg. Antagonizing the effect of angiotensin II led to an earlier and more marked fall in GFR, indicating an important role for angiotensin II in the autoregulation of GFR.

in normal dogs as the renal artery pressure is lowered from 125 to 85 mm Hg. The ability to autoregulate eventually fails and the GFR begins to decline as the renal artery pressure falls to 70 mm Hg.

Angiotensin II plays an important role in the autoregulation of GFR by preferentially constricting the efferent glomerular arteriole, thereby maintaining the intraglomerular pressure. If, however, the effect of angiotensin II is blocked by an angiotensin II antagonist or its production is diminished by the administration of an ACE inhibitor, then the reduction in GFR begins at a higher pressure and is more pronounced (Fig. 11.2).

Patients who have greater than a 75% narrowing of one or both renal arteries are often hypertensive, as the angiotensin II formed within the kidney during the autoregulatory response can also enter the systemic circulation and induce vasoconstriction. An ACE inhibitor will usually partially or completely reverse the hypertension in this setting. It will, however, tend to impair autoregulation, thereby lowering the GFR. This effect will not significantly raise the plasma creatinine concentration in patients with a unilateral lesion, since filtration will be maintained in the contralateral, nonstenotic kidney. However, acute renal failure can occur in some patients with bilateral renal artery stenosis or unilateral stenosis in a solitary kidney.

It should be emphasized that, although the risk is greatest with an ACE inhibitor, any antihypertensive agent can lead to acute renal failure if the stenoses are severe. As shown in Figure 11.2, the ability to autoregulate GFR in normal dogs occurs over a certain range of renal perfusion pressures; reducing the pressure below this level will lower the GFR even in the presence of angiotensin II.

Nonsteroidal Anti-inflammatory Drugs

Effective volume depletion of any cause leads to enhanced secretion of angiotensin II and norepinephrine, both of which are potent renal vasoconstrictors. Angiotensin II and norepinephrine also stimulate the renal production of vasodilator prostaglandins, particularly prostacyclin and PGE_2 by the glomeruli. As a result of these hormonal interactions, excessive vasoconstriction (with consequent reductions in renal blood flow and GFR) is generally prevented.

This relationship assumes clinical importance because of the widespread use of nonsteroidal anti-inflammatory drugs (NSAIDs), which reduce prostaglandin synthesis by inhibiting the enzyme cyclooxygenase. NSAIDs have little effect on renal function in normal subjects in whom angiotensin II, norepinephrine, and renal prostaglandin production are relatively low. However, NSAID can lead to acute renal failure when given to patients with true volume depletion (as with diuretic therapy), congestive heart failure, or hepatic cirrhosis. In these settings, exaggerated renal vasoconstriction occurs as the compensatory prostaglandin response to increased release of angiotensin II and nore-pinephrine is blocked.

The selective cyclooxygenase-2 inhibitors have been shown to result in fewer gastrointestinal side effects, but the consequences on renal hemodynamics and renal function are similar to traditional NSAIDs. Therefore, these drugs should also be avoided in patients with renal insufficiency, volume depletion, congestive heart failure, or hepatic cirrhosis.

Acute Tubular Necrosis

There are two major types of ATN: postischemic and toxic (Table 11.1). Regardless of the mechanism, ATN is associated with two major histologic changes *and normal glomeruli*:

■ Tubular necrosis with denuding of the epithelial cells; the tubular injury tends to be most prominent in the proximal tubules and in the thick ascending limb of the loop of Henle.
■ Occlusion of the tubular lumens by cellular debris and casts and, with hemolysis or rhabdomyolysis, by precipitation of heme pigments.

It is now appreciated that complex mechanisms involving the vasculature and renal tubular epithelium converge in ischemic ATN to cause the dramatic reduction in GFR that is the hallmark of this injury (10% of normal GFR). Figures 11.3 and 11.4 summarize the major events contributing to the renal failure. Furthermore, the anatomy of the nephron renders certain tubular segments susceptible to ischemic injury. Although the kidneys receive 20% of cardiac output, the renal medulla normally

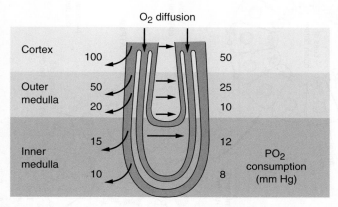

FIGURE 11.3.   Development of hypoxia (with the tissue PO_2 falling below 10 mm Hg) in the renal medulla due to the exchange of oxygen between the descending and ascending limbs of the vasa recta capillaries (*straight arrows*) and oxygen consumption by the medullary cells (*curved arrows*).

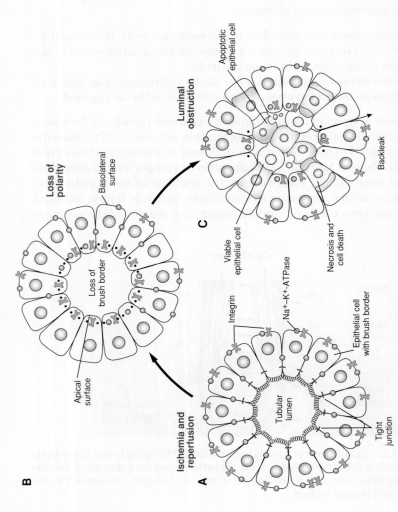

FIGURE 11.4. Following ischemia and reperfusion, morphological changes occur in the proximal tubules, including loss of polarity, loss of the brush border, loss of tight junctions, and redistribution of integrins and Na^+-K^+-ATPase to the apical surface. Calcium and reactive oxygen species may also have a role in these morphological changes, in addition to subsequent cell death resulting from necrosis and apoptosis. Both viable and nonviable cells are shed into the tubular lumen, resulting in the formation of casts and luminal obstruction with backleak contributing to the reduction in the GFR.

exists on the brink of hypoxia, due in part to high metabolic activity required for transport processes and low blood flow to this segment. The hairpin configuration of the vasa recta capillaries (essential for normal operation of the countercurrent mechanism) results in the exchange of oxygen between the oxygen-rich blood leaving the cortex and entering the descending capillary limb and the oxygen-poor blood draining the inner medulla in the ascending capillary limb (Fig. 11.3). The net effect is that the PO_2 bathing the cells of the thick ascending limb of the loop of Henle is normally as low as *10 to 20 mm Hg*. It might therefore be expected that the tubular cells in the medulla would be most susceptible to ischemic injury. Both animal and human studies have suggested that, in many cases of postischemic ATN, there is preferential injury to the thick ascending limb and the terminal segment of the proximal tubule that ends in the outer medulla.

Pathogenesis

Vascular Abnormalities. With acute ischemic injury, there is loss of renal autoregulation and a paradoxical increase in vasoconstriction resulting from increased cystosolic and mitochondrial calcium concentrations. Outer medullary congestion is another prominent finding of acute renal ischemia that may contribute to worsening hypoxia. Endothelial damage from increased oxidant injury has also been proposed to play a role and oxidant injury may lead to a decrease in endothelial cell nitric oxide synthase (eNOS) and vasodilatory prostaglandins.

Tubular Abnormalities. How tubular abnormalities in ischemic ATN mediate the fall in GFR is not completely understood but involves numerous mechanisms (Figs. 11.4 and 11.5). Studies have documented shedding of proximal brush border membranes and viable epithelial cells into the urine. With ischemic injury, abnormalities of the cytoskeleton have been demonstrated that result in translocation of the Na^+–K^+-ATPase from the basolateral to the apical membrane. This loss of vectorial sodium transport could explain the decrease in tubular sodium reabsorption that occurs in this condition. Hypoxia induced activation of cysteine proteases such as calpain may play a role in the Na^+–K^+-ATPase translocation. In addition, accumulation of cellular debris results in intratubular obstruction and the finding of dilated tubules on renal biopsy. The resulting elevation in intraluminal tubular pressure can disrupt epthithelial cell tight junctions and integrin-mediated adhesion causing backleak of glomerular ultrafiltrate into the circulation. The decrease in proximal tubule sodium chloride reabsorption that results from these processes will lead to increased delivery to the macula densa and activate tubuloglomerular feedback to reduce GFR. Since the afferent arteriole is

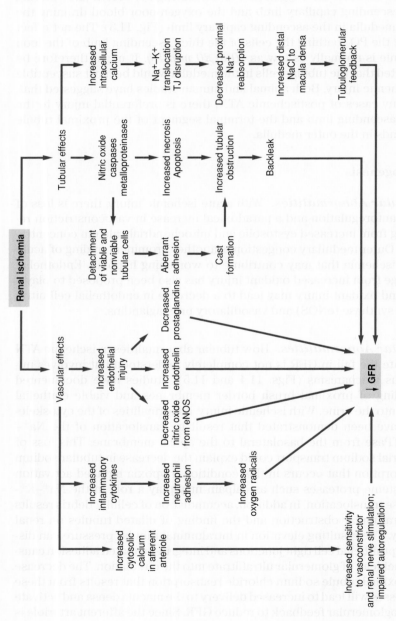

FIGURE 11.5. Vascular and tubular processes leading to reduced GFR in ischemic ATN. Vascular and tubular processes leading to reduced glomerular filtration rate (GFR) in ischemic acute tubular necrosis (ATN). eNOS, endothelial nitric oxide synthase; TJ, tight junction.

vasoconstricted with ischemic injury, this may be sufficient to explain the very low GFR.

Inflammation. Hypoxia induces release of inflammatory cytokines including TNFα and IL-18 resulting in increased neutrophil adhesion and increased free oxygen radicals. Inducible NOS (iNOS) is induced with ischemia leading to increased NO levels and the scavenging of NO by oxygen radicals produces peroxynitrite that causes tubular damage.

 In some nephrons, the cellular injury is severe enough to impair sodium reabsorption but not severe enough to induce backleak. How might reduced sodium chloride reabsorption in the proximal tubule and loop of Henle contribute to the decline in GFR in ATN? Consider the mechanisms by which the GFR is normally regulated.

Treatment and Prevention

Although it is often possible to identify patients at risk for developing ATN and major advances in understanding the pathogenesis have been achieved, effective therapeutic strategies remain elusive. Supportive care with dialysis and correction of electrolyte and metabolic disturbances remain the mainstay of therapy. Numerous potential strategies have been tried but *not* been found to be effective in patients with ischemic ATN (although several have demonstrated efficacy in animals models). These unsuccessful strategies include (1) loop diuretics to inhibit metabolic demands and promote cell preservation, (2) forced diuresis to wash out cellular debris, and (3) ANP, mannitol, dopamine, calcium channel blockers to modulate renal hemodynamics.

Aminoglycoside-Induced Acute Tubular Necrosis

The major causes of nephrotoxic ATN are listed in Table 11.1. Probably, the most common and pathogenetically best understood is the renal failure that may follow prolonged administration of an aminoglycoside antibiotic such as gentamicin or tobramycin. It has been estimated, for example, that an elevation in the plasma creatinine concentration of more than 0.5 to 1.0 mg/dL occurs in 10% to 20% of patients treated with these drugs. ATN can occur even if plasma drug levels are closely monitored, although the risk is clearly greater in those patients with high peak drug levels.

Pathogenesis

The aminoglycosides are freely filtered across the glomerulus; most of the drug is then excreted with a small amount being taken up by and stored in the tubular cells, particularly those in the proximal tubule. Experimental studies suggest that intracellular aminoglycoside accumulation persists for as long as 4 to 6 weeks after therapy is discontinued.

The number of cationic amino groups (NH_3^+) per molecule appears to be an important determinant of nephrotoxicity. Neomycin (six per molecule), gentamicin (five), and tobramycin (five) produce the most renal injury; streptomycin (three) the least.

The role of molecular charge seems to be related to binding of the cationic drug to receptors in the apical and subcellular membranes. At the apical membrane, the aminoglycoside may bind to anionic phospholipids, thereby promoting drug entry into the tubular cell. Within the cell, the aminoglycoside accumulates within lysosomes, an effect that may also be dependent upon charge. Inhibition of lysosomal functions (such as decreased synthesis of the proteolytic enzymes cathepsin B and cathepsin L) may then be responsible for the associated cellular injury.

The likelihood of developing renal failure is dependent upon the dose and the duration of therapy. The plasma creatinine concentration does not usually begin to rise until the aminoglycoside has been given for at least 7 days in patients who are otherwise well. However, the latent period may fall to as little as 2 days if there is concurrent renal ischemia (due to volume depletion or hypotension) or sepsis with endotoxinemia.

Prevention

Careful monitoring of drug levels and minimizing the duration of drug therapy are at present the primary methods used to reduce the incidence of aminoglycoside nephrotoxicity. Studies indicate that aminoglycoside nephrotoxicity can be minimized by giving the entire dose once a day (4 mg/kg in one study) rather than in three divided doses (1.33 mg/kg each). Once-daily therapy results in very high peak plasma and urinary concentrations; the latter exceeds the reabsorptive capacity of the proximal tubule so that most of the drug is excreted, not taken up by the tubular cells. In contrast, reabsorption is not saturated with divided-dose therapy and drug uptake by the proximal cells is much greater over the course of the day.

Contrast Nephropathy

This is a common and often preventable form of toxic tubular injury since it is the only clinical circumstance where the exact timing of exposure is known beforehand. Development of contrast nephropathy in hospitalized patients is associated with increased morbidity and mortality.

Pathogenesis

The mechanism of injury is thought to be a combination of direct vasoconstrictive effects of the contrast agent with tubular toxicity mediated by generation of free radicals. Risk factors for developing contrast

nephropathy include existing renal insufficiency, especially if a consequence of diabetic nephropathy, advanced heart failure or other cause
of reduced renal perfusion (such as hypovolemia), high total dose of
contrast agent, and perhaps underlying multiple myeloma, especially if
associated with hypercalcemia

Prevention
The best treatment of contrast-induced renal failure is prevention. The
risk can be lowered through the use of intravenous fluids, lower doses
of contrast, the use of "isosmolar" agents, the avoidance of repetitive
studies that are closely spaced, and the avoidance of volume depletion
and NSAID use. In recent years, the use of the antioxidant acetylcysteine
has generally been used for prevention, and some recent studies have
suggested better outcomes with bicarbonate-based fluid replacement (vs.
saline).

Clinical Course

Postischemic or nephrotoxic ATN is associated with a progressive elevation in the plasma creatinine concentration, which may stabilize if the
injury is not severe or continue to rise until dialysis is required. The renal failure typically begins on the day of the insult with hypotension or
the administration of a radiocontrast agent; in comparison, the onset is
delayed with aminoglycoside therapy.

   The rate of rise in the plasma creatinine concentration is generally
above 0.5 mg/dL per day in patients with ATN. The maximum rate if there
is essentially *no GFR* is approximately from 2 to 2.5 mg/dL per day.

   Recovery usually requires the regeneration of tubular cells, mediated
in part by the activation of growth response genes and the release of
growth factors. The recovery process can be accelerated in experimental
animals; as examples, the administration of insulin-like growth factor I or
epidermal growth factor can enhance tubular regeneration and the rate
of improvement in renal function. The applicability of this observation
to humans is uncertain, since growth factors are not clinically available.

   Assuming that the underlying insult has been removed or corrected,
the GFR rises and, as a result of the increased filtered creatinine load, the
plasma creatinine concentration begins to fall within 3 to 21 days. The
interval is shorter with a mild, self-limited injury and longer with a severe
and persistent injury. For example, patients with continued infection may
have recurrent episodes of renal ischemia and prolonged renal failure,
while patients with uncomplicated contrast nephropathy typically show
peak creatinine concentrations at 3 to 5 days and then begin to improve.

   Recovery of renal function is usually preceded by a progressive increase in urine output that is an indicator of the enhanced number of
functioning nephrons. Most patients return to their previous baseline

plasma creatinine concentration, although careful measurements of GFR will often reveal some degree of permanent injury. In patients with prolonged ATN (>6 weeks), only partial recovery may be seen and some will remain dialysis dependent.

CASE DISCUSSION The patient presented at the beginning of the chapter had a fall in urine output and elevations in the BUN and creatinine concentration following major abdominal surgery that was complicated by episodes of hypotension. The differential diagnosis in this setting is prerenal disease versus ATN. The urinalysis, high urine sodium concentration, high FENa, and urine osmolality of 320 mOsm/kg are all compatible with ATN.

The 1.1-mg/dL elevation in the plasma creatinine concentration occurring so soon after surgery suggests that the decline in GFR is relatively severe. It is therefore likely that the great majority of nephrons are poorly functioning or nonfunctioning at the time laboratory tests were obtained.

Since the patient is seen in the first few hours after the onset of postischemic ATN, furosemide (a loop diuretic) is given in an attempt to increase the urine output. Although this will make fluid management of the patient easier, there is no evidence that administration of diuretics will change the course of recovery. Patients who are oliguric (<400 mL of urine per day) have suffered a more severe injury and have a poorer prognosis than nonoliguric patients. Increasing urine output with the use of diuretics does not change the prognosis. The spontaneous recovery (or increase) in urine output usually preceeds improvements in GFR and reductions in serum creatinine.

ANSWERS TO QUESTIONS

1 Sodium balance can be maintained as the GFR falls by lowering the rate of tubular reabsorption. If, for example, the fractional excretion of sodium (FENa) is 0.6% at a normal GFR, then sodium excretion will remain constant at a GFR that is 20% of normal if the FENa increases fivefold to 3%. Increased ANP, decreased activity of the renin–angiotensin–aldosterone system, and pressure natriuresis due to volume expansion–induced hypertension all may contribute to the decline in sodium reabsorption. (These hormonal systems are reviewed in Chapter 2.)

Potassium balance, on the other hand, is maintained by increased collecting tubule potassium secretion. This process is stimulated by a rise in the plasma potassium concentration and by aldosterone (see Chapter 7). Note that the rate of aldosterone release cannot be predicted in renal disease, since it will tend to be suppressed by volume expansion and enhanced by hyperkalemia.

2 The relationship between the plasma creatinine concentration and the GFR can be predicted only in the steady state when creatinine production and excretion are equal and the plasma creatinine concentration is stable. The GFR cannot be predicted the day after surgery, since it is not known if the patient is in a steady state. For example, the GFR could be below 5 mL/min and the plasma creatinine concentration will continue to rise each day because excretion remains below the rate of production.

If, however, the plasma creatinine concentration is stable for several days, then the steady state is present. In this setting, the product of the GFR and the plasma creatinine concentration must be constant. This product reflects the amount of creatinine filtered and excreted, which, in the steady state, is equal to the relatively constant amount of creatinine produced. Thus,

$$20 \times 4 = 6 \times \text{new GFR}$$

$$\text{New GFR} = 13.3 \text{ mL/min}$$

3 In obstruction, as in other renal diseases, the urine output is equal to the difference between the GFR and tubular reabsorption. Complete obstruction results in no urine output, but the output is not predictable in patients with partial obstruction. Although the GFR may be markedly reduced, tubular reabsorption also may be diminished due to both the adaptations described in the answer to Question 1 and tubular injury induced by the elevated intratubular pressure. Thus, an output of 1500 mL/day does not exclude the presence of partial urinary tract obstruction.

4 Reduced sodium chloride reabsorption in the proximal tubule and loop of Henle will increase the delivery of chloride to the macula densa. This will activate the tubuloglomerular feedback system (see Chapter 1), which will lower the nephron filtration rate until macula densa delivery has returned toward normal. If this compensatory decline in GFR did not occur, the reabsorptive capacity of the distal and collecting tubules might be overwhelmed, leading to potentially fatal sodium and water losses. Thus, some investigators have called ATN "acute renal success," since systemic hemodynamics are preserved.

SUGGESTED READINGS

Abuelo JG. Normotensive ischemic acute renal failure. N Engl J Med 2007; 357:797–805

Arroyo V, Guevara M, Gines P. Hepatorenal syndrome in cirrhosis: pathogenesis and treatment. Gastroenterology 2002;122:1658.

Asif A, Epstein M. Prevention of radiocontrast-induced nephropathy. Am J Kidney Dis 2004;44:12.

Lameire N, Van Biesen W, Vanholder R. Acute kidney injury. Lancet 2008;372:1863–1865.

Miller TR, Anderson RJ, Linas SL, et al. Urinary diagnostic indices in acute renal failure: a prospective study. Ann Intern Med 1978;89:47.

Racussen LC, Fivush BA, Li YL, et al. Dissociation of tubular cell detachment and tubular cell death in clinical and experimental "acute tubular necrosis." Lab Invest 1991;64:546.

Ricci Z, Cruz D, Ronco C. The RIFLE criteria and mortality in acute kidney injury: a systematic review. Kidney Int 2008;73:538–546.

Shrier RW, Wang W, Poole B, et al. Acute renal failure: definitions, diagnosis, pathogenesis and therapy. J Clin Invest 2004;114:5–14.

Thadhani R, Pascual M, Bonventre JV. Acute renal failure. NEJM 1996;334:1448–1460.

12

PROGRESSION OF CHRONIC RENAL FAILURE

CASE PRESENTATION

A 38-year-old woman has chronic glomerulonephritis due to IgA nephropathy. She presented with intermittent episodes of gross hematuria, but her disease has been overtly quiescent for the past 4 years. During this time, her plasma creatinine concentration has gradually risen from 1.3 to 2.2 mg/dL. This has been accompanied by a progressive elevation in protein excretion (from 1.3 to 3.2 g/day), but the urine sediment has remained inactive, with only a few cells being seen.

Physical examination is unremarkable except for a borderline high blood pressure of 140/90. There is no edema.

OBJECTIVES

By the end of this section, you should have an understanding of each of the following issues:

■ The adaptive responses by the kidney to loss of functioning nephrons, regardless of cause.
■ The potential importance of intraglomerular hypertension and hypertrophy in producing secondary glomerular injury that is independent of the activity of the primary kidney disease.
■ The risk factors for, and the clinical findings in, the kidney disease associated with diabetes mellitus (diabetic nephropathy).
■ The therapeutic modalities that may slow disease progression in humans, irrespective of the underlying disease.

Introduction

There are currently over 500,000 patients in the United States with end-stage kidney disease (prevalence) either undergoing chronic dialysis (72%) or with a functional kidney transplant (28%); each year, new cases (incidence) are added to this number. This treatment is not only exceedingly costly but also ineffective in terms of outcome and quality of life. Thus, the annual Medicare cost for treatment of patients with end-stage kidney disease in 2005 was $32 billion, the annual mortality rate in patients with end-stage disease and on dialysis exceeded 20%, the mean number of comorbid conditions in dialysis patients was about 4 per year, and the mean number of days spent in the hospital was about 15. In the great majority of cases, progression to end-stage kidney disease occurs slowly over a period of several to many years. The most common causes of progressive chronic kidney failure are diabetic nephropathy, chronic glomerular diseases, polycystic kidney diseases, and primary forms of vascular injury, including the so-called "hypertensive nephrosclerosis."

Although it has been appreciated for a long time that many patients with chronic kidney disease inexorably progress, it had been thought that continued activity of the underlying disease (which was often untreatable) played a major role. It now seems clear, however, that the prominent glomerular, vascular, and tubulointerstitial changes that are typically associated with progressive disease may be induced in part by secondary *disease-independent* functional, structural, and metabolic adaptations. Experimental and clinical observations suggest that treatment aimed at these secondary factors, rather than the primary disease, may slow or even prevent the decline in glomerular filtration rate (GFR) that is seen in this setting.

Consider, for example, the course of events in chronic pyelonephritis due to vesicoureteral reflux in young children (see Chapter 10). Recurrent or persistent infection in this disorder leads to classic pyelonephritic scars primarily involving the tubules and interstitium. The loss of functioning nephrons leads to prominent compensatory enlargement of glomeruli in better preserved areas in an attempt to maintain the GFR. Focal and segmental sclerosis of capillaries in these glomeruli ensues over a period of years, often with entrapment of plasma-derived proteins, which results in hyalinosis. This lesion has been called *focal and segmental glomerulosclerosis with hyalinosis*, and it may be difficult to distinguish this lesion by light microscopy alone from similar glomerular abnormalities observed in the idiopathic nephrotic syndrome due to primary or idiopathic focal glomerulosclerosis (see Chapter 9). Of particular importance, when the scarring process in chronic pyelonephritis has reached a critical level of kidney damage, the rate of progression of these glomerular lesions does not appear to be diminished by surgical correction of the reflux and prevention of further kidney infection with antimicrobial agents.

Thus, *primary tubulointerstitial, vascular, and glomerular diseases eventually show secondary glomerular injury* manifested morphologically as secondary or adaptive focal and segmental glomerulosclerosis and clinically by slowly increasing proteinuria, hypertension, and a gradual elevation in the plasma creatinine concentration. This sequence of events has been documented in many chronic tubulointerstitial disorders (such as papillary necrosis due to analgesic abuse), in children in whom glomerular hypertrophy results from being born with too few functioning nephrons (as in unilateral kidney agenesis and oligomeganephronia), in patients with cystic diseases, in patients with primary glomerular diseases, in a subgroup of patients with morbid obesity, in patients with diabetes mellitus, and in patients with vascular diseases that result in focal scarring of the kidney parenchyma due to ischemia or underperfusion (postpartum acute kidney failure, scleroderma, antiphospholipid syndrome, etc.).

Glomerular hypertrophy and increased filtration per nephron are also seen in some metabolic disorders early in their course, before overt kidney injury has occurred. Examples include diabetic nephropathy (which is discussed below), the kidney damage seen in patients with the metabolic syndrome, and glycogen storage diseases. These conditions are associated with progressive glomerulosclerosis similar to that described previously, and it has therefore been proposed that the hemodynamic and structural changes are at least partially responsible for this type of kidney injury.

This chapter will review the experimental findings that have helped to better define the nature of these adaptations and then present the human data suggesting that treatment aimed at reversing the hemodynamic changes slows the rate of progressive glomerular injury, proteinuria, and loss of GFR.

Remnant Kidney Model of Focal Glomerulosclerosis

Many of the current concepts on the mechanisms responsible for secondary or adaptive focal and segmental glomerulosclerosis have been derived from the *remnant kidney* model in the rat. In this model, one kidney is usually removed and two-thirds of the other is infarcted by ligation of segmental arterial branches. Thus, a five-sixths nephrectomy is essentially performed, leaving behind a remnant of normal kidney tissue consisting of about one-third of one kidney. Although initially used to study the mechanisms by which the kidney responds to nephron loss, it was noted that these animals usually developed end-stage kidney failure within 4 to 6 months. Histologic examination of kidney tissue revealed widespread focal global and segmental glomerulosclerosis in the nephrons of the initially normal remnant kidney.

No cause for the glomerular injury was apparent, raising the possibility that the associated functional and structural adaptations might have played an important role. How these changes occur is incompletely understood, but endocrine and other humoral mediators are thought to be responsible. Regardless of the mechanism, it has been presumed that the response to nephron loss in this experimental model is similar to that seen in humans with any form of progressive kidney disease.

Functional Adaptations

A substantial reduction in the number of functioning nephrons in the rat (i.e., five-sixths nephrectomy) and other experimental animals leads to systemic hypertension and to an increase in the single nephron glomerular filtration rate (SNGFR) in the remaining nephrons; the magnitude of the latter change roughly correlates with the extent of nephron loss.

The elevation in SNGFR results in large part from a marked reduction in glomerular arteriolar resistance; this vasodilation is uneven and results in a greater distention of the afferent than the efferent arteriole. Afferent dilation induces two major changes in the remnant kidney when compared to sham-operated rats with two intact kidneys (Fig. 12.1, upper panel):

■ An elevation in intraglomerular pressure (and hence in the transcapillary hydraulic pressure gradient, ΔP), since more of the systemic pressure is transmitted to the glomerulus.
■ A marked increase in effective kidney plasma flow, Q_A.

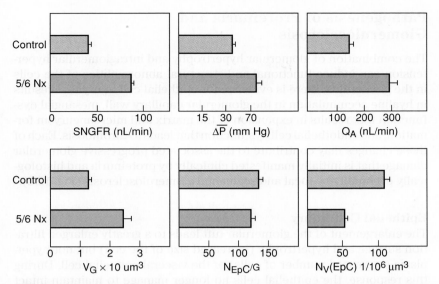

FIGURE 12.1.   Hemodynamic and structural adaptations in the rat following subtotal nephrectomy (5/6 Nx). *Upper panel:* Glomerular arteriolar vasodilation (afferent much greater than efferent) led to increases in single nephron plasma flow rate (Q_A) and a rise in the mean transcapillary hydraulic pressure gradient (ΔP). The latter is equal to the difference between the hydraulic pressure in the glomerular capillary and in Bowman's space. These adaptations result in an approximately twofold elevation in single nephron glomerular filtration rate (SNGFR). *Lower panel:* The hemodynamic changes are associated with a sizable increase in glomerular tuft volume (V_G) with corresponding expansion of the surface area available for filtration. The level of hypertrophy, however, is not uniform, since there is not a similar degree of hyperplasia of the visceral epithelial cells. The number of epithelial cells (N_{EpC}) remains unchanged since these terminal cells do not undergo cell division, which results in a reduction in the density of these cells within the enlarged volume of the glomerular tuft [$N_v(EpC)$].

Concurrent systemic hypertension induced by the nephron loss will exacerbate these hemodynamic changes by further increasing glomerular pressure and plasma flow.

Structural Adaptations

These hemodynamic compensations are associated with significant structural changes. As illustrated in the lower panel in Figure 12.1, kidney hypertrophy in the remnant leads to an increase in the volume of the glomerular tuft, without a corresponding increase in the number of highly differentiated and terminal visceral epithelial cells. This results in a reduction in the cell density of the epithelium within the enlarged tuft, a change that is thought to be an important factor in the ensuing glomerular injury.

Pathogenesis of Proteinuria and Glomerulosclerosis

The combination of glomerular hypertrophy and intraglomerular hypertension can induce functional and structural abnormalities of the cells in the glomerulus; there is evidence for epithelial cell injury that results in hyaline accumulation in the glomerular capillary wall, mesangial dysfunction that results in expansion of the matrix and microaneurysm formation, and endothelial cell dysfunction that leads to thrombosis. Each of these changes may contribute to the associated progressive glomerular damage that is initially manifested clinically by proteinuria and histologically eventually by focal and segmental glomerulosclerosis (Fig. 12.2).

Epithelial Cell Injury

The enlargement of the glomerular tuft leads to a greatly enlarged filtration surface and hypertrophy (increased size of the cell) but not hyperplasia (increased number of cells) of the visceral epithelial cell. During this response, the epithelial cells no longer manage to maintain intact all interdigitating foot processes and filtration slit diaphragms. These changes are very isolated in the beginning and are manifested by focal epithelial cell simplification that results in segmental effacement or "fusion" of foot processes in some capillaries; other parts of the greatly expanded capillary surface show more severe injury such as focal loss and even denudation of the epithelial cells. As described in Chapter 9, the slit diaphragms between the intact epithelial cell foot processes are part of the small pore system of filtration and represent a major

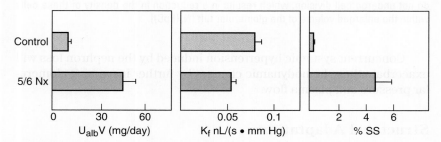

FIGURE 12.2. Structural and functional maladaptations following subtotal nephrectomy (5/6 Nx) in the rat. The permselectivity of the glomerular capillary wall is impaired, leading to significant albuminuria ($U_{alb}V$). The ultrafiltration coefficient K_f, which is a measure of the number of small pores allowing the filtration of water and small solutes, has fallen. This change is most likely a reflection of two factors: the simplification and effacement of foot processes over large areas of the glomerular capillary wall and the development of segmental sclerosing lesions with obsolescence of capillaries and hyaline deposition in the glomeruli. % SS, the percentage of glomeruli with segmental sclerosis.

component of the resistance to the filtration of water; they also greatly affect the trafficking of macromolecules such as albumin across the glomerular capillary wall. Thus, distortion and loss of the slit diaphragms and denudation of the capillary wall will lead to an increased local flow of ultrafiltrate and increased convection of albumin. Protein excretion increases only in those nephrons with damaged visceral epithelium (see also Chapter 9; Fig. 9.6). The result of these structural changes is loss of hydraulic conductivity (K_f), proteinuria, and eventually focal and segmental glomerulosclerosis; these functional changes can be considered an expression of the "insufficiency" of the glomerular visceral epithelial cell to maintain its structural integrity following the hemodynamic and structural adaptations described earlier.

Hyaline Accumulation and Mesangial Expansion

Those areas in which the epithelial cell has been denuded are freely open to filtration, leading to an increased flux of water, small solutes, and some macromolecules across the glomerular capillary wall. This increase in permeability plus the associated intraglomerular hypertension will favor the accumulation of very large plasma proteins (e.g., fibrin, IgM, and activated complement components) in the subendothelial space, since they are too large to pass through the glomerular basement membrane. This amorphous, *hyaline* material will eventually lead to narrowing and complete occlusion of the capillary lumens, a process that may be exacerbated by concurrent increases in mesangial matrix and cellularity that are induced by an increase in macromolecule entry into the mesangial space.

Microaneurysm Formation

The combination of the increase in the glomerular capillary radius (due to enlargement of the glomerular tuft) and the elevation in the intraglomerular pressure can produce a significant rise in the *tension* exerted on the glomerular capillary wall. This increase in tension may eventually exceed the tensile strength of the fibrillary structures that connect the mesangial cells to the glomerular basement membrane (GBM) at the level of the neck of the capillaries (see right panel of Fig. 9.3), leading to rupture of these structures and the formation of a microaneurysm that affects several capillary loops connected to the same (defective) mesangial area. These microaneurysms usually thrombose due to exposure of circulating platelets to matrix components, and a local inflammatory response is triggered. Eventually, these lesions organize within a few weeks, leaving behind collapsed capillaries with entrapped cellular debris, representing an area of segmental and sometimes nodular sclerosis. The influx of macrophages into the mesangium and an increased delivery or local generation of cytokines and growth factors may also result in overproduction of matrix by the mesangial cell. This process will also

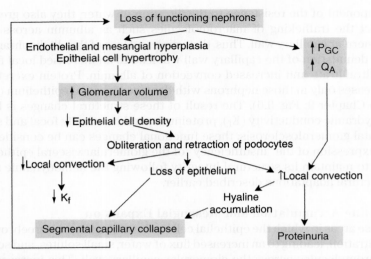

FIGURE 12.3. Flow diagram summarizing the events leading to progressive glomerulosclerosis and proteinuria in the subtotal nephrectomy model of chronic kidney failure. The loss of filtering nephrons leads to functional and structural adaptations that result in a positive feedback loop that can eventually destroy most of the nephrons.

contribute to the expansion of the mesangium, often resulting in nodular glomerulosclerosis. These lesions are particularly prominent in diabetic glomerulosclerosis.

Endothelial Cell Dysfunction

Thrombi within the glomerular capillaries are often seen in experimental animals with five-sixths nephrectomy; they are the result of endothelial cell dysfunction. How this occurs is not completely understood, but increased shear stress induced by intraglomerular hypertension and hyperperfusion may cause the endothelial cells to lose their natural thromboresistance, resulting in an increase in platelet adhesion to the cell surface. This loss of thromboresistance of the endothelium has been demonstrated in cultured cells exposed to increased shear stress and turbulent flow conditions.

SUMMARY

The relative importance of any one of the changes listed previously is uncertain. Nevertheless, the aggregate effect is segmental capillary collapse and glomerulosclerosis, manifested clinically by proteinuria and progressive kidney failure (Fig. 12.3). Furthermore, this sequence leads to a positive feedback loop. The loss of some nephrons will induce more pronounced hypertrophy and hypertension in the remaining glomeruli, thereby increasing their risk of secondary glomerular injury.

It is important to remember that the development of glomerulosclerosis is independent of the activity of the underlying disease. Furthermore, reversing the intraglomerular hypertension may minimize the severity of these deleterious changes or even prevent them from occurring, as will be discussed below.

Vascular and Tubulointerstitial Damage

Although glomerulosclerosis is the most prominent change in the remnant kidney, both vascular and tubulointerstitial injury also occur. The increased pressure and flow through the arterial system may also result in additional endothelial cell dysfunction, leading to thrombosis and accumulation of cell debris and connective tissue in the subintima. Systemic hypertension can also cause hypertrophy of smooth muscle cells in the media and, if the hypertension is severe, fibrinoid necrosis of the wall. These vascular changes result in additional injury of the parenchyma due to ischemia and hypoperfusion.

Tubular atrophy and interstitial fibrosis are also common in animals with progressive kidney failure. This process is probably also related, at least in part, to the progressive glomerulosclerosis. Given the unique distribution pattern of the peritubular microcirculation, the lack of blood flow through the efferent arteriole of a damaged or sclerosed glomerulus will result not only in atrophy of that entire nephron but also in ischemia of tubular elements in close proximity but unrelated to the sclerosed glomerulus. The affected tubules can be located in the cortex or in the medulla, the latter in the case of sclerosis that affects juxtamedullary glomeruli. Several additional factors have also been postulated to contribute to the tubulointerstitial damage observed in experimental animals and in patients with progressive kidney disease:

■ **Calcium phosphate deposition**—A fall in GFR leads to initial phosphate retention and secondary calcium phosphate deposition in the tissues (see Chapter 13). An increase in calcium phosphate content in the kidney can be demonstrated in humans before the plasma creatinine concentration is above 1.5 mg/dL.

■ **Local ammonia accumulation**—The tubules as well as the glomeruli must hypertrophy in the remnant kidney. If, for example, the daily acid load remains constant and the number of nephrons is reduced by five-sixths nephrectomy, then each nephron must increase ammonia production and ammonium excretion sixfold if acid–base balance is to be maintained. In general, only a three- to fourfold increase can be achieved so that animals and patients with a marked loss of functioning nephrons develop metabolic acidosis (see Chapter 6). The local accumulation of some of this excess ammonia can directly activate complement via amidation, a process that induces accumulation of macrophages resulting in tubulointerstitial inflammation and eventually fibrosis. This process can be ameliorated in experimental animals with partial nephrectomy by administration of sodium bicarbonate.

■ **Proteinuria as a direct driving force of tubulointerstitial injury**—Direct tubular injury can also be induced by the generation of oxygen-reactive species, a result of the increased iron that reaches the tubule cells through increased filtration of transferrin. It has also been postulated that several lipid precursors (fatty acids) that reach the tubule cell via the filtered and reabsorbed albumin would contribute to the generation of potent chemotactic agents, driving an inflammatory process at this level that is independent of the glomerular changes already discussed. Macrophages are considered to be the source of cytokines and growth factors, including TGFβ, which is postulated to contribute to the increased deposition or decreased degradation of matrix components and scar collagen. Hence, it has been suggested that measures that reduce proteinuria, such as angiotensin-converting enzyme (ACE) inhibitors, angiotensin II receptor blockers, and other selected antihypertensive agents, or agents that affect the initial inflammatory response or the scarring process, would result in a beneficial effect on the tubule and on the interstitium that are independent of the effects on the glomerulus.

Prevention of Secondary Glomerular Injury

These experimental studies in the rat may have important therapeutic implications, since treatment aimed at reversing the intraglomerular hypertension and hypertrophy or the degree of proteinuria and interstitial inflammation may slow the rate of, or even prevent, secondary glomerulosclerosis. Two major forms of therapy have been utilized: dietary protein restriction and antihypertensive therapy, preferably with an ACE inhibitor or angiotensin II receptor blockers.

Dietary Protein Restriction
The GFR in animals and humans varies directly with dietary protein intake. Ingesting a protein load, for example, can acutely raise the GFR by 15% to 40% in normal subjects. This can be considered an appropriate response, since it will facilitate the excretion of potentially toxic protein metabolites. How it occurs is not clear, but amino acids may increase the secretion of an as yet unidentified renal vasodilating hormone. On the other hand, restricting protein intake might be expected to lower the GFR and intraglomerular pressure. When administered to rats with a remnant kidney, a low-protein diet prevents the intraglomerular hypertension and hypertrophy, reduces the degree of proteinuria, largely prevents segmental glomerulosclerosis, and prolongs kidney survival.

Antihypertensive Therapy

An equivalent benefit can be achieved when the intraglomerular pressure is lowered by antihypertensive therapy. However, the degree of kidney protection is in part dependent upon the antihypertensive agents that are used. ACE inhibitors decrease the formation of angiotensin II. The latter preferentially increases resistance of the efferent glomerular arteriole. Thus, lowering angiotensin II levels will lead to a more pronounced efferent dilation, a change that will directly reduce the intraglomerular pressure. This regimen may also minimize glomerular hypertrophy, since angiotensin II can act as a growth promoter.

Administration of an ACE inhibitor is clearly beneficial in the remnant kidney. In comparison, antihypertensive therapy with triple therapy consisting of a combination of hydrochlorothiazide (a diuretic), reserpine (a sympathetic blocker), and hydralazine (a direct vasodilator) results in preferential afferent arteriolar dilation. Although the systemic blood pressure is reduced with this regimen, more of the arterial pressure is transmitted to the glomeruli, thereby preventing a fall in intraglomerular pressure. Hence, triple therapy provides no protection against progressive proteinuria and glomerulosclerosis (Fig. 12.4).

The efficacy of other antihypertensive drugs, such as the calcium channel blockers, is less certain, since a beneficial effect is dependent upon the drug resulting in a reduction in intracapillary pressure; it is now established that the nondihydropyridine calcium channel blockers have a significant antiproteinuric effect and may be "renoprotective," while the dihydropyridines have no effect on proteinuria. This topic will be discussed in more detail in the section on the use of antihypertensive agents in humans.

Lipid-Lowering Therapy

Although beyond the scope of this discussion, chronic kidney failure of any cause is often associated with the gradual development of hyperlipidemia. These changes are much more prominent in the nephrotic syndrome, where the plasma cholesterol concentration may be markedly elevated, exceeding 500 mg/dL in some cases. In addition to promoting systemic atherosclerosis, it has been shown that the increased lipid levels can also contribute to the glomerular injury, perhaps via a process analogous to atherosclerosis. Lowering the plasma lipid concentration with hypolipidemic drugs has been shown to minimize both the degree of proteinuria and segmental sclerosis in the remnant kidney model.

Other factors are also thought to contribute to the progression of kidney disease and require therapeutic interventions; these factors include high circulating or local levels of aldosterone and corticosteroids, altered prostanoid metabolism, anemia, hyperhomocysteinemia, and currently

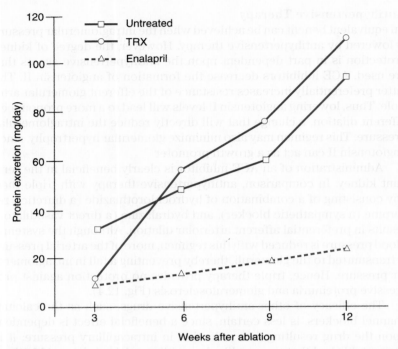

FIGURE 12.4. Change in daily protein excretion over time following subtotal nephrectomy (or ablation) in untreated rats that were hypertensive and in rats in which the hypertension was corrected by the administration of enalapril, an angiotensin-converting enzyme (ACE) inhibitor, or triple therapy with hydrochlorothiazide, reserpine, and hydralazine (TRX). Untreated and TRX-treated animals had increasing glomerulosclerosis (not shown). These abnormalities were almost entirely prevented by enalapril.

unidentified racial and genetic factors that accelerate or predispose to chronic kidney failure.

Experimental Diabetic Nephropathy

One criticism voiced earlier against the previously mentioned experimental studies is that the remnant kidney is an extreme situation and that it may not be a realistic model of human chronic kidney disease. The numerous trials performed to date in patients with progressive kidney diseases have proven that these concerns were largely unfounded. As a result, diabetic nephropathy in the rat has also been extensively evaluated. Via an uncertain mechanism, renal vasodilation and hypertrophy, an increased GFR, and intraglomerular hypertension are all induced by the metabolic abnormalities associated with hyperglycemia and/or insulin deficiency. These changes occur early in the disease before nephron loss has occurred; they are initially reversible with an intensive insulin regimen instituted to normalize the metabolic abnormality and the plasma glucose concentration.

Therapeutic studies in experimental diabetes mellitus have essentially replicated the results in the remnant kidney. Despite giving only enough insulin to prevent severe hyperglycemia, a low-protein diet, administration of an ACE inhibitor, or hypolipidemic therapy reduces the degree of proteinuria and segmental glomerulosclerosis in animals. Once again, triple therapy appears to be ineffective to reduce proteinuria and progressive glomerulosclerosis compared to an ACE inhibitor. Thus, treating the hemodynamic, metabolic, and structural adaptations is beneficial, even if the underlying disease is not entirely corrected, as in diabetes mellitus.

Human Studies

The applicability of these experimental findings to progressive chronic kidney disease in humans is currently well established. Large definitive trials have shown a beneficial effect from therapies aimed at minimizing or preventing secondary or adaptive and disease-independent glomerular injury. Although there are few studies on slowing progression by treating hyperlipidemia and metabolic acidosis, it is probably desirable to treat these problems to minimize atherosclerosis, renal bone disease, and muscle wasting (see Chapters 6 and 13).

The following discussion will center on the following questions:

- Is the remnant kidney model applicable to human disease?
- What are the clinical implications of hypertrophy of the remaining functioning nephrons?
- What are the clinical characteristics of diabetic nephropathy, a common cause of slowly progressive chronic kidney failure?
- What data are at present available on the efficacy of dietary protein restriction (which also includes phosphate restriction) and antihypertensive therapy?
- Might there be a preferential benefit from the use of ACE inhibitors as opposed to other antihypertensive agents?
- Is there an additional benefit to be gained from the use of a combination of an ACE inhibitor, an angiotensin II receptor blocker, and other inhibitors or antagonists of the renin–angiotensin–aldosterone system?

Kidney Response to Nephron Loss

It has been known for some time that compensatory hypertrophy and hyperfiltration occurs in humans following nephron loss. For example, surgical removal of one kidney may be performed for a number of reasons,

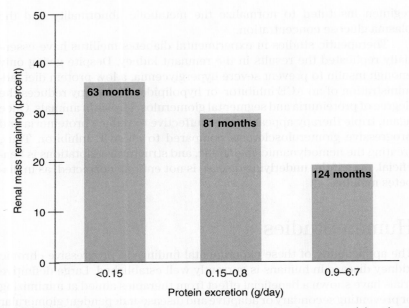

FIGURE 12.5. Degree of proteinuria in patients who have undergone partial nephrec-tomy in a solitary kidney according to amount of kidney mass remaining and duration of follow-up. Patients with less than 20% of the total kidney mass remaining appear to be at greatest risk for developing clinically significant proteinuria after 10 years.

including malignancy and donation for kidney transplantation. Although 50% of the kidney mass has been removed in this setting, the GFR usually falls by only 20% to 30%. Thus, the nephrons in the remaining kidney must have increased their individual filtration rates by approximately 50%.

The long-term implications of these changes are clearly an impor-tant issue. Monitoring of kidney transplant donors has revealed only a slight increase in the incidence of proteinuria and hypertension at 10 to 15 years. However, a recent study looked at more marked loss of kidney mass in patients undergoing *partial nephrectomy in a solitary kidney* (usually for cancer). As shown in Figure 12.5, the degree of protein-uria that was seen was dependent upon both the duration and degree of nephron loss. Patients who had less than 20% to 30% of their total kid-ney mass remaining for more than 10 years, a situation not unusual in many patients with kidney tumors, were most likely to have relatively heavy proteinuria. Kidney biopsy in this setting showed focal and seg-mental glomerulosclerosis, similar to that in the animal models, and some patients progressed to end-stage kidney disease. Thus, the human re-sponse to nephron loss is "dose dependent" and appears to be similar to that in animals; proteinuria is again the earliest clinical marker of hemodynamically mediated glomerular injury.

Effect on Evaluation of Patients with Chronic Kidney Disease

In addition to possibly promoting secondary glomerular injury, the compensatory hyperfiltration following nephron loss also can interfere with the clinical evaluation of the course of the underlying kidney disease. Serial monitoring of both the GFR (via measurement of the plasma creatinine concentration) and the urinalysis are the most common modalities used to assess disease activity. As described in Chapter 1, increased creatinine secretion by the tubules can minimize the elevation in plasma creatinine concentration that should follow a reduction in GFR. Similarly, hyperfiltration in remaining nephrons may mask significant and even persistent nephron loss due to ongoing but subclinical kidney diseases.

The potential importance of the latter phenomenon has been demonstrated in patients with immune complex–mediated glomerulonephritis due to systemic lupus erythematosus that was refractory to conventional therapy. An experimental regimen of total lymphoid irradiation (to diminish immune activity) successfully induced *clinical remission* of both the kidney and extrarenal disease: After 3 years, the GFR was stable (at about 45 mL/min) and protein excretion had fallen by 80%; however, the kidney disease continued to progress during this period as documented by yearly kidney biopsies. As depicted in Figure 12.6, the percentage of glomeruli that were completely scarred (or sclerotic) increased from 15% to almost 60%. This scarring presumably reflected healing of glomeruli previously damaged by inflammation during the period of active disease. Despite the loss in functioning nephrons, the total GFR was unchanged because the remaining glomeruli hypertrophied, reaching a volume almost twice the upper limit of normal. This increase in size must have been accompanied by an elevation in filtration rate in these individual nephrons. Over time, these enlarged glomeruli might be susceptible to hemodynamically mediated injury even if the underlying lupus remains inactive.

Diabetic Nephropathy

Diabetic nephropathy is currently the single most common cause of kidney disease in patients coming to dialysis. It is estimated, for example, that 30% to 40% of patients with type 1 insulin-dependent diabetes mellitus (IDDM) will develop kidney failure during their lifetime. This disorder is characterized clinically by slowly progressive proteinuria and by glomerular lesions characterized by a progressive increase in mesangial matrix and eventual capillary collapse, nodular glomerulosclerosis, and loss of glomerular filtration. Since only a fraction of patients with diabetes mellitus develop end-stage kidney disease, factors other than the metabolic abnormalities must play a critical role in the predisposition to diabetic nephropathy.

It is clear that hyperglycemia and/or insulin deficiency play a major role in the pathogenesis of diabetic nephropathy, at least in part by

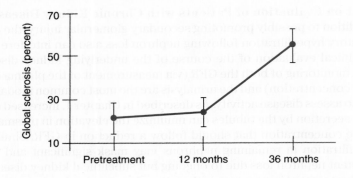

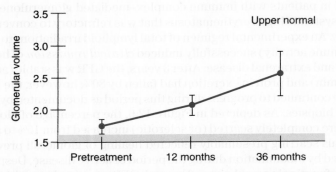

FIGURE 12.6. Effect of total lymphoid irradiation (TLI) on glomerular morphology in patients with lupus nephritis who had a stable glomerular filtration rate (GFR) (45 to 50 mL/min) and an 80% reduction in protein excretion. The number of sclerosed glomeruli increased from 15% before TLI to almost 60% 3 years later (*top panel*). This did not lead to a fall in GFR because of a marked increase in glomerular size (and presumably filtration) in those glomeruli that were preserved (*bottom panel*).

inducing glomerular hyperfiltration, capillary hypertension, and glomerular hypertrophy as described in the animal models previously. Roughly 50% of patients with IDDM have a GFR that is 25% to 50% greater than normal in the earliest stages of the disease. This change is detectable in the first year, and patients with an initial GFR above 140 to 150 mL/min (normal equals 90 to 125 mL/min) appear most likely to develop diabetic nephropathy. The factors responsible for the glomerular hyperfiltration in recently diagnosed diabetics are incompletely understood, but increased release of insulin-like growth factor I (which induces both renal vasodilation and hypertrophy) may be important.

The earliest clinical manifestation of diabetic nephropathy is *microalbuminuria*, which usually develops in susceptible subjects with IDDM within 8 to 15 years after the onset of the disease. Microalbuminuria refers to an increase in albumin excretion above 30 mg/day (normal is less than 20 mg/day). This abnormality is detectable years before the dipstick for protein becomes positive. The dipstick is a relatively insensitive test for early glomerular disease, since it does not become positive until total protein excretion is greater than 300 to 500 mg/day (normal is less than 150 mg/day).

Type 2 Diabetes Mellitus

For reasons that are not well understood, both hyperfiltration and clinical kidney disease are generally slightly less common in patients with type 2 non–insulin-dependent diabetes mellitus (NIDDM). There are, however, exceptions, such as the Pima Indians in the southwest United States. The incidence of diabetic nephropathy in Pima Indians with NIDDM approaches 50%. Affected patients have a higher GFR than matched controls, and increased albumin excretion can be demonstrated within 3 years of the onset of the disease, much shorter than the 8- to 15-year latent period in IDDM. Thus, there appears to be an increased susceptibility to glomerular injury in Pima Indians that may at least in part be genetically determined.

Effect of Strict Glycemic Control

Suboptimal glycemic control is clearly a risk factor for diabetic nephropathy. Intensive insulin therapy (either multiple daily injections or a continuous subcutaneous insulin pump) has allowed a near-normal plasma glucose concentration to be maintained throughout the day in patients with type 1 diabetes. This regimen can reverse the initial glomerular hyperfiltration, and the development of microalbuminuria can be delayed. Intensive therapy also appears to be effective if begun after the onset of microalbuminuria, as albumin excretion can be gradually reduced over a 2-year period. In comparison, strict glycemic control does not appear to be effective in slowing the rate of loss of GFR in patients with overt and well-established nephropathy, which is defined as having a positive dipstick for protein. This observation indicates the importance of other, perhaps hemodynamic factors in the progression of this disorder. The efficacy of modalities such as protein restriction and antihypertensive therapy will be described below.

Kidney Function at Onset of Overt Disease

There is one last finding that must be appreciated in this disorder. Diabetic patients predisposed to develop kidney disease may begin with a supernormal GFR of 150 to 170 mL/min. As progressive glomerular injury leads to dipstick-positive proteinuria, there is a concomitant 30% to 50% reduction in GFR to 90 to 100 mL/min. Conversely, a diabetic patient seen for the first time who presents with a GFR of 100 mL/min (similar to that in the normal general population) will have a normal plasma creatinine concentration. These patients already have advanced glomerulosclerosis on biopsy and, if left untreated, will progress to end-stage kidney disease within 3 to 7 years. The combination of a normal plasma creatinine concentration and protein excretion that might be less than 1.0 g/day may lead the physician to conclude erroneously that this is mild kidney disease. Although probably true in most other disorders, this is clearly not the case for diabetic kidney disease.

Efficacy of Dietary Protein Restriction

Dietary protein restriction and antihypertensive therapy are the two major modalities that have been applied to humans in an attempt to slow the rate of disease progression in patients with chronic kidney disease. Although the following discussion will present some of the findings that suggest these regimens may be beneficial, we cannot be certain of all the mechanism by which this occurs in patients. The animal models described previously suggest that a reduction in intraglomerular pressure may be important, but it is not known if this applies entirely to humans in whom intraglomerular hemodynamics cannot be measured directly as was done in the experimental animals.

Many of the trials reported thus far comparing a low-protein diet to a regular diet have involved a relatively small number of patients. Some of these studies have shown benefit whereas others have shown a trend toward a better outcome that was not statistically significant. The latter observation could represent a beta error (a false-negative result) in that the lack of statistical significance was a result of the small number of patients rather than lack of improvement with therapy. One large multicenter study, the MDRD (Modification of Diet in Renal Disease) study, showed only a relatively modest benefit of the low-protein diet on the rate of progression of the kidney failure; however, a very interesting biphasic response was noted in the group on a protein-restricted diet: There was a greater initial decline in GFR in the first 4 months (that may well have been a reflection of the reduction in intracapillary pressure brought about by the low-protein diet), followed by a slower rate of decline of the GRF over the ensuing 32 months of observation when compared to the group on the control diet. Thus, if one ignores the initial rapid fall in GFR in the group on a low-protein diet, the rate of the fall in GFR over the remainder of the observation period was clearly reduced in the group on a low-protein diet compared to the group that consumed a diet with a higher protein content (on average, 2.8 vs. 3.9 mL/min loss of GFR per year). The long-term follow-up analysis of this study revealed a benefit of the low-protein diet on kidney failure and all-cause mortality at 6 years; this effect was lost, however, at 12 years after completion of the study, probably due to a decrease in adherence to the otherwise less palatable low-protein diet.

Several meta-analyses have evaluated the effect of protein restriction on the rate of progression of kidney failure. The most recent review published in 2006 suggests that a low-protein diet (0.3 to 0.6 g/kg per day) compared to a standard protein diet (>8 g/kg per day) was associated with a decreased risk of need for renal replacement therapy or death during the follow-up.

Response in Diabetic Nephropathy

Although only few results with dietary protein restriction are available in overt diabetic nephropathy, Figure 12.7 depicts the findings of two smaller studies of affected patients with IDDM who had an initial GFR that was usually between 40 and 50 mL/min. As can be seen, the GFR fell by 0.6 to 1.0 mL/min/month in the control groups at 18 to 36 months, while the rate of progression was reduced by approximately 75% in protein-restricted groups. A larger prospective study showed a similar decline in GFR in the protein-restricted group, and in the group on the control diet, the incidence of death or onset of end-stage kidney disease was significantly reduced with protein restriction.

If these results can be extrapolated over a longer period of time, they allow us to estimate the true benefit of the low-protein diet to the patient. Dialysis is generally begun when the GFR is less than 7 mL/min. Thus, a patient with a GFR of 45 mL/min who loses 12 mL/min/year

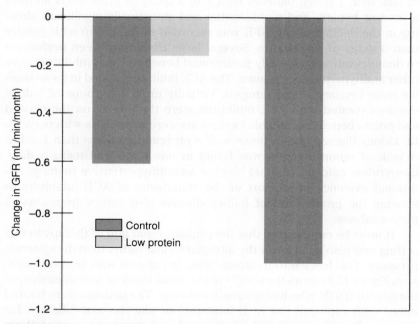

FIGURE 12.7. Effect of dietary protein restriction on the rate of decline in glomerular filtration rate in two different studies of patients with diabetic nephropathy. Reducing protein intake slowed the rate of disease progression by approximately 75%.

(1 mL/min/month) would require dialysis in roughly 3 years. In comparison, on a low-protein diet, dialysis would be necessary in 12 years, a delay in the need for replacement therapy of *9 years*, if the rate of loss of GFR were slowed by 75% to 3 mL/min/year (0.25 mL/min/month). This theoretical benefit would be even greater if treatment were begun earlier in the disease when the dipstick for protein was positive but the GFR was still in the normal range.

Efficacy of Antihypertensive Therapy

Hypertension is a risk factor for a worse prognosis in almost any form of chronic kidney disease, in addition to the devastating effect on the cardiovascular system. This observation alone, however, does not prove that hypertension accelerates progression, since the elevation in blood pressure could also be a marker for more severe kidney disease.

Several large trials have looked at the efficacy of antihypertensive therapy in slowing the rate of progression in nondiabetic chronic kidney disease. The MDRD study mentioned previously also addressed the issue of aggressive versus conventional blood pressure control and progression of kidney failure. The more aggressive treatment was associated with no apparent benefit in patients with a protein excretion rate of less than 1 g/day, patients with 1 to 3 g/day of proteinuria showed a modest benefit, and a substantial and statistically significant slowing in the decline of the GFR was recorded in the group with greater than 3 g/day of proteinuria. Several large trials have been performed to demonstrate a potentially preferential benefit of ACE inhibitors over other antihypertensive regimen. The ACE inhibitors tested in these studies were benazepril and ramipril. Virtually in all subgroups of kidney diseases treated with ACE inhibitors were the effects on the chosen end points beneficial; notable exceptions were in patients with polycystic kidney disease and in those with a proteinuria of less than 1 g/day. A lack of renoprotection was found in one large trial using a dihydropyridine calcium channel blocker as antihypertensive therapy. Additional evidence in support of the superiority of ACE inhibitors in slowing the progression of kidney disease also comes from several meta-analyses.

It must be emphasized that the primary *renal* aim of therapy in this setting may also be to lower the intraglomerular rather than the systemic pressure. This has led to treatment even in patients who are normotensive. Figure 12.8 shows the results of one small study of normotensive patients with IDDM who had microalbuminuria. The patients were treated either with captopril (an ACE inhibitor) or placebo and followed for 4 years. Albumin excretion fell in the captopril group and none of 21 patients progressed to overt, dipstick-positive proteinuria. In comparison, albumin excretion rose in the placebo group, 30% of whom progressed.

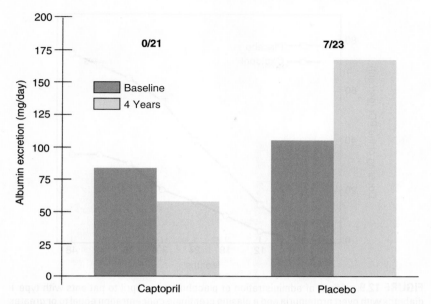

FIGURE 12.8. Effect of 4-year treatment with captopril (an angiotensin-converting enzyme inhibitor) or placebo on albumin excretion in normotensive diabetics with microalbuminuria. Captopril lowered albumin excretion and no patient progressed to overt dipstick-positive proteinuria. In comparison, albumin excretion increased and progression occurred in 7 of 23 patients in the placebo group.

It is of interest that there was little difference in systemic blood pressure between the two groups, suggesting that the primary effect of captopril was on the kidney.

The results of a larger trial in established diabetic nephropathy are shown in Figure 12.9. Patients were randomized to captopril or placebo, and other antihypertensive drugs were added to patients in the placebo group as necessary. Both regimens lowered the blood pressure to the same degree, but the rate of progressive kidney injury was slowed by approximately 50% in the captopril group.

Several studies have also explored the question of ACE inhibition versus angiotensin II receptor blockers. These studies showed an equivalent beneficial effect on proteinuria and on the decline of the GFR. However, the combination of ACE inhibition and angiotensin II receptor blockade in some studies offered the greatest antiproteinuric effect. Only one major study evaluated the effect of the combination therapy on disease progression. Although at first glance this study was very promising, concerns about the reliability of data and an increased incidence of adverse effects have significantly dampened the enthusiasm for this type of therapy.

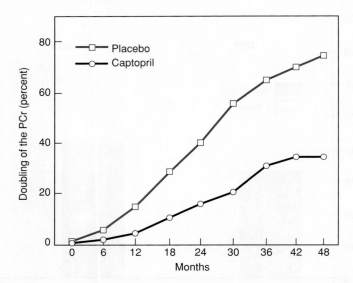

FIGURE 12.9. Effect of administration of placebo or captopril to patients with type 1 diabetes with overt proteinuria and a plasma creatinine concentration equal to or greater than 1.5 mg/dL. Likelihood of a doubling of the plasma creatinine concentration (PCr) was reduced by more than 50% in the captopril group.

All of these human studies are outrageously expensive; public funds through the National Institutes of Health are often unavailable, and many of them are sponsored and financed entirely by the manufacturers of the drugs. Hence, these studies can be flawed in that they often lack a direct comparison between competing agents (e.g., ACE inhibition vs. angiotensin receptor blockade), resulting in studies that extol the virtues of a newer, more expensive agent over older yet very effective and cheaper alternatives. This raises not only scientific but often also serious ethical concerns.

Reduction in Protein Excretion

The decline in protein excretion in Figure 12.8 may have more general implications for evaluating the efficacy of any given therapy and potentially new drugs in chronic kidney disease. Studies in animals and mathematical models of macromolecular permeability suggest that protein filtration through size-selective defects in an abnormally permeable glomerular capillary wall varies directly with the fraction of GFR that filters through the abnormal or large pore system, and this fraction, in turn, is a direct function of the glomerular capillary pressure. Thus, a reduction in protein excretion with antihypertensive therapy in humans may reflect, at least in part, a desired reduction in intraglomerular pressure.

These observations have led to the hypothesis that the likelihood of long-term benefit can be assessed by measuring changes in protein excretion, which has effectively been viewed as a surrogate marker of progression. In particular, a fall in protein excretion in the short term may be associated with a better renal prognosis over longer periods of time.

The following summarizes the results of many studies in chronic kidney disease, most of which were performed in patients with diabetic nephropathy:

- ACE inhibitors and angiotensin II receptor blockers almost uniformly reduce protein excretion. The only other drugs that appear to be as effective are the nondihydropyridine calcium channel blockers diltiazem and verapamil. There also appears to be a benefit from the combined use of an ACE inhibitor and angiotensin receptor blocker over single therapy with these agents, at least for the protein excretion rate.
- Diuretics and β-blockers have less predictable antiproteinuric activity; they usually have little or no effect on protein excretion (Fig. 12.9), although some studies have found a response similar to the ACE inhibitors.
- The dihydropyridine calcium channel blockers, such as nifedipine, either have no effect on or may actually *increase* protein excretion.

What actions could nifedipine have on glomerular arteriolar resistance to allow protein excretion to increase despite a reduction in the systemic blood pressure?

SUMMARY AND CASE DISCUSSION   Experimental studies and many large trials in patients with kidney diseases or diabetic nephropathy have dramatically altered our approach to the patient with progressive chronic kidney disease. Treatment in the past was only aimed at the underlying kidney disease; now, therapy is also aimed at the secondary hemodynamic, structural, and metabolic changes that typically occur. These adaptations are disease independent; as a result, dietary protein restriction and therapeutic modalities such as the administration of an ACE inhibitor and/or angiotensin II receptor blockers may be broadly effective, even if the underlying disease cannot be effectively treated.

Large trials have clearly shown the efficacy of this approach. Many physicians already recommend therapy with an ACE inhibitor and modest restriction of protein intake to patients with evidence of progressive kidney disease, such as a patient with type 1 diabetes with overt proteinuria. Some physicians will also begin therapy in IDDM when there is persistent microalbuminuria, since this is the earliest clinical sign of diabetic nephropathy. Unfortunately, there are also many patients with chronic kidney disease or diabetic nephropathy currently under medical care who are not receiving this type of therapy due to poor understanding or complete ignorance of the basic pathophysiological principles among health care providers.

One of the fundamental aims of therapy in this setting is to lower the intraglomerular pressure, which may be elevated independent of the systemic pressure. Thus, there is no requirement of the patient to have systemic hypertension to begin therapy with an ACE inhibitor, an angiotensin II receptor blocker, or a nondihydropyridine calcium channel blocker. Although we cannot currently measure or estimate the intraglomerular pressure in patients, a reduction in protein excretion is most likely a reflection of the desired intrarenal response and is currently used as a valid surrogate marker for progressive kidney damage.

The case presented at the beginning of the chapter represents another setting in which secondary factors are likely to be important and in which an ACE inhibitor and a low-protein diet might be beneficial. Although the patient has a primary glomerular disease, IgA nephropathy, a slowly progressive elevation in the plasma creatinine concentration and increasing proteinuria are occurring at a time when the benign urine sediment suggests that there is little active glomerular inflammation.

ANSWERS TO QUESTIONS

1 The rise in protein excretion suggests that the intraglomerular pressure has increased despite the fall in systemic pressure. This could occur either by dilation of the afferent glomerular arteriole (thereby allowing more of the systemic pressure to be transmitted to the glomerulus) or by constriction of the efferent arteriole. Studies in animals suggest that afferent dilation is the primary effect of nifedipine.

SUGGESTED READINGS

Anderson S, Rennke HG, Brenner BM. Therapeutic advantage of converting enzyme inhibitors in arresting progressive renal disease associated with systemic hypertension in the rat. J Clin Invest 1986;77:1993.

Atkins RC, Briganti EM, Lewis JB, et al. Proteinuria reduction and progression to renal failure in patients with type 2 diabetes mellitus and overt nephropathy. Am J Kidney Dis 2005;45:281.

Brenner BM. Nephron adaptation to renal injury or ablation. Am J Physiol 1985;249:F324.

Brenner BM, Cooper ME, de Zeeuw D, et al. Effect of losartan on renal and cardiovascular outcomes in patients with type 2 diabetes and nephropathy. N Engl J Med 2001;345:861.

Brunner HR. ACE inhibitors in renal disease. Kidney Int 1992;42:463.

Diabetes Control and Complications Trial Research Group. Effects of intensive treatment of diabetes on the development and progression of long-term complications in insulin-dependent diabetes mellitus. N Engl J Med 1993;329:977.

Dworkin LD, Burstein JA, Parker M, et al. Calcium antagonists and converting enzyme inhibitors reduce renal injury by different mechanisms. Kidney Int 1993;43:808.

Hostetter TH. Prevention of end-stage renal disease due to type 2 diabetes. N Engl J Med 2001;345:910.

Jacobson H, Klahr S. Chronic renal failure: pathophysiology; management. Lancet 1991;338:419,423.

Klahr S, Levey AS, Beck GJ, et al. The effect of dietary protein restriction and blood pressure control on the progression of chronic renal disease. N Engl J Med 1994;330:877.

Lewis EJ, Hunsicker LG, Bain RP, et al. The effect of angiotensin-converting enzyme inhibition on diabetic nephropathy. N Engl J Med 1993;329:1456.

Lewis EJ, Hunsicker LJ, Clarke WR, et al. Renoprotective effect of the angiotensin-receptor antagonist irbesartan in patients with nephropathy due to type 2 diabetes. N Engl J Med 2001;345:851.

Meyer TW, Anderson SA, Rennke HG, et al. Reversing glomerular hypertension stabilizes established glomerular injury. Kidney Int 1987;31:752.

Rennke HG, Klein PS. Pathogenesis and significance of non-primary focal and segmental glomerulosclerosis. Am J Kidney Dis 1989;13:443.

Zeller K, Whittaker E, Sullivan L, et al. Effect of restricting dietary protein and progression of renal failure in patients with insulin-dependent diabetes mellitus. N Engl J Med 1991;324:78.

13

SIGNS AND SYMPTOMS OF CHRONIC RENAL FAILURE

CASE PRESENTATION

A 34-year-old woman has had insulin-dependent diabetes mellitus for 23 years. She has developed a number of diabetic microvascular complications including retinopathy, peripheral neuropathy, and nephropathy. Proteinuria was first noted 7 years ago when a dipstick for protein was positive on a routine urinalysis. Since that time, protein excretion has progressively increased to 5.6 g/day and her plasma creatinine concentration has risen from 1.0 to 7.3 mg/dL. She now complains of increasing fatigue but her appetite remains good. Her medications include insulin, a diuretic and an angiotensin-converting enzyme inhibitor for hypertension, and calcium carbonate as a phosphate binder.

Physical examination reveals a well-appearing, slightly pale woman in no acute distress. Positive findings include a blood pressure of 150/90, decreased visual acuity bilaterally with evidence of microaneurysms and exudates on fundoscopic examination, 2+ (moderate) peripheral edema extending up to the mid-calf, and decreased vibration sense and deep tendon reflexes.

Laboratory data reveal the following:

BUN	= 85 mg/dL (9–25)
Creatinine	= 7.3 mg/dL (0.8–1.4)
Sodium	= 140 mEq/L (136–142)
Potassium	= 5.7 mEq/L (3.5–5)
Chloride	= 106 mEq/L (98–108)
Total CO_2	= 15 mEq/L (21–30)
Calcium	= 9.6 mg/dL (9–10.4)
Phosphate	= 5.8 mg/dL (3.0–4.5)
Hemoglobin	= 9 g/dL (13–15)

OBJECTIVES

By the end of this section, you should have an understanding of each of the following issues:

- The different mechanisms by which uremic symptoms might be produced.
- The role of parathyroid hormone and vitamin D in the normal regulation of calcium and phosphate balance.
- The impairments in mineral metabolism that occur in chronic renal failure and how this leads to bone disease.
- The importance of erythropoietin deficiency in the development of anemia and the therapeutic implications of erythropoietin replacement.
- The basic principles of diffusion and ultrafiltration with dialytic therapy for end-stage renal disease.

Pathogenesis of Uremia

A variety of signs and symptoms begin to appear as renal dysfunction becomes more severe. A partial list of the most common complications is in Table 13.1, which shows that virtually every organ system may be involved. These signs and symptoms are collectively referred to as the *uremic state* or simply *uremia*.

The pathogenesis of the different uremic symptoms is understood to a variable degree. In general, however, four major mechanisms are involved: diminished excretion of electrolytes and water, reduced excretion of organic solutes (also called *uremic toxins*), decreased renal hormone synthesis, and compensation of renal failure leading to maladaptive changes (trade-off hypothesis; see below).

TABLE 13.1

Major Signs and Symptoms of Uremia

System	Sign or Symptom
Musculoskeletal	Renal osteodystrophy Muscle weakness Decreased growth in children Amyloid arthropathy due to β_2-microglobulin deposition
Hematologic	Anemia Platelet dysfunction
Electrolytes	Hyperkalemia Metabolic acidosis Edema Hyponatremia Hyperphosphatemia Hypocalcemia Hyperuricemia
Neurologic	Encephalopathy Peripheral neuropathy Seizures
Cardiopulmonary	Hypertension Pericarditis Congestive heart failure Edema
Endocrine	Carbohydrate intolerance due to insulin resistance Hyperlipidemia Sexual dysfunction, including infertility in women
Gastrointestinal	Anorexia, nausea, vomiting Protein calorie malnutrition
Dermatologic	Pruritus

The remainder of this chapter will briefly review these mechanisms and then discuss in some detail three uremic complications for which the pathophysiology is relatively well understood: renal osteodystrophy (bone disease), anemia, and hypertension. It will conclude with a brief review of the basic principles of dialysis, which is used to treat the symptoms of uremia.

Diminished Excretion of Electrolytes and Water

One of the primary functions of the kidney is to excrete the electrolytes and water generated from dietary intake. The excretion of these substances is usually equal to the difference between filtration and tubular reabsorption, although the excretion of hydrogen and potassium primarily involves tubular secretion. As has been mentioned in several of the preceding chapters, urinary excretion of a particular substance (such as sodium) can be maintained in the presence of a marked reduction in glomerular filtration rate (GFR) via a parallel reduction in the degree of tubular reabsorption. The net effect is that more of this substance is excreted per functioning nephron. If, for example, three-quarters of nephrons have been lost, then *each remaining nephron must excrete four times as much sodium* (as well as other solutes and water) if balance is to be maintained at the same level of dietary intake.

Steady State in Chronic Renal Failure

These adaptations are generally so efficient that the steady state (in which intake and urinary excretion are roughly equal) for sodium, potassium, and water can usually be maintained even though the GFR may be reduced by more than 80%. As an example, edema due to sodium retention is infrequent in mild to moderate chronic renal disease in the absence of the nephrotic syndrome.

 Review the adaptations—hormonal and otherwise—that would allow sodium balance to be maintained in chronic renal failure by decreasing tubular sodium reabsorption.

The ability to compensate by increasing hydrogen and ammonium secretion per nephron is somewhat more limited. Each functioning nephron must excrete more ammonium as the number of functioning nephrons is reduced. The *signal* for this response is probably a small and at first clinically undetectable decline in the plasma bicarbonate concentration that occurs after the initial loss of nephrons. This slight extracellular acidemia will induce a fall in pH in the renal tubular cells that constitutes at least part of the stimulus to increase both ammonium production and hydrogen secretion (see Chapter 6).

The degree to which the plasma bicarbonate concentration will fall depends upon the sensitivity of the system. As shown in Figure 6.1, for example, the administration of an acid load to lower the plasma bicarbonate concentration by 4 to 5 mEq/L in normal subjects results in a fourfold increase in ammonium excretion to approximately 160 mEq/day. Although the sensitivity may be different in chronic renal disease, a small reduction in the plasma bicarbonate concentration that is initially within the normal range is required to increase ammonium excretion *per nephron*.

However, a fourfold increase appears to represent the maximum response that the tubular cells can achieve, even in normal subjects. Thus, if dietary intake and therefore the daily acid load are relatively constant, retention of some hydrogen ions must occur every day once more than three-fourths of the nephrons have been lost. At this time, there will be a more pronounced fall in the plasma bicarbonate concentration, which usually remains above 12 mEq/L since most of the retained acid is buffered in bone and in the cells. However, continuous buffering over a prolonged period has potentially deleterious effects. Buffering by bone carbonate leads to the dissolution of bone mineral as bone calcium is released into the extracellular fluid; buffering by skeletal muscle is associated with enhanced muscle breakdown, possibly leading to loss of lean body mass and muscle weakness.

Similar limitations to the renal adaptation apply to other electrolytes. With potassium, for example, increased potassium excretion per nephron is driven in part by transient potassium retention leading to an initially small rise in the plasma potassium concentration. As a result, the plasma potassium concentration will increase slowly with progressive renal failure until the daily potassium load can no longer be excreted due to near end-stage renal disease or due to the superimposition of another disorder such as hyporeninemic hypoaldosteronism (see Chapter 7).

The problem of phosphate retention will be discussed in detail below. As will be seen, phosphate plays a major role in the pathogenesis of the secondary hyperparathyroidism and bone disease commonly associated with advanced chronic renal failure.

All of these compensatory mechanisms ultimately fail in end-stage renal disease. The number of functioning nephrons at this time is so small that urinary excretion can no longer be maintained at a level equal to intake. Clinical manifestations include edema, hyponatremia (due to free water retention), hyperkalemia, metabolic acidosis, and hyperphosphatemia. Numerous medications are provided to help offset these metabolic consequences of near end-stage renal disease, but eventually renal replacement therapy with dialysis or renal transplantation is required for patient survival.

Intact Nephron Hypothesis

Initial studies in animals and patients with chronic renal failure assumed that damaged nephrons functioned abnormally. However, in a series of elegant experiments, it was demonstrated that nephrons continued to function appropriately in proportion to their GFR. An example of the "intact nephron" hypothesis is shown in Figure 13.1. Unilateral renal disease was induced in animals and the function of the diseased and

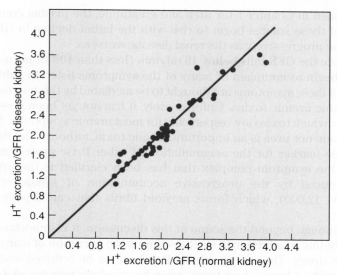

FIGURE 13.1. Relation between net acid (H$^+$) excretion per unit of glomerular filtration rate (GFR) in damaged and normal kidneys under varying acid–base conditions in experimental animals with unilateral renal disease. The slope of the *solid line,* which is the line of equivalence, indicates that acid excretion per GFR (to factor for the number of functioning nephrons) is essentially the same in both kidneys.

normal kidney compared. When factored for GFR, a presumed reflection of the number of functioning nephrons, net acid excretion (mostly as ammonium), was virtually equivalent in the two kidneys. The human correlate of this experiment was described above (Fig. 6.1). The approximately fourfold increase in ammonium excretion per GFR in patients with chronic renal failure is equivalent to the maximum response seen in normal subjects given an acid load.

In summary, damaged nephrons generally continue to function appropriately. The eventual inability to excrete water and electrolytes is primarily due to too few functioning nephrons rather than due to failure of nephron function.

Reduced Excretion of Organic Solutes

The kidney excretes a variety of organic solutes, the most commonly measured being urea and creatinine. Many organic solutes are excreted primarily by glomerular filtration, although there may be some contribution from reabsorption or tubular secretion. The excretion of these solutes differs in an important way from that of water and electrolytes in that there is generally *no active regulation involved.* Thus, as has been mentioned in Chapter 1 for urea and creatinine, the plasma concentrations of these solutes begin to rise with the initial decline in GFR and increase progressively as the renal disease worsens.

Once the GFR falls below 10 mL/min (less than 10% of normal), patients begin to complain of many of the symptoms listed in Table 13.1. Many of these symptoms are thought to be mediated by the accumulation of organic uremic toxins. Unfortunately, it has not yet been possible to identify which toxins are responsible for most uremic symptoms. Neither creatinine nor urea is an important uremic toxin, although the BUN is a valuable marker for the accumulation of other toxic protein metabolites. One symptom complex that has been clarified is the arthropathy induced by the progressive accumulation of β_2-microglobulin (mol wt 12,000), which forms amyloid fibrils that can deposit in the tissues.

Although beyond the scope of this discussion, it is important to appreciate that a reduction in GFR also limits the excretion of many water-soluble drugs. Thus, drug doses often have to be reduced and, when appropriate, plasma drug levels must be carefully monitored. One exception to this general rule is diuretic therapy. In view of the diminished number of functioning nephrons, the diuretic dose typically has to be increased to produce an effective diuresis (see Chapter 4).

Decreased Renal Production of Hormones

The kidneys normally produce a variety of hormones including renin, prostaglandins, kinins, calcitriol (1,25-dihydroxycholecalciferol, the most active metabolite of vitamin D), and erythropoietin. As will be reviewed below, decreased production of calcitriol and erythropoietin in renal failure plays a central role in the development of renal osteodystrophy and anemia, respectively.

Trade-off Hypothesis

The maintenance of fluid and electrolyte balance in progressive renal failure requires a variety of adaptations. One example is increased release of atrial natriuretic peptide (ANP) in an attempt to maintain sodium balance. This adaptation is well tolerated because hypersecretion of ANP has no important side effects.

The consequences are different with the hypersecretion of parathyroid hormone (PTH). Although this response tends to maintain the plasma calcium and phosphate concentrations, there is a *trade-off* because excess PTH may itself be toxic. The most well-recognized complication is hyperparathyroid bone disease, but PTH may also contribute to a number of other problems in the uremic patient, including anemia, pruritus, sexual dysfunction, and encephalopathy. How this might occur is incompletely understood but alterations in calcium metabolism are thought to be involved.

Another maladaptive trade-off is described in the previous chapter (12). As nephrons are lost, the remaining nephrons increase their filtration rate (in part via a rise in intraglomerular pressure) and undergo structural hypertrophy in an attempt to maximize the total GFR. Over a period of years, however, the intraglomerular hypertension can lead to progressive glomerulosclerosis that is independent of the activity of the underlying disease.

Renal Osteodystrophy

Almost all patients with chronic renal failure will develop alterations in bone. These changes are initially asymptomatic but bone pain and pathologic fractures can occur in more advanced disease. Before discussing the pathogenesis of this disorder, it is helpful to review the roles of PTH and vitamin D in the normal regulation of calcium and phosphate balance. The kidney maintains overall calcium balance by excreting the calcium that is absorbed from the gut but not utilized for bone formation; this is similar to the renal excretion of dietary sodium, potassium, and water. However, regulation of the plasma calcium concentration is primarily regulated by a second process: changes in the distribution of calcium between bone stores and the extracellular fluid.

Hormonal Regulation of Calcium and Phosphate Homeostasis

Maintenance of the plasma calcium and phosphate concentrations is mediated to an important degree by PTH and vitamin D.

Parathyroid Hormone

As illustrated in Figure 13.2, PTH acts to increase the plasma calcium concentration in the following three ways:

■ It stimulates bone resorption in the presence of permissive amounts of calcitriol (1,25-dihydroxycholecalciferol, the most active metabolite of vitamin D), thereby releasing both calcium and phosphate into the extracellular fluid.
■ It enhances calcium and phosphate absorption from the gut by promoting the renal synthesis of calcitriol.
■ It promotes active calcium reabsorption in the distal tubule (see Fig. 1.3).

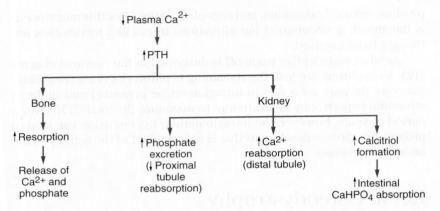

FIGURE 13.2. Effects of parathyroid hormone on calcium and phosphate metabolism. The primary stimulus to PTH secretion, hypocalcemia, is shown; this is consistent with the major action of PTH, which is to raise the plasma calcium concentration. Overall, there is little effect on plasma phosphate concentration.

PTH has an additional important renal action, decreasing proximal phosphate reabsorption by diminishing the activity of the sodium–phosphate cotransporter in the apical membrane; this transporter mediates the first step in phosphate reabsorption, the entry of filtered phosphate into the cells (see Fig. 1.1).

The net effect is that PTH *raises the plasma calcium concentration while having little effect on the plasma phosphate concentration* as changes in phosphate handling in bone, the intestine, and the kidney tend to balance out. The primary physiologic stimulus to PTH secretion is *hypocalcemia;* the varied actions of PTH will tend to correct this problem by increasing the plasma calcium concentration toward normal.

Vitamin D

The synthetic pathways involved in the activation of vitamin D are illustrated in Figure 13.3. Vitamin D_3 (cholecalciferol) is a fat-soluble steroid that is present in the diet and can also be synthesized in the skin in the presence of ultraviolet light. Vitamin D_3 is converted in the liver to calcifediol (25-hydroxycholecalciferol) and then in the kidney (primarily in the proximal tubule) either to the active metabolite calcitriol (1,25-dihydroxycholecalciferol) or to 24,25-dihydroxycholecalciferol, the function of which is not well defined. The hepatic production of calcifediol is primarily substrate dependent and is not under physiologic regulation. In comparison, the renal synthesis of calcitriol varies according to physiologic needs.

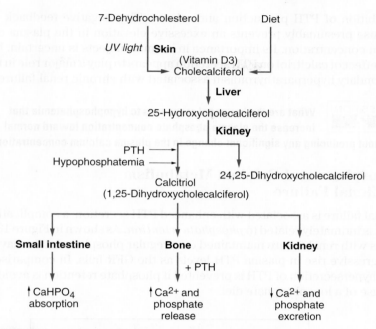

FIGURE 13.3. Metabolic activation of vitamin D_3 and its effects on calcium and phosphate balance. Both the plasma calcium and phosphate concentrations are elevated, thereby promoting bone formation and preventing hypocalcemia or hypophosphatemia.

Calcitriol has the following major actions on calcium and phosphate handling:

- It increases the absorption of calcium and phosphate from the gut.
- It acts in concert with PTH to enhance bone resorption, releasing calcium and phosphate into the extracellular fluid.
- It may decrease urinary calcium and phosphate excretion.

The net effects are elevations in both the plasma calcium and phosphate concentrations (in contrast to PTH, which raises only the plasma calcium concentration). It is therefore appropriate that the main physiologic stimuli to calcitriol production are *hypocalcemia* (acting via increased secretion of PTH) and *hypophosphatemia*, since the actions of calcitriol will tend to correct these abnormalities. These stimuli are also consistent with the two major functions of calcitriol: maintaining the availability of calcium and phosphate for new bone formation, and preventing symptomatic hypocalcemia or hypophosphatemia. In fact, calcitriol is the main hormonal regulator of phosphate homeostasis.

Calcitriol has one additional action on calcium metabolism. It attaches to specific receptors in the parathyroid gland, leading to partial inhibition of PTH production and release. This negative feedback response presumably prevents an excessive elevation in the plasma calcium concentration. Its importance in normal subjects is uncertain, but the effect of calcitriol on PTH secretion appears to play a major role in the secondary hyperparathyroidism associated with chronic renal failure.

 What are the hormonal responses to hypophosphatemia that increase the plasma phosphate concentration toward normal without producing any significant change in the plasma calcium concentration?

Phosphate and Calcium Metabolism in Renal Failure

Renal failure is associated with enhanced PTH secretion, a complication that is intimately related to *phosphate retention*. As shown in Figure 13.4, dogs with renal failure maintained on a regular phosphate intake have a progressive rise in plasma PTH levels as the GFR falls. In comparison, the hypersecretion of PTH is prevented if phosphate retention is avoided by use of a low-phosphate diet.

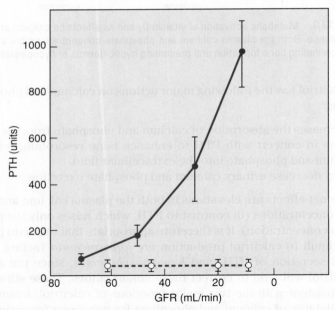

FIGURE 13.4. Relationship between plasma PTH levels and glomerular filtration rate in two groups of dogs. One group (*closed circles*) was maintained on a regular 1200-mg/day phosphorus diet and developed progressive hyperparathyroidism as the GFR fell. A second group (*open circles*) was maintained on a low (100 mg/day) phosphorus diet to prevent phosphorus retention; these dogs did not development hyperparathyroidism even when the GFR was very low.

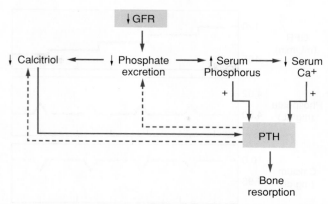

FIGURE 13.5. Summary of disturbances in calcium, phosphate, and parathyroid hormone (PTH) metabolism with renal failure. *Solid lines* show stimulatory effects mediated by the change. *Dotted lines* indicate feedback that compensates for dysregulation. GFR, glomerular filtration rate.

The following hypothesis has been proposed to explain the relationship between phosphate and the development of secondary hyperparathyroidism (Figs. 13.5 and 13.6). The initial fall in GFR will reduce the filtered phosphate load, thereby decreasing phosphate excretion. This will lead to phosphate retention and a small rise in the plasma phosphate concentration if intake is unchanged. The excess phosphate may then drive the following reaction to the right:

$$Ca^{2+} + HPO_4^{2-} \leftrightarrow CaHPO_4$$

The ensuing small reduction in the plasma calcium concentration will stimulate the release of PTH, which, by increasing calcium release from bone and phosphate excretion in the urine, will return both the plasma calcium and phosphate concentrations toward normal. However, the price to maintain this adaptation is persistent hyperparathyroidism.

The role of transient hypocalcemia as the primary stimulus to PTH secretion has been challenged by experimental studies demonstrating that the administration of calcium to maintain a normal plasma calcium concentration does not prevent the development of hyperparathyroidism. An alternative, and not mutually exclusive, theory has been proposed to explain how phosphate retention might lead to the hypersecretion of PTH. As mentioned above, hypophosphatemia is one of the two major stimuli to calcitriol production. On the other hand, the initial elevation in the plasma phosphate concentration seen as the GFR falls should diminish calcitriol synthesis. The ensuing reduction in plasma calcitriol levels can then promote PTH release by removing the normally inhibitory effect of calcitriol on the parathyroid gland. Clinical evidence in support

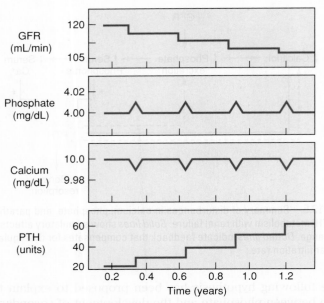

FIGURE 13.6. Hypothetical model for the development of secondary hyperparathyroidism in progressive chronic renal failure. Each decrement in GFR leads to transient phosphate retention; the ensuing elevation in the plasma phosphate concentration leads to a small reduction in the plasma calcium concentration. The latter stimulates the release of PTH, which, via its varied actions, initially is able to return both the plasma calcium and phosphate concentrations to normal. However, the price is persistent hyperparathyroidism.

of a central role for calcitriol deficiency is the observation that the intravenous administration of calcitriol to patients on maintenance dialysis can dramatically reduce PTH secretion, an effect that cannot be achieved by raising the plasma calcium concentration with calcium supplementation.

Although the relative contributions of hypocalcemia, calcitriol deficiency, and perhaps other factors remains uncertain, the degree of hyperparathyroidism increases with each further decrement in GFR (Figs. 13.5 and 13.6). This progressive elevation in PTH levels produces increasing inhibition of proximal phosphate reabsorption. In normal subjects, the fraction of the filtered phosphate that is reabsorbed ranges from 80% to 95% depending upon dietary intake. This value falls to as low as 15% in severe renal failure (GFR below 20 to 30 mL/min).

At this point, PTH is unable to reduce phosphate reabsorption further, resulting in persistent hyperphosphatemia. Furthermore, PTH may actually increase the plasma phosphate concentration in this setting due to continued phosphate release from bone.

Renal Bone Disease and Treatment of Hyperphosphatemia

Prolonged hyperparathyroidism leading to enhanced bone resorption can produce a characteristic bone disease called *osteitis fibrosa cystica*. The diagnosis of this disorder is usually established by its radiologic findings, which include skeletal demineralization, resorption of the lateral ends of the clavicles, and subperiosteal resorption of the phalanges. Bone cysts and, more commonly, spontaneous fractures and tendon ruptures are responsible for the symptoms that can occur.

Hyperparathyroidism can also predispose to the development of *metastatic calcifications* in which calcium phosphate precipitates out of the plasma and is deposited in arteries (possibly leading to ischemic symptoms), soft tissues, and the viscera. This complication is most likely to occur when the product of the plasma calcium and phosphate concentrations (in mg/dL) exceeds from 60 to 70. This is well above the calcium–phosphate product of approximately 30 seen in normal subjects with respective plasma calcium and phosphate concentrations of roughly 9.5 and 3 mg/dL.

Excess PTH plays an essential role in the pathogenesis of metastatic calcifications, both by maintaining a relatively normal plasma calcium concentration (despite the hyperphosphatemia and calcitriol deficiency) and, as noted above, by raising the plasma phosphate concentration in advanced renal failure as phosphate release from bone is no longer counteracted by adequate phosphate excretion in the urine.

Treatment of Hyperphosphatemia

The complications associated with hyperparathyroidism can be prevented or minimized by lowering PTH release. Given the central role of phosphate retention (as shown in Fig. 13.4), therapy is primarily aimed at maintaining the plasma phosphate concentration between 4.5 and 5.5 mg/dL (which represents the high-normal or slightly elevated range). Studies in patients with chronic renal failure have shown that correction of hyperphosphatemia can at least partially reverse the hypocalcemia, calcitriol deficiency, and excess PTH secretion. Calcitriol, particularly, if given in high doses intravenously, can also reverse the hyperparathyroidism via a direct suppressive effect on the parathyroid gland.

Phosphate retention can be minimized or prevented by limiting its intestinal absorption via either a low-phosphate diet (which is often associated with problems in patient compliance) or the administration of a phosphate binder. At present, calcium-based binders (as carbonate or acetate salts) are most widely used; the calcium in these preparations form insoluble calcium phosphate salts in the intestinal lumen that cannot be absorbed as long as they are taken with meals. However, hypercalcemia can develop, and there is growing concern for increased cardiovascular complications associated with the large calcium intake required to control serum phosphorous in patients with chronic renal failure.

Magnesium hydroxide is an effective phosphate binder but is associated with hypermagnesemia in patients with reduced GFR. Aluminum hydroxide was the treatment of choice to bind phosphate, but accumulates in tissue and bone and results in vitamin D–resistant osteomalacia, bone and muscle pain. As a result, newer phosphate binders have been developed that include sevelamer chloride, sevelamer carbonate, and lanthanum carbonate. There are potential advantages and disadvantages to the long-term use of these newer phosphate binders, but they all must be taken with meals to be maximally effective. Due to side effects and cost, many patients require a combination of phosphate binders to be effective.

Hypertension

Hypertension eventually occurs in 85% to 90% of patients with chronic renal failure. In approximately 80% of cases, volume expansion is primarily responsible for the elevation in blood pressure, and fluid removal with diuretics or dialysis will either normalize the blood pressure or make it much easier to control with antihypertensive medications (Fig. 13.7). Increased renin release with the subsequent generation of angiotensin II appears to be an important determinant of hypertension in most of the remaining patients. Some of these patients have a primary vascular disease, such as hypertensive nephrosclerosis or vasculitis. In other cases, it is presumed that disordered renal architecture leads to focal areas of renal ischemia and enhanced renin release.

Treatment of the hypertension in chronic renal failure is aimed at correcting both of these abnormalities. Although diuretic therapy is the agent of choice in patients who are volume expanded (as evidenced clinically by edema), an angiotensin-converting enzyme (ACE) inhibitor is also frequently given in an attempt to slow the rate of progression of secondary glomerular injury (see Chapter 12). An ACE inhibitor is most likely to be protective if given relatively early in the course before extensive irreversible injury has occurred.

Potential Role of Pressure Natriuresis

It is useful to consider the function of the relationship between sodium balance and hypertension in patients with renal disease. Normal subjects given a sodium load excrete the excess sodium by suppressing the release of renin and increasing that of ANP. Patients with chronic renal failure have a similar problem, since sodium excretion per nephron must be

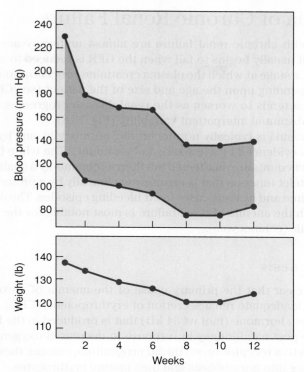

FIGURE 13.7.   Volume-dependent, previously resistant hypertension in a patient with chronic renal failure. Fluid removal led to a gradual reduction in the blood pressure from very high levels to normal without further antihypertensive medications.

increased due to the reduction in the number of functioning nephrons. In this setting, inhibition of the renin–angiotensin–aldosterone system may not occur because of focal renal ischemia and the direct hyperkalemic stimulus to adrenal aldosterone release (see Chapter 7).

The combination of renal disease and persistent secretion of angiotensin II and aldosterone makes sodium excretion less efficient. As a result, sodium retention will initially occur if intake remains relatively constant, leading to an elevation in blood pressure that is initially mediated by a volume expansion–induced rise in cardiac output. As described in Chapter 2, enhanced renal perfusion pressure directly increases sodium excretion via the phenomenon of *pressure natriuresis*. Thus, volume-mediated hypertension in chronic renal disease may be essential to maintain sodium balance. This represents another example of the trade-off hypothesis described above, as hypertension is the price for the prevention of progressive sodium accumulation.

Anemia of Chronic Renal Failure

Patients with chronic renal failure are almost uniformly anemic. The hematocrit usually begins to fall when the GFR is reduced to about 40% of normal, a stage at which the plasma creatinine concentration can vary widely depending upon the age and size of the patient (see Chapter 1). The anemia tends to worsen as the renal disease progresses, although there is substantial interpatient variability (Fig. 13.8).

The anemia is typically normochronic, normocytic, and hypoprolif-erative (as evidenced by a low reticulocyte count). The white blood cell and platelet counts are unaffected but there is commonly a qualitative de-fect in platelet function that is manifested clinically by a prolongation in bleeding time and in some cases overt bleeding episodes. The peripheral smear with the anemia of renal failure is most notable for the presence of burr cells (echinocytes).

Pathogenesis

It is now clear that the primary cause of the anemia of chronic renal disease is inadequate renal secretion of erythropoietin (EPO). EPO is a glycoprotein hormone (mol wt 34 kD) that is produced in the fetal liver and in the post natal kidney in response to decreased oxygen delivery. EPO binds to a receptor on erythroid progenitors, causing these cells to differentiate into normoblasts and then mature erythrocytes.

Anemia normally induces a compensatory increase in EPO re-lease, a response that is blunted or absent in renal failure due to the

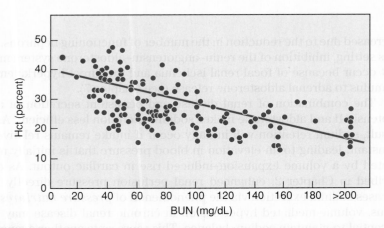

FIGURE 13.8. Relationship between the hematocrit (Hct) and the blood urea nitrogen (BUN) in 152 patients with chronic renal disease. The degree of anemia tends to vary directly with the severity of the renal failure although there is substantial interpatient variability.

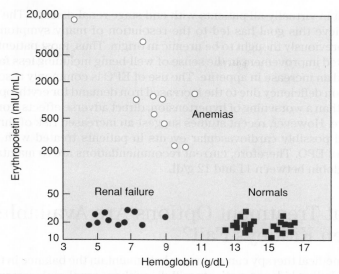

FIGURE 13.9. Relationship between plasma erythropoietin (EPO) levels and the hematocrit in patients with renal failure (*open circles*) and those with anemia and normal renal function (*closed symbols*). At an equivalent degree of anemia, EPO levels are appropriately increased in nonrenal anemia but not in patients with renal failure.

reduction in functioning renal mass (Fig. 13.9). The intrarenal site of EPO production still remains uncertain; it has been proposed that the peritubular capillary endothelial cells play a major role. The renal oxygen sensor is probably a heme protein that, in the presence of decreased oxygen delivery, undergoes a conformational change that induces increased EPO mRNA levels.

In addition to EPO deficiency, other factors may also contribute to the anemia in selected patients. These include the following:

■ A modest reduction in red cell survival of uncertain etiology.
■ Possible EPO resistance due to retention of unidentified uremic toxins or to hyperparathyroidism-induced bone marrow fibrosis.
■ Iron deficiency resulting from blood loss, including repeated blood drawing.
■ Inflammation or infection causing the "anemia of chronic disease" that appears to represent disordered iron utilization.
■ Other nutritional or vitamin deficiencies such as B12 and folate.

Treatment

The widespread availability of recombinant human EPO has revolutionized the management of patients with renal failure. In a dose-dependent fashion (either intravenously or subcutaneously), EPO can correct the anemia in virtually all patients with end-stage renal disease. The ability to achieve this goal has led to the resolution of many symptoms that were previously thought to be uremic in origin. Thus, most patients note a marked improvement in the sense of well-being including less fatigability and an increase in appetite. The use of EPO is commonly associated with iron deficiency due to the increased iron demand for erythropoiesis. Other than a worsening of hypertension, direct adverse effects from EPO are rare. However, recent studies suggest an increased risk of thrombosis and possibly cardiovascular events in patients treated with higher doses of EPO. Therefore, current recommendations are to maintain the hemoglobin between 11 and 12 g/dL.

What Treatment Options Are Available When Kidneys Fail?

Once medical therapy can no longer help maintain the balance in the setting of failing kidneys, patients will die without renal replacement therapy. Replacement options include renal transplantation or one of two dialysis options. Renal transplantation from either a cadaveric or living donor is the treatment of choice when available. Although renal transplantation does not cure the underlying renal disease and is associated with potential serious side effects from surgery and from immunosuppressive medications (infection and cancer), survival and quality of life with a successful transplant are superior to dialysis. A detailed description of renal transplantation is beyond the scope of this book. Dialysis is used for patients waiting for a transplant and for patients unable to safely undergo renal transplantation. Dialysis will remove fluid, potassium, and uremic toxins in an attempt to relieve edema, severe hyperkalemia, or uremic symptoms such as anorexia, lethargy, pericarditis, or paresthesias due to a peripheral neuropathy. In comparison, marked but asymptomatic elevations in the BUN and plasma creatinine concentration are generally not the indications to institute dialysis.

There are two major methods of dialysis: hemodialysis and peritoneal dialysis. For hemodialysis, a catheter is placed into a large vein, or an arteriovenous fistula is created in the forearm so that blood can be pumped at a rate of 300 to 500 mL/min into a dialysis cartridge (Fig. 13.10). Within the cartridge, the patient's blood is separated by a semipermeable membrane from a constantly replenished volume of dialysis solution (or dialysate). After flowing through the cartridge, the cleansed blood is returned to the patient.

With peritoneal dialysis, the peritoneal membrane is used as the dialyzing membrane. Dialysate is infused into the peritoneum through a soft, indwelling catheter that is normally taped to the skin when not in use. The dialysate is allowed to dwell for 4 to 6 hours (or overnight),

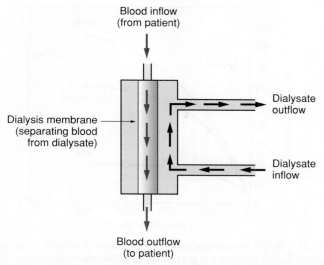

Blood inflow
(from patient)

Dialysis membrane
(separating blood
from dialysate)

Dialysate
outflow

Dialysate
inflow

Blood outflow
(to patient)

FIGURE 13.10. Schematic representation of blood and dialysate flow through a hemodialysis cartridge.

and is then drained. This cycle is followed by the instillation of fresh dialysate.

Both forms of dialysis perform two functions: Solutes are removed by diffusion from the plasma into the dialysate, and fluid is removed by utilizing favorable hydrostatic or osmotic gradients. The following discussion will emphasize the principles of hemodialysis although the same concepts apply to peritoneal dialysis.

Solute Diffusion

Dialysate is an artificial solution with a composition designed to maximize the rate of removal of uremic toxins and other retained substances. Thus, the sodium concentration is generally similar to that in the plasma; the potassium concentration is low (since most patients are hyperkalemic), and there is no phosphate, uric acid, urea, or creatinine. The calcium and bicarbonate concentrations are usually higher than that of uremic plasma, since these patients often have hypocalcemia and metabolic acidosis.

Given the concentration gradients that are created, urea, creatinine, potassium, phosphate, and uric acid diffuse out of the plasma into the dialysate, while calcium and bicarbonate (or another organic anion that is metabolized to bicarbonate, such as acetate) move in the opposite direction. The rate at which this occurs is dependent on three major factors:

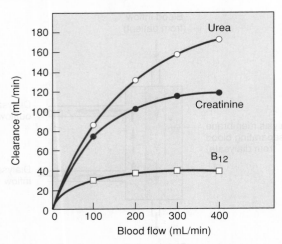

FIGURE 13.11. Solute clearances during hemodialysis in relation to solute size and blood flow rate. Solute clearance is greater with smaller molecules—urea > creatinine > vitamin B_{12}—and is directly related to blood flow rate. Solute diffusion out of the blood diminishes the favorable concentration gradient for further diffusion. However, this gradient can be maintained by the delivery of new undialyzed blood.

- The rate of blood flow and the rate of dialysate flow. The diffusion of solutes out of the plasma will lower the plasma concentration and raise the dialysate concentration, thereby lowering the gradient for further diffusion. Delivery of new blood and dialysate will maintain maximum gradients for continued diffusion (Fig. 13.11).
- The permeability of the dialysis membrane, with more permeable membranes increasing solute clearance.

As shown in Figure 13.11, the creatinine clearance with a standard hemodialysis membrane may exceed 100 mL/min while the urea clearance can approach 200 mL/min. In comparison, larger molecules such as vitamin B_{12} (mol wt 1355) are more slowly cleared. Although these clearance rates are equal to or even exceed that of two normal kidneys, patients on maintenance hemodialysis are only dialyzed from 3 to 4 hours, 3 days per week; this is in contrast to normal kidneys that are active 168 hours per week. Thus, the net effect of hemodialysis is only a small fraction of what is achieved by normal renal function. For example, if the creatinine clearance by hemodialysis is similar to that with normal kidneys but the patient is only dialyzed for 7% ($12 \div 168$) of one week, then the net clearance will be 7% of normal or approximately 7 mL/min.

Somewhat similar considerations apply to peritoneal dialysis. Patients are essentially being dialyzed all the time because there is always fluid dwelling in the peritoneum (except during the periods that fluid is draining out or running in). However, the clearance rate per time is much lower than that with hemodialysis in part because peritoneal blood flow is an order of magnitude lower than the flow rate into the dialyzer with hemodialysis. Thus, the clearance is again only a small fraction of that achieved by normal kidneys.

Efficacy of Dialysis

The net effect is that the BUN and plasma creatinine concentration in a chronically hemodialyzed patient are roughly from 70 to 100 mg/dL and from 10 to 15 mg/dL, respectively, when measured immediately before dialysis. Nevertheless, a sufficient quantity of uremic toxins is removed to alleviate most symptoms that are due to toxin accumulation, such as nausea, pericarditis, and the early signs of peripheral neuropathy. Some of the symptoms that appeared to persist in the past, such as weakness and easy fatigability, were probably due to persistent anemia since they are largely corrected by EPO administration.

There are, however, some problems that are not corrected by dialysis:

- Phosphate does not rapidly diffuse across the dialysis or peritoneal membrane. As a result, the tendency to hyperphosphatemia will persist and patients must continue to be treated with phosphate binders.
- Dialysis cannot correct problems related to decreased hormone production, such as calcitriol deficiency or anemia due to EPO deficiency. Some patients do have a small rise in hematocrit that is presumably due to removal of inhibitors of erythropoiesis but most of the anemia is due to lack of EPO.
- Hypertension due to volume expansion can be corrected, but an elevation in blood pressure induced by enhanced renin secretion will not be reversed.
- β_2-microglobulin, which is part of the class I HLA antigens that are present on virtually all cells in the body, is a relatively large molecule (mol wt 12,000) that is not well dialyzed. As a result, it progressively accumulates in patients on maintenance dialysis, potentially leading to the tissue deposition of β_2-microglobulin as amyloid fibrils that can induce a symptomatic arthropathy involving the carpal tunnel, shoulder, and other areas.

Fluid Removal

Diffusion of solutes will not remove the excess fluid that accumulates in the absence of adequate renal function. This is a particular problem with hemodialysis, since there are from 2 to 3 days between dialyses. The dialysis membrane functions in a similar fashion to a peripheral capillary in that fluid movement across it is determined by the membrane permeability and by the balance of Starling's forces (see Chapter 4). The rate of fluid removal (called ultrafiltration) with hemodialysis is usually regulated by altering the transmembrane hydrostatic pressure gradient. This is most often achieved by applying a variable degree of negative pressure to the dialysate side of the membrane. The greater the fluid that needs to be removed, the higher the negative pressure setting is on the dialysis machine. An alternative in patients with massive fluid overload is to use a larger, more permeable dialysis membrane, thereby increasing the rate of fluid removal. In contrast, neither the peritoneal membrane permeability nor the hydraulic pressures can be regulated with peritoneal dialysis. In this setting, fluid removal is achieved by increasing the osmolality of the dialysate, most often by adding glucose. A standard peritoneal dialysis solution may contain 1.5% glucose (1.5 g per 100 mL) in addition to electrolytes as mentioned above. This solution is hypertonic to plasma since the glucose concentration of 1500 mg/dL is more than 10 times the normal plasma glucose concentration. On average, from 400 to 500 mL is removed with each dwell. Four dwells per day will therefore remove 1600 to 2000 mL, which should be roughly equal to water intake. Using a more concentrated solution (e.g., 2.5% glucose) will remove more fluid in a patient with excessive fluid gain.

Solute Removal

Either method of fluid removal also results in solute removal. As plasma water is lost, frictional forces between solvent and solutes (solvent drug) pull solutes through the dialysis or peritoneal membrane. This mechanism of solute removal is called *convective mass transfer* as compared to diffusive loss described above (and illustrated in Fig. 13.11).

Solute loss by convection is determined by the rate of fluid removal but, in contrast to diffusion, does not depend upon a favorable concentration gradient. In view of the high membrane permeability to small solutes (e.g., urea, sodium, and potassium), the fluid that is removed by convection has virtually the same small solute concentrations as the plasma. As a result, urea or creatinine loss by convection will lower the total body burden of these compounds but will not lower their plasma concentrations. Thus, convection is not an effective way to relieve uremic symptoms because it *does not reduce the concentration of uremic toxins.*

Furthermore, the total quantity of solutes removed is much less than that seen with diffusion. Clearance by convection is equal to the rate of fluid removal, since the dialysate and plasma concentrations are roughly equal. The average rate of fluid removal (and therefore the solute clearance) is from 5 to 10 mL/min during hemodialysis. This is much lower than the clearance rates achieved by diffusion: 100 and 200 mL/min for creatinine and urea, respectively (Fig. 13.10).

In summary, solute loss by convection is a byproduct of fluid removal. It cannot, however, substitute for dialysis by diffusion as a means to remove uremic toxins.

| **CASE DISCUSSION** | The patient presented at the beginning of the chapter has chronic renal failure due to diabetic nephropathy. |

She also has many of the electrolyte complications that have been discussed in this chapter: hyperkalemia, edema, a high anion gap metabolic acidosis, hyperphosphatemia, hypertension, and anemia. The peripheral neuropathy is primarily due to the diabetes, since more advanced renal failure is generally required before uremic neuropathy is seen.

Therapy can be directed toward each of these problems:

- A loop diuretic for both the edema and the hypertension.
- A low-potassium diet and, if this is ineffective, a cation exchange resin for hyperkalemia.
- Sodium bicarbonate for the metabolic acidosis once most of the edema has been removed. Correction of the acidemia may also lower the plasma potassium concentration by driving potassium into the cells (see Chapter 7).
- An increased dose of calcium carbonate to lower the plasma phosphate concentration.

EPO can also be given to raise the hematocrit. Targeting her hemoglobin to 11g/dl would help her fatigue and improve oxygen delivery. However, to date there is no evidence for favorable cardiovascular outcomes with correction of anemia to normal levels.

ANSWERS TO QUESTIONS

1 A reduction in GFR will initially lead to a decrease in the filtered sodium load and, if tubular reabsorption did not change, a decline in sodium excretion. The ensuing sodium retention will reduce the activity of the renin–angiotensin–aldosterone system and enhance the secretion of ANP, both of which will tend to inhibit sodium reabsorption and raise the level of excretion back to the level of sodium intake. If these hormonal responses are inadequate, then pressure natriuresis will also come into play. Extracellular fluid volume expansion due to sodium retention will tend to raise the systemic blood pressure; transmission of this pressure to the kidney will then promote urinary sodium excretion (see Chapter 2).

2 Hypophosphatemia directly increases renal calcitriol production, thereby enhancing intestinal calcium and phosphate absorption and bone resorption. The ensuing rise in the plasma calcium concentration will suppress PTH release, an effect that will reduce urinary phosphate excretion by removing the normal inhibitory effect of PTH. The intestinal, bone, and renal changes will all raise the plasma phosphate concentration toward normal. An undesired elevation in the plasma calcium concentration is prevented by the fall in PTH secretion.

SUGGESTED READINGS

Andress DL, Norris KC, Coburn JW, et al. Intravenous calcitriol in the treatment of refractory osteitis fibrosa of chronic renal failure. N Engl J Med 1989;321:274–279.

Block GA, Martin KJ, de Francisco AL, et al. Cinacalcet for secondary hyperparathyroidism in patients receiving hemodialysis. N Engl J Med 2004;350(14):1516–1525.

Bricker NS, Fine LG, Kaplan M, et al. "Magnification phenomenon" in chronic renal disease. N Engl J Med 1978;299:1287.

Guyton AC. Blood pressure control—special role of the kidneys and body fluids. Science 1991;252:1813.

Hruska KA, Teitelbaum SL. Renal osteodystrophy. N Engl J Med 1995;333(3):166–174.

Meyer TW, Hostetter TH. Uremia. N Engl J Med 2007;357:1316–1325.

van der Putten K, Braam B, Jie KE, et al. Mechanisms of disease: erythropoietin resistance in patients with both heart and kidney failure. Nat Clin Pract Nephrol 2008;4:47–57.

Figure Credits

FIGURE 1.1.	Modified from O'Callaghan CA, Brenner BM. The Kidney at a Glance. Malden, MA: Blackwell Publishers, 2000.
FIGURE 1.2.	Modified from O'Callaghan CA, Brenner BM. The Kidney at a Glance. Malden, MA: Blackwell Publishers, 2000.
FIGURE 1.3.	Modified from O'Callaghan CA, Brenner BM. The Kidney at a Glance. Malden, MA: Blackwell Publishers, 2000.
FIGURE 1.4.	Modified from O'Callaghan CA, Brenner BM. The Kidney at a Glance. Malden, MA: Blackwell Publishers, 2000.
FIGURE 1.5.	Modified from O'Callaghan CA, Brenner BM. The Kidney at a Glance. Malden, MA: Blackwell Publishers, 2000.
FIGURE 1.6.	Modified from O'Callaghan CA, Brenner BM. The Kidney at a Glance. Malden, MA: Blackwell Publishers, 2000.
FIGURE 1.7.	From Rose BD. Clinical Physiology of Acid–Base an Electrolyte Disorders, 3rd Ed. New York: McGraw-Hill, 1989:52.
FIGURE 1.8.	Adapted from Hall JE, Guyton AC, Jackson TE, et al. Am J Physiol 1977; 233:F366.
FIGURE 1.9.	Modified from O'Callaghan CA, Brenner BM. The Kidney at a Glance. Malden, MA: Blackwell Publishers, 2000.
FIGURE 1.10.	From Shemesh O, Golbetz H, Kriss JP, et al. Kidney Int 1985;28:830. Modified with permission from Kidney International.
FIGURE 2.3.	From Zimmerman EA, Robinson AG. Kidney Int 1976;10:12. Modified with permission from Kidney International.
FIGURE 2.4.	From Robertson GL, Aycinena P, Zerbe RL. Am J Med 1982;72:339; and from Dunn FL, Brennan TJ, Nelson AE, et al. J Clin Invest 1973;52:3212. Modified with permission of the American Society for Clinical Investigation.
FIGURE 2.5.	Modified with permission from UpToDate, © 2005.
FIGURE 2.7.	From Hall JE, Granger JP, Smith MJ, et al. Hypertension 1984;6(Suppl. 1): I-183. Modified with permission from the American Heart Association.
FIGURE 2.8.	From Sagnella GA, Markandu ND, Buckley MG, et al. Am J Physiol 1989; 256:R1171.
FIGURE 2.9.	From Sagnella GA, Markandu ND, Buckley MG, et al. Am J Physiol 1989; 256:R1171.
FIGURE 2.10.	From Rabelink TJ, Koomans HA, Hené RJ, et al. Kidney Int 1990;38:942. Modified with permission from Kidney International.
FIGURE 3.1.	From Edelman I, Leibman J, O'Meara MP, et al. J Clin Invest 1958;37:1236. Modified with permission from the American Society for Clinical Investigation.
FIGURE 3.2.	From Arieff AI, Llach F, Massry SG. Medicine 1976;55:121.
FIGURE 3.3.	Redrawn from Verbalis JG, Gullans SR. J Am Soc Nephrol 1990;1:709.
FIGURE 3.5.	Modified with permission from Sterns RH. Ann Intern Med 1987;107:656.
FIGURE 3.6.	Modified with permission from Robertson GL, Aycinena P, Zerbe RL. Am J Med 1982;72:339.
FIGURE 3.7.	Modified with permission from Pollock AS, Arieff AI. Am J Physiol 1980; 239:F195.
FIGURE 3.8.	Modified from Rose BD, Post TW. Clinical Physiology of Acid–Base and Electrolyte Disorders, 5th Ed. New York: McGraw-Hill, 2001:289.

FIGURE 3.9.   Modified with permission from Rose BD, Post TW. Clinical Physiology of Acid–Base and Electrolyte Disorders, 3rd Ed. New York: McGraw-Hill, 1989:659.

FIGURE 4.2.   Data from Ichikawa I, Rennke HG, Hoyer JR, et al. J Clin Invest 1983;71:91.

FIGURE 4.3.   Modified from Koomans HA, Kortlandt W, Geers AB, et al. Nephron 1985; 40:391.

FIGURE 4.4.   From Watkins L Jr, Burton JA, Haber E, et al. J Clin Invest 1976;57:1606. Modified with permission from the American Society for Clinical Investigation.

FIGURE 4.5.   Modified from Cohn JN. Am J Med 1973;55:131.

FIGURE 4.6.   Data from Lenz K, Hortnagl H, Druml W, et al. Gastroenterology 1991;101: 1060.

FIGURE 4.7.   Data from Brater DC, Day B, Burdette A, et al. Kidney Int 1984;26:183.

FIGURE 4.9.   Modified from Maronde RF, Milgrom M, Vlachakis MD, et al. J Am Med Assoc 1983;249:237.

FIGURE 4.10.   Data from Pockros PJ, Reynolds TJ. Gastroenterology 1986;90:1827.

FIGURE 5.1.   Modified from O'Callaghan CA, Brenner BM. The Kidney at a Glance. Malden, MA: Blackwell Publishers, 2000.

FIGURE 5.2.   Modified from O'Callaghan CA, Brenner BM. The Kidney at a Glance. Malden, MA: Blackwell Publishers, 2000.

FIGURE 5.3.   From Slatopolsky E, Hoffsten P, Purkerson M, et al. J Clin Invest 1970;49:988. Modified with permission from the American Society for Clinical Investigation.

FIGURE 5.4.   Modified from Fuller GR, MacLeod MB, Pitts RF. Am J Physiol 1956;182:111.

FIGURE 5.5.   Modified from O'Callaghan CA, Brenner BM. The Kidney at a Glance. Malden, MA: Blackwell Publishers, 2000.

FIGURE 6.1.   From Welbourne T, Weber M, Bank N. N J Clin Invest 1972;51:1852. Modified with permission from the American Society for Clinical Investigation.

FIGURE 6.3.   Modified from Batlle DC, Higon M, Cohen E, et al. NEJM 1998;318:594–599.

FIGURE 7.1.   Modified from Rosa RN, Silva P, Young JB, et al. N Engl J Med 1980;302:431.

FIGURE 7.3.   Modified with permission from Rabelink TJ, Koomans HA, Hené RJ, et al. Kidney Int 1990;38:942.

FIGURE 7.5.   Modified from Young DB, Paulsen AW. Am J Physiol 1983;244:F28.

FIGURE 7.6.   Modified from Surawicz B. Am Heart J 1967;73:814.

FIGURE 8.1.   Modified from www.uptodate.com.

FIGURE 8.2.   Modified from Miles B, Paton A, deWardener H. Br Med J 1954;2:904.

FIGURE 9.4.   Modified with permission from Bohrer MP, Baylis C, Humes HD, et al. J Clin Invest 1978;61:72.

FIGURE 9.5.   Modified with permission from Carrie BJ, Salyer WR, Myers BD. Am J Med 1981;70:262.

FIGURE 11.2.   Modified from Epstein M, Berk DP, Hollenberg NK, et al. Am J Med 1970; 49:175.

FIGURE 11.3.   Modified from Brezis M, Rosen S, Silva P, et al. Kidney Int 1984;26:375.

FIGURE 11.4.   Modified from Shrier RW, Wang W, Poole B, et al. Acute renal failure: definitions, diagnosis, pathogenesis and therapy. J Clin Invest 2004;114: 5–14.

FIGURE 11.5.   Original illustration in Thadhani R, Pascual M, Bonventre JV. Acute renal failure. N Engl J Med 1996;334;1448–1460. Modified from Shrier RW, Wang W, Poole B, et al. Acute renal failure: definitions, diagnosis, pathogenesis and therapy. J Clin Invest 2004;114:5–14.

FIGURE 12.9.   Data from Lewis EJ, Hunsicker LG, Bain RP, et al. The effect of angiotensin-converting enzyme inhibition on diabetic nephropathy. N Engl J Med 1993; 329:1456.

Index

Note: Page numbers in *italics* denote figures; those followed by a t denote tables.